C000067915

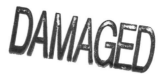

Immune and Inflammatory Responses in the Nervous System

Second Edition
(Molecular and Cellular Neurobiology)

Whilst every effort has been made to ensure that the contents of this book are as complete, accurate and up to date as possible at the date of writing, Oxford University Press is not able to give any guarantee or assurance that such is the case. Readers are urged to take appropriate qualified medical advice in all cases. The information in this book is intended to be useful to the general reader, but should not be used as a means of self-diagnosis or for the prescription of medication.

Immune and Inflammatory Responses in the Nervous System

Second Edition

Nancy Rothwell
School of Biological Sciences
University of Manchester
UK

and

Sarah Loddick
School of Biological Sciences
University of Manchester
UK

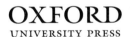

OXFORD
UNIVERSITY PRESS

OXFORD
UNIVERSITY PRESS

Great Clarendon Street, Oxford OX2 6DP

Oxford University Press is a department of the University of Oxford.
It furthers the University's objective of excellence in research, scholarship,
and education by publishing worldwide in

Oxford New York

Auckland Bangkok Buenos Aires Cape Town Chennai
Dar es Salaam Delhi Hong Kong Istanbul Karachi Kolkata
Kuala Lumpur Madrid Melbourne Mexico City Mumbai Nairobi
São Paulo Shanghai Taipei Tokyo Toronto

Oxford is a registered trade mark of Oxford University Press
in the UK and in certain other countries

Published in the United States
by Oxford University Press Inc., New York

© Oxford University Press, 2002

The moral rights of the author have been asserted

Database right Oxford University Press (maker)

First edition published by BIOS Scientific publishers Limited, 1995
Second edition published by Oxford University Press, 2002

All rights reserved. No part of this publication may be reproduced,
stored in a retrieval system, or transmitted, in any form or by any means,
without the prior permission in writing of Oxford University Press,
or as expressly permitted by law, or under terms agreed with the appropriate
reprographics rights organization. Enquiries concerning reproduction
outside the scope of the above should be sent to the Rights Department,
Oxford University Press, at the address above

You must not circulate this book in any other binding or cover
and you must impose this same condition on any acquirer

A catalogue record for this title is available from the British Library

Library of Congress Cataloging in Publication Data
(Data available)

ISBN 0 19 850980 4 (Hbk)

10 9 8 7 6 5 4 3 2 1

Typeset by Newgen Imaging Systems (P) Ltd., Chennai, India
Printed in Great Britain
on acid-free paper by
Biddles Ltd, Guildford and King's Lynn

Preface

It is now seven years since the first edition of *Immune Responses in the Nervous System* was published. At that time the book reviewed a relatively new topic of emerging interest. Its popularity (somewhat of a surprise to the authors) probably reflected a growing curiosity about the field of neuroimmunology and how immune responses contribute to CNS disease.

A great deal has happened in this field since 1995. This new edition is re-titled to cover inflammatory responses, includes several chapters covering new topics and each chapter has been fully rewritten rather than simply updated, by leading experts.

Anthony and Campbell discuss the marked and surprising differences in brain responses to inflammatory stimuli between juvenile and adult animals and their potential clinical significance. Many chapters include information in new techniques, which have led to advances in the field. In particular, Banati describes the use of PET imaging to visualize activated microglia. The prominent role of non-neuronal cells is highlighted in most chapters. Verkhratsky and Jones specifically discuss the role of glial cells and Johansson's chapter considers the contribution of endothelial and perivascular cells and how the blood–brain barrier participates in CNS infection. Disruption to the blood–brain barrier commonly occurs in CNS disease, but events in the periphery can also markedly influence CNS expression of inflammatory molecules (see Chapter by Luheshi and Konsman).

A major focus of the book is on the contribution of infection and inflammatory molecules to diseases of the CNS including cerebral ischaemia (del Zoppo and Hallenbeck), traumatic brain injury (Morganti-Kossman), demyelinating diseases (Cuzner and Woodroofe) and Alzheimer's (Rogers). Cytokines feature prominently as mediators of CNS immune responses (Loddick and Rothwell) and as potential therapeutic targets. Widner considers transplantation strategy for experimental and therapeutic modification of CNS disease and inflammation.

The vast array of information presented here is accompanied by many unanswered questions about the mechanisms and mediators of immune and inflammatory responses and about effective clinical therapies. There is now intense interest from both academic and industrial communities, in identifying inflammation as a potential treatment of CNS diseases. This interest is undoubtedly influenced by the fact that for many of these diseases such as stroke, head injury, Alzheimer's and multiple sclerosis there are few, if any, effective therapies. Perhaps further understanding of CNS immune and inflammatory responses will help to rectify this important need.

Sarah Loddick
Nancy Rothwell

Contents

List of Contributors

Anthony, Daniel C.
Molecular Neuropathology Laboratory
University of Southampton
School of Biological Sciences
Biomedical Sciences Building
Southampton SO16 7PX, UK

Banati, Richard B.
MRC Cyclotron Unit
Imperial College School of Medicine
Hammersmith Hospital
Du Cane Road
London W12 0NN, UK

Campbell, Sandra J.
Molecular Neuropathology Laboratory
University of Southampton
School of Biological Sciences
Biomedical Sciences Building
Southampton SO16 7PX, UK

Cuzner, M. Louise
Department of Neuroinflammation
Institute of Neurology
University College London
Queen Square
London WC1N 3BG, UK

del Zoppo, Gregory J.
Department of Molecular &
Experimental Medicine
The Scripps Research Institute
10550 North Torrey Pines Road
La Jolla CA 92037, UK

Hallenbeck, J. M.
Stroke Branch
National Institutes of Neurological
Disorders and Stroke
National Institutes of Health
Bethesda MD
USA

Johansson, Barbro B.
Division of Experimental Brain Research
Wallenberg Neuroscience Center
BMC A13
SE-22184 Lund
Sweden

Jones O. T.
School of Biological Sciences
1.124 Stopford Building
University of Manchester
Oxford Road
Manchester M13 9PT, UK

Konsman, J-P.
Laboratory of Integrative Neurobiology
INRA-INSERM Unit 394
Institut François Magendie
33077 Bordeaux
France

Kossmann, Thomas
Department of Trauma
The Alfred Hospital
Monash University
Commercial Road
Melbourne
Victoria 3181
Australia

Kovelowski, Carl J.
Sun Health Research Institute
10515 W Santa Fe Drive
Sun City AZ 85351
USA

Loddick, Sarah
School of Biological Sciences
1.124 Stopford Building
University of Manchester
Oxford Road
Manchester M13 9PT, UK

Luheshi, Giamal N.
The Douglas Hospital Research Centre
McGill University
6875 Boulevard LaSalle
Verdun, Quebec
Canada H4H 1R3

Morganti-Kossmann, M. C.
Senior Neuroscientist
Department of Trauma
The Alfred Hospital
Monash University
Commercial Road
Melbourne
Victoria 3181
Australia

Rancan, Mario
Division of Trauma Surgery
Department of Surgery
University Hospital
Zurich
Switzerland

Rogers, Joseph
President & Senior Scientist
Sun Health Research Institute
10515 W Santa Fe Drive
Sun City AZ 85351
USA

Rothwell, Nancy
School of Biological Sciences
1.124 Stopford Building

University of Manchester
Oxford Road
Manchester M13 9PT, UK

Stahel, Philip F.
Dept of Trauma & Reconstructive
  Surgery
University Hospital Benjamin Franklin
The Free University of Berlin
Germany

Strohmeyer, Ron
Sun Health Research Institute
10515 W Santa Fe Drive
Sun City AZ 85351
USA

Verkhratsky, Alex
School of Biological Sciences
1.124 Stopford Building
University of Manchester
Oxford Road
Manchester M13 9PT, UK

Widner, Håkan
Department of Neurology
Lund University Hospital
SE-22185 Lund
Sweden

Woodroofe, Nicola
Biomedical Research Centre
School of Science & Mathematics
Sheffield Hallam University
Sheffield S1 1WB, UK

List of Abbreviations

Aβ	beta amyloid peptide
AD	Alzheimer's disease
APP	amyloid precursor protein
BBB	blood brain barrier
C5a	complement 5a
CINC	cytokine induced neutrophil chemoattractant
CNS	central nervous system
EAE	experimental allergic encephalomyelitis
FDG	$[^{18}F]$ fluorodeoxyglucose
fMLP	formyl-met-leu-phe
GABA	gamma-aminobutyric acid
GAGs	glycosaminoglycans
ICAM	intercellular adhesion molecule
IFN-γ	interferon gamma
IL-1β	interleukin-1 beta
IL-6	interleukin-6
IL-15	interleukin-15
IP-10	interferon inducible protein-10
LFA-1	lymphocyte function associated antigen
LPS	lipopolysaccharide
LTB$_4$	leukotriene B$_4$
MBP	myelin basic protein
MBR	mitochondrial benzodiazepine receptor
MCAO	middle cerebral artery occlusion
MCP	monocyte chemoattractant protein
MHC	major histocompatibility complex
MIP	macrophage inflammatory protein
MRI	magnetic resonance imaging
MRS	MR spectroscopy
MS	multiple sclerosis
NIF	neutrophil inhibitory factor
NMDA	N-methyl-D-aspartate
NSAID	non steroidal anti-inflammatory drug
PAF	platelet activating factor
PBBS	peripheral benzodiazepine binding site
PD	Parkinson's disease
PECAM	platelet and endothelial cell adhesion molecule
PET	positron emission tomography
PGE$_2$	prostaglandin E$_2$

RANTES	regulated upon activation normal T-cells expressed and secreted
SPECT	single photon emission tomography
T8	thoracic level 8
TNFα	tissue necrosis factor alpha
tPA	tissue plasminogen activator
VCAM	vascular cellular adhesion molecule
VLA-4	very late antigen-4
ZO-1	zonale occludens

Chapter 1

Developmental influences on inflammation in the brain

Daniel C. Anthony and Sandra J. Campbell

1.1 Introduction

As any parent knows, minor head injuries seem to be a feature of early childhood, but when damage resulting from comparable injuries in adults and children is assessed, it is seen to be more severe in children (Sharples *et al.* 1995). Thus, development can influence the nature of the inflammatory response in the central nervous system (CNS) to injury or disease and may influence clinical outcome. In the brain parenchyma, where there is little scope for functional repair, it is clear that mechanisms have evolved to tightly regulate the acute inflammatory response, and in particular to restrict the recruitment of specific leucocyte populations. This is likely to be a protective measure to guard against the potentially damaging consequences of an uncompromising inflammatory response in the brain. However, the evidence that is emerging suggests that at either end of the age spectrum the mechanisms that protect the mature CNS appear to be compromised.

1.2 The unusual nature of the inflammatory response in the brain

In non-CNS tissues, the acute leucocyte-independent phase of the vascular response is mediated by molecules such as histamine, bradykinin, platelet activating factor (PAF), and neurogenic mediators, all of which produce vasodilatation and local oedema (Wedmore and Williams 1981). However, microinjection of high concentrations of PAF (Andersson *et al.* 1992) or capsaicin (Markowitz *et al.* 1987) into the brain parenchyma of rodents does not produce the same vascular reactions. The response to cell death is also atypical in the brain. Acute neuronal degeneration in the adult brain caused by excitotoxic injury (Andersson *et al.* 1991) or during either retrograde or anterograde (Wallerian) degeneration (Lawson *et al.* 1994) in the CNS does not elicit an acute leucocyte response. Retrograde degeneration of the facial nerve results in microglial proliferation in the facial nucleus in the absence of leucocyte recruitment (Graeber *et al.* 1998). In contrast, Wallerian degeneration of peripheral nerves results in a more dramatic infiltration of monocytes from the circulation (Perry *et al.* 1995).

The atypical nature of the inflammatory response within the brain parenchyma is, perhaps, best demonstrated by the microinjection of endotoxin (lipopolysaccharide (LPS)) or the proinflammatory cytokine interleukin-1β (IL-1β) into the murine brain parenchyma, which fails to produce the oedema or recruit significant numbers of neutrophils (Andersson *et al.* 1992) that would be expected following a similar challenge in non-CNS tissues. Injection of LPS or IL-1β also demonstrates an important distinction between different compartments of the CNS. Despite the absence of acute inflammation in the parenchyma, there is a florid inflammatory response in the meninges and the choroid plexus.

1.3 The influence of the blood–brain barrier on brain inflammation

The blood–brain barrier (BBB) is part of the regulatory system that controls the micro-environment of the brain by preventing the free entry of solutes from the blood. In peripheral tissues there are relatively large gaps between adjacent endothelial cells, but in the brain continuous tight junctions join endothelial cells. There is a common perception that the tight junctions between the endothelial cells pose a potentially impenetrable barrier to leucocytes attempting to exit the vasculature and that cells can only travel across a damaged endothelium. This notion has dogged research into diseases such as multiple sclerosis, where disease activity and concomitant tissue destruction is often considered to be directly related to the number of gadolinium enhancing lesions (lesions displaying BBB breakdown). It is clear from a growing number of studies that the permeability to solutes and the permeability of cells with regard to the BBB are not the same. The sparse leucocyte recruitment observed in response to neuronal cell death cannot be attributed to the presence of the BBB. For example, lesions made by kainic acid (a glutamate receptor agonist) injection lead to BBB breakdown, but do not cause acute neutrophil recruitment (Bolton and Perry 1998). When the BBB is once again intact (measured by the exclusion of plasma proteins or the tracer horseradish peroxidase), monocytes are able to cross the BBB and enter the tissue. These observations show that damage or breakdown of the BBB is not itself sufficient for neutrophil or monocyte recruitment, even when cell degeneration products are present within the tissue (Bell and Perry 1995). The fact that monocytes cross the intact barrier a few days later should not be surprising since we know that they do so under normal conditions.

1.4 Resident leucocytes in the CNS

As in peripheral tissues, the brain contains a resident set of bone marrow derived mono-nuclear phagocytes that include the microglia in the parenchyma, perivascular macro-phages, and macrophages in the meninges and choroid plexus. Lawson *et al.* estimated that there are approximately the same number (3.5 million) of microglia in the mouse brain as there are resident macrophages in the mouse liver (Lawson *et al.* 1990). Macrophages are detected in the CNS as early as embryonic day 12 in the mouse, which is prior to the formation of the cerebral vasculature and there is evidence that monocytes continue to enter the brain until the early postnatal period. The mechanism that drives monocyte recruitment to the developing brain is not known. It was thought that the recruitment of monocytes might be related to the pattern of neuronal apoptosis in the developing CNS, but the temporal and spatial pattern of monocyte recruitment to the brain does not coincide with neuronal cell death.

During embryogenesis, the BBB is present, but is not as impermeable to solutes as in the postnatal period. In adult animals, it is clear that macrophages in the meninges turnover relatively rapidly, but so too do the perivascular macrophages. Local division maintains the microglial population, but there is also some influx of monocytes (Lawson *et al.* 1992).

Circulating monocytes labelled with intravenous colloidal carbon are found in the CNS parenchyma (Flugel *et al.* 2001). Thus, monocytes are able to enter the developing brain not only when the BBB is immature, but also as it develops its adult characteristics. In the normal adult rodent CNS, the expression of adhesion molecules on the cerebral endothelium is virtually undetectable by highly sensitive immunocytochemistry. Thus the mechanisms that give rise to the recruitment of monocytes under non-pathogenic conditions is unknown. It is not even clear whether the cells cross the endothelium through the tight junctions or by some other mechanism. The unusual phenotype of the resident tissue macrophages in the brain, (microglia), may, at least in part, account for some of the refractory nature of the inflammatory response in the brain (Perry *et al.* 1998). Microglial cells normally express few of the cell surface antigens that are usually expressed on other tissue macrophages, such as MHC class II, and it is clear that microglia do not have the ability to initiate a primary T cell response (Matyszak and Perry 1996). Indeed, it appears that microglia can suppress T cell activation (Ford *et al.* 1996). However, once activated they quickly respond by up-regulating their expression of many of these antigens, which has made it difficult to distinguish resident microglia from recruited macrophages. It remains unclear, however, whether microglia, once activated, are able to produce the full gamut of cytokines and proteases made by tissue macrophages elsewhere in the body.

Unlike most other tissues, the brain contains very few mast cells or dendritic cells. In a survey of the distribution of mast cells in different murine tissues, mast cells were not seen in the spinal cord, brain, optic nerve, or eyes at any stage of development, but they were found in most other organs (Majeed 1994). Dendritic cells are absent from the brain parenchyma, but can be found in the meninges and choroid plexus (Matyszak and Perry 1997). In certain immune-mediated lesions within the CNS, dendritic cells can be found in the brain parenchyma and may contribute to the chronicity of disease, but the absence of dendritic cells from the normal brain is likely to be a major contributor to the altered immunological response to foreign antigens within the brain parenchyma. For example, tissue grafted into the adult brain can survive in the absence of immunosuppressive therapy (see Chapter X).

In pathogen free laboratory rodents, very few T cells are found within the brain parenchyma. However, if activated T cells, which are involved in immune surveillance, are delivered intravenously, some of them will enter the CNS parenchyma independently of their antigen specificity across an intact adult BBB. Laboratory rodents live in well-defined and commonly pathogen-free environments, but humans are continually exposed to antigens that might activate T cells and larger numbers of trafficking leucocytes are to be expected. Indeed, the common observation that there are significant numbers of T-lymphocytes in the perivascular space is a good indicator of this. Thus, the evidence that it is not the presence or absence of the intact BBB *per se* that limits the traffic of leucocytes into the CNS means that some other factors must account for the atypical inflammatory response observed in the brain.

1.5 The refractory nature of the brain

It is clear that cytokines are readily produced *in vivo* in the brain in response to pro-inflammatory stimuli such as mechanical injury (Woodroofe *et al.* 1991) or LPS (Konsman *et al.* 2000). Tumour necrosis factor-α (TNFα) and IL-1β are expressed in the brain in models of ischaemia and traumatic injury (Feuerstein *et al.* 1994; Liu *et al.* 1994; Fan *et al.* 1995; Yabuuchi *et al.* 1994*b*), and also in response to stimuli such as LPS which gives rise to minimal leucocyte infiltration (Breder *et al.* 1988; Quan *et al.* 1994; Higgins and Olschowka 1991). Furthermore, both type I and type II receptors for IL-1β (Cunningham *et al.* 1992; Parnet *et al.* 1994; Yabuuchi *et al.* 1994*a*; Ericsson *et al.* 1995) and the TNFα p55 and p75 receptors (Benigni *et al.* 1996; Akassoglou *et al.* 1998) are expressed in the brain and may be upregulated during inflammatory responses (Laye *et al.* 1996; Cunningham and De Souza, 1993; Lucas *et al.* 1997). Overall, these studies have indicated that the origin of the resistant phenotype of the brain to leucocyte recruitment must lie beyond the production of proinflammatory cytokines.

An essential requirement for leucocyte recruitment from the circulation is the expression of adhesion molecules on the endothelium. The arrest of freely flowing leucocytes and their subsequent rolling along the endothelium is thought to be mediated by the selectins, which bind to carbohydrate ligands (Vestweber and Blanks 1999). The processes of firm adhesion and transmigration further require the expression of CD11/CD18 integrins such as very late antigen-4 (VLA-4) and lymphocyte function-associated antigen (LFA-1) on the leucocyte and their cognate ligands, members of the immunoglobulin family of transmembrane glycoproteins such as intercellular adhesion molecule-1 (ICAM-1), vascular cell adhesion molecule (VCAM) and platelet-endothelial cell adhesion molecule (PECAM), on the endo-thelium (Gahmberg *et al.* 1998; Gahmberg *et al.* 1997; Issekutz and Issekutz 1993). In the brain, all the principal adhesion molecules involved in leucocyte recruitment are rapidly induced following proinflammatory challenges. ICAM-1 and VCAM are readily up-regulated on brain endothelium following injury, as are E- and P-selectin after the intra-striatal injection of IL-1β in adult animals, where there is no appreciable subsequent leucocyte recruitment (Bernardes-Silva *et al.* 2001). However, in injuries where the resistant characteristic of the brain parenchyma is compromised and neutrophil recruitment occurs, administration of the P-selectin blocking antibodies will inhibit neutrophil recruitment by 90 per cent compared to control. Surprisingly, E-selectin antibody blockade has no effect on neutrophil recruitment to the brain parenchyma in these cases. Thus the refractory nature of the brain parenchyma cannot be attributed to the absence of adhesion molecules or to the absence of cytokine expression or to the presence of the BBB, but may be related to the lack of appropriate chemoattractants.

A number of mediators have been shown to induce leucocyte migration including activ-ated serum components such as complement protein 5a (C5a), PAF, eicosanoids such as prostaglandin-E$_2$ (PGE$_2$), leukotriene B$_4$ (LTB$_4$), bacterial-derived peptides (formyl-met-leu-phe (fMLP)), LPS and cytokines (Bokoch 1995; Allavena *et al.* 1997). When injected *in vivo* into the periphery they often produce non-specific inflammatory infiltrates consisting of neutrophils, monocytes, and lymphocytes. However, it is the chemokines, which are induced by cytokines, that are thought to be responsible for determining the composition of an inflammatory infiltrate seen under particular conditions. Until their discovery about 12 years ago, the mechanism by which the appropriate leucocyte population was recruited to a lesion remained unclear. Indeed, despite our growing understanding of the way in which leucocytes are able to roll and adhere to the endothelium, it is still not clear how, and at what stage, chemokines are presented to leucocytes on the endothelium. The chemokines are a family of small inducible proteins, which comprise about 50 members at present, whose effects are restricted to specific leucocyte populations (Howard *et al.* 1999). The CXC family of chemokines in general have potent chemotactic activity for neutrophils, while the C–C family attract monocytes and lymphocytes but not neutrophils (Miller and Krangel 1992). To determine whether chemokines *per se* can overcome the intrinsic resistance of the brain parenchyma, we micro-injected MIP-2 (a CXC chemokine), MCP-1, RANTES, or IP-10 (CC chemokines) into the parenchyma of the mouse brain (Bell *et al.* 1996; Anthony *et al.* 1998). Following the injection of 1 µg MIP-2 there was a marked recruitment of neutrophils to the CNS parenchyma in the absence of any other stimulus. MCP-1 provoked monocyte recruitment to the parenchyma, although IP-10 and RANTES were ineffective in provoking leucocyte entry (Bell *et al.* 1996). Neutrophil recruitment to the brain parenchyma in response to CXC chemokine expression in the brain has also been demonstrated in transgenic mice where the CXC chemokine, N51/KC, was expressed from a myelin basic protein promoter (Tani *et al.* 1996). MCP-1 has also been expressed in a transgenic mouse under the control of the MBP promoter (Fuentes *et al.* 1995). These mice exhibited F4/80 and Mac-1-positive monocyte recruitment to perivascular CNS sites. However, in all these cases it is likely that the amount of chemokine present in the brain was well above a physiologically relevant quantity and, while these studies show that single chemokines appear to be competent on their own to provoke leucocyte migration into the brain, they also raise the question of whether a bolus injection of chemokine or even persistent transgenic expression produces the same response as the *in vivo* production of chemokines by resident CNS cells in inflammatory conditions. Quantitative Taqman RT-PCR and ELISA studies indicate that the level of chemokine induction within the CNS is comparable within both permissive (meninges) and refractory (parenchyma) compartments of the CNS in response to pro-inflammatory challenge. This leaves unresolved the question of the mechanism by which the brain parenchyma resistant to leucocyte recruitment.

1.6 Inflammation in the CNS is deleterious

Although there is minimal acute neutrophil or monocyte recruitment in response to excitotoxin-mediated neuronal degeneration or challenge with LPS or proinflammatory cytokines, neutrophils and monocytes are not always excluded from the brain. Indeed, they are found in large numbers in the brain parenchyma after traumatic lesions (Clark *et al.* 1994), ischaemic lesions (Matsuo *et al.* 1994), and, in rodents, during the 'window of susceptibility' after injection of IL-1β into the brain parenchyma (see below), following which large numbers of neutrophils are recruited to the brain parenchyma (Anthony *et al.* 1997). Microglial activation and the recruitment of monocytes is often a prominent feature of chronic neurodegenerative disease. While others maintain that the presence of phagocytic cells within lesions in the CNS is likely to promote regeneration (Schwartz *et al.* 1999), the balance of evidence strongly supports the view that the presence of neutrophils or macrophages (or activated microglia) is deleterious.

Microglia are highly sensitive to alterations in the CNS microenvironment and are readily activated by stimuli involving injury or infection to the CNS, such as neuronal degeneration, but also respond to disturbances in electrical activity or osmotic changes (Gehrmann *et al.* 1993; Lawson *et al.* 1993). K^+ and Cl^- channels are thought to be involved in the regulation of microglial phenotype (Kettenmann *et al.* 1990; Brown *et al.* 1998). Activation of microglia is accompanied by an up-regulation of surface markers such as LFA-1, CD4, amyloid precursor protein (APP), MHC classes I and II, and ED1, a change to an amoeboid morphology from a highly ramified morphology and an increased phagocytic capacity. It may also lead to cytokine secretion, respiratory burst, and nitric oxide production, chemotaxis and proliferation (Zielasek and Hartung 1996). Thus although resting microglia are unlike most peripheral tissue macrophages, they are readily activated in response to proinflammatory stimuli and can contribute to the initiation of an inflammatory response. Activated microglia and recruited macrophages have the potential to secrete a broad spectrum of molecules, some of which may be neuroprotective, whilst others may exacerbate the lesion. An example demonstrating the contribution of microglia to acute neurodegeneration can be found in transgenic mouse studies where tissue plasminogen activator (tPA) has been knocked out conferring resistance to excitotoxic agents (Chen and Strickland 1997; Tsirka et al. 1995). Following kainic acid injection in wild-type animals, the microglia secrete tPA which converts plasminogen to plasmin (Anthony and Perry 1998). One of the substrates of plasmin is extracellular network of laminin, which surrounds the CA1 pyramidal neurones. The degradation of laminin appears to contribute to the neurodegenerative process by destabilizing neurones. These studies show that secretory products of microglia can significantly contribute to the outcome of an acute insult to the brain.

Perhaps the most direct evidence that the presence of neutrophils is detrimental, comes from experiments employing a middle cerebral artery occlusion (MCAO) model of focal stroke for 2 h where neutrophil recruitment to the lesions was inhibited with neutrophil inhibitory factor (rNIF) (Jiang et al. 1995) or with a depleting anti-neutrophil monoclonal antibody (RP3) (Matsuo et al. 1994). Therapy with either rNIF or RP3 halved the infarct volume in the frontoparietal cortex supplied by the middle cerebral artery. In both studies, neutrophil accumulation in the ischaemic brains of treated rats was significantly reduced compared to that in control animals, and the number of neutrophils within the infarcted tissue correlated with the size of the area of infarction. Zhang et al. have shown that the infarct volume in an MCAO model of focal stroke can be significantly reduced post-ischaemically with anti-CD11b and anti-CD18 monoclonal antibodies that block neutrophil recruitment. Myeloperoxidase activity was also significantly reduced, which is a marker of neutrophil recruitment (Zhang et al. 1995). Neutrophil recruitment into the CNS parenchyma, as in other tissues, leads to extravasation of plasma proteins. The mechanisms by which the binding of neutrophils to endothelium leads to extravasation is not well understood, but recent experiments show that the endothelium is an active participant. The junctions between endothelial cells forming the BBB are both tight junctions and adherens junctions. Our in vivo studies have examined the changes in endothelial junctions when neutrophils are adherent. There is increased phosphorylation of tyrosine residues, and the expression of the tight junction protein, zonale occludens-1 (ZO-1) (Bolton et al. 1998), so prominent in normal vasculature, is lost. It is unclear whether ZO-1 is redistributed within the endothelial cell cytoplasm or the epitope recognized by the antibody undergoes some modification such as phosphorylation. The picture is emerging from both in vitro and in vivo studies that cross-linking of cell surface adhesion molecules initiates an intracellular signalling cascade that leads to changes in the cytoskeleton, disassembly of the junctional complex and ultimately an increase in vessel permeability.

1.7 Developmental influences on the inflammatory response in the CNS

The inflammatory response in neonatal rats (P0) is reminiscent of the inflammatory response to an equivalent challenge in adult animals. However, a window exists in young rodents during which the brain parenchyma is susceptible to acute inflammatory challenges, which is not the case in adult animals. This is especially clear following an inflammatory challenge with IL-1β, which initiates an intense acute neutrophil-mediated inflammatory response in the brains of young rats (P21) and mice (P7) that is not seen in adults (Anthony et al. 1997; Lawson and Perry 1995). Thus all the signals necessary to support typical leucocyte recruitment are present in the brain in juvenile animals and the brain becomes able to restrict leucocyte immigration during subsequent postnatal development. Differential neutrophil recruitment during rat development appears to be generalized to a number of different stimuli, including IL-1β, the excitotoxins kainic acid and N-methyl-D-aspartate (NMDA) (Bolton and Perry 1998). The exact mechanism of this age-related susceptibility to brain inflammation remains to be defined; if paralleled in humans it may account for the higher risks of permanent brain damage following head injury in children.

Given that the injection of chemokines into the brain parenchyma can overcome the intrinsic resistance of the brain, we investigated whether the failure of IL-1β to induce neutrophil recruitment in adult animals compared to juvenile animals might be accounted for by inadequate expression of the neutrophil chemoattractant cytokines (CINC). The results were surprising (Anthony et al. 1998). A competitive RT-PCR assay was used to determine the level of acute mRNA expression for the rat CXC chemokines CINC-1 and CINC-3, following intrastriatal injection of rat recombinant IL-1β. The assay revealed a rapid increase in CINC-3 and CINC-1 mRNA (up to 10 000 fold) and protein both in adult and juveniles treated with IL-1β, whereas these CINCs were virtually undetectable in saline-treated controls. Thus, despite our previous demonstrations of a more intense IL-1β-induced neutrophil recruitment and BBB breakdown in juvenile rats, the experiments described above indicate that the expression of CXC chemokines, particularly CINC-1, occurs rapidly and at much the same level in the brains of adults and juveniles. Consequently, we examined whether, like IL-1β, the intrastriatal administration of CXC chemokines would provoke different patterns of responses in adult and juvenile brains. Striking age-related differences were observed in the effects of both recombinant rat CINC-1 and recombinant CINC-3. CINC-1 induced marked plasma extravasation and neutrophil recruitment as early as 4 h following its administration to juvenile rat brain, whereas adult rats showed significantly less neutrophil recruitment and plasma extravasation at this time. CINC-3 also produced a more intense response in juvenile rats, although in comparison to CINC-1 the onset of neutrophil recruitment and plasma extravasation induced by CINC-3 was delayed. Given the similarity of the CINC-1 and the CINC-3 proteins it is hard to account for the difference in recruitment profile. As with IL-1β, the plasma extravasation induced by both CINC-1 and CINC-3 was also neutrophil-dependent, as demonstrated by its inhibition following the depletion of circulating neutrophils using an anti-neutrophil anti-serum. Overall, these results suggest that although the intrinsic resistance of the brain can be overcome by CXC chemokine administration, there appear to be further downstream events mediating neutrophil recruitment that are absent from the adult animal. There may also be as-yet-unidentified inhibitory molecules present in the adult brain parenchyma.

We have discovered one notable difference between adult and juvenile animals in their response to CNS injury, which, surprisingly, occurs outside the CNS (unpublished observations). The focal microinjection of IL-1β into the brain parenchyma of a rat induces the rapid synthesis of CINC-1 mRNA and protein in the liver (see Fig. 1.1). If the stimulus generated in the CNS is sufficient, CINC-1 protein is released from the liver into the blood where it drives the mobilization of neutrophils. The administration of CINC-1 neutralizing antibodies can completely block neutrophil mobilization in this model—a surprising outcome given the plethora of neutrophil chemoattractants that have been described. The acute hepatic response to the intrastriatal injection of IL-1β is more marked in juvenile animals

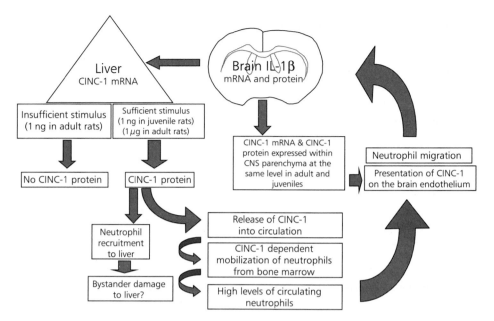

Fig. 1.1. The hepatic response to focal inflammation in the brain. Two hours after the focal injection of IL-1β into the striatum of rats, CINC-1 mRNA and protein are synthesized in the liver if the stimulus is sufficient. CINC-1 expression in the liver is sufficient to recruit neutrophils although it is unknown whether the presence of neutrophils in the liver causes damage. CINC-1 protein is released from the liver into the blood and drives the mobilization of neutrophils from the bone marrow. IL-1β in the brain parenchyma results in CINC-1 expression in the brain parenchyma at similar levels in both adults and juveniles after 4 h. The CINC-1 may be presented on the brain endothelium to attract the increased number of circulating neutrophils allowing their capture and subsequent diapedesis into the brain.

than in adult animals. Precisely how this novel phenomenon affects the differential neutrophil recruitment observed in adult and juvenile animals is currently under study. The ratio of local chemokine production and systemic chemokine production using *in vivo* models has been demonstrated to be a critical factor dictating local neutrophil recruitment (Call *et al.* 2001; Blackwell *et al.* 1999). Thus hepatic chemokine release is likely to influence neutrophil recruitment to the brain.

The inflammatory response in neonatal rats and mice, which resembles the inflammatory response in adult animals, may also be influenced by other factors that are extrinsic to the CNS. The absence of neutrophil recruitment in neonatal animals may reflect deficits in neonatal neutrophil function. Neonatal neutrophils appear to be more refractory to proinflammatory stimuli than neutrophils in adult animals. While neonatal neutrophils express fMLP receptors and produce LTB4 at normal levels, they exhibit decreased motility and decreased respiratory burst activity to classical neutrophil chemoattractants (Anderson *et al.* 1981; Kikawa *et al.* 1986). These findings highlight the fact that developmental changes outside the CNS are likely to have a bearing on the outcome of CNS injury and disease.

In addition to developmental differences in the inflammatory response in the brain parenchyma, it would appear that there is a rostro-caudal susceptibility gradient to pro-inflammatory stimuli in the CNS. In previous studies, we have shown that the inflammatory response induced by stereotactic injection of proinflammatory cytokines (IL-1β and TNFα) (Schnell *et al.* 1999*b*), or following a traumatic injury (Schnell *et al.* 1999*a*) is far more pronounced in the spinal cord (T8) than in the striatum. Traumatic injury to the spinal cord in humans is accompanied by an especially florid, neutrophil-rich, inflammatory cell infiltrate and neuronal cell death is often a prominent sequelae. Others have shown that the regulation of class II MHC after a local injection of IFN-gamma is site-specific (Phillips *et al.* 1999). As compared to hippocampus, the brainstem shows enhanced class II expression at lower IFN-gamma doses, and reaches a higher plateau. Furthermore, in rats immunized with a normal neural antigen (MBP), the stereotaxic injection of IFN-gamma into the hippocampus or into the brainstem gave rise to several-fold more T cells in the brainstem than in the hippocampus. The mechanisms by which the inflammatory response is controlled in different parts of the CNS is poorly understood. The differential induction and presentation of the chemokines may account for the variations observed in the inflammatory response at different sites in the CNS and at different stages in development.

An interesting possibility that remains unexplored, which may contribute to the refractory nature of the brain and variations in the inflammatory response observed in different parts of the CNS, is variation in glycosaminoglycans (GAGs) that are present on endothelial cells in the CNS. The charge on vascular endothelial cells, which is determined, in part, by the nature of GAGs present on the luminal surface, is important in regulating permeability, and cellular traffic and has been shown *in vitro* to be related to the age of cells (dos Santos *et al.* 1996). The charge on brain endothelia is higher than that observed on endothelia derived from the aorta (dos Santos *et al.* 1996), where florid neutrophil recruitment is observed following proinflammatory challenge. It remains to be determined whether age-related differences exist in GAG composition *in vivo*, which might affect leucocyte traffic across the BBB in response to injury. Chemokines are hypothesized to bind to GAGs *in vivo* through their C-terminal α-helix and remain active (Webb *et al.* 1993) thus providing a solid phase gradient to attract passing leucocytes. Chemokines show selective binding to different GAGs, which suggests that the tissue-specific or organ-specific expression of endothelial proteoglycans could play a role in determining the effectiveness of presentation of individual chemokines to circulating leucocytes; this may also be true in the CNS. Andjelkovic *et al.* have shown that specific and distinct binding sites for the chemokines MIP-1α and MCP-1 exist on brain microvessels (Andjelkovic *et al.* 1999). The distribution pattern of the CINC binding sites in the CNS may also play a significant role in influencing these phenomena.

1.8 Immune-mediated disease and development

The archetypal chronic immune-mediated inflammatory disease in the CNS is multiple sclerosis (MS). MS is widely believed to have an autoimmune aetiology in which the immune system attacks the CNS. This results in focal lesions, predominantly in fibre tracts, with breakdown of the BBB, T-cell, and macrophage infiltrate, and myelin and axon damage. The animal model most widely used to study aspects of the pathology of MS is experimental allergic encephalomyelitis (EAE) (Daniel *et al.* 1983). In this disease model, susceptible strains of rodents are injected subcutaneously with CNS antigens in adjuvant, which activates a subset of CNS antigen-specific T cells that have escaped the induction of tolerance. From 7–10 days after immunization, animals develop clinical signs: weight loss, a limp tail, and hind-limb paralysis. Tolerance to CNS antigens appears to be age dependent, which may reflect the developmentally regulated expression of different CNS antigens (MBP for example). Thus windows appear to exist when animals are particularly prone to disease induction (Huseby *et al.* 2001). In general, aged rodents are resistant to the development of EAE, but the altered responsiveness appears to be a function of altered T cell activity in ageing animals rather than changes in the properties of the CNS. It is of interest to note that the severity of an inflammatory response in the CNS of adults can be conditioned early in development. The treatment of neonatal rats with glucocorticoids leads to increases in the severity and incidence of EAE in adulthood (Bakker *et al.* 2000). Again this phenomenon is thought to be related to alterations in T cell function rather than any change to the CNS. The exposure of rodents, at different stages of development, to CNS antigens can dramatically alter their susceptibility to EAE in adulthood. However, these experiments are beyond the scope of this chapter.

1.9 Inflammatory response in ageing animals

The peripheral inflammatory response is modified by the ageing process. Circulating levels of TNFα, IL-6, and cytokine inhibitors have been found to be elevated in aged, though healthy, individuals. Infections in the elderly are associated with prolonged inflammatory activity and a prolonged febrile response, suggesting that the acute phase response is also altered by ageing. Chronic neurodegenerative diseases such as Alzheimer's disease (AD), Parkinson's disease (PD) and the prion diseases are not usually associated with inflammation, but recent data suggests this aspect of the pathogenesis has been overlooked. Within the CNS, the microglia are activated in these chronic neurodegenerative diseases, which are more common in the elderly. The inflammatory response, dominated by activated microglia, may simply be a consequence of the ongoing neurodegeneration, or it may contribute to the evolution of the pathology and exacerbate it. Epidemiological evidence suggests that inflammation is a contributory factor in AD since persons taking non-steroidal anti-inflammatory drugs (NSAIDs) show delayed onset or slowed progression of the disease (Breitner *et al.* 1995). Possible support for the role of inflammation in AD comes from *in vitro* studies in which it has been demonstrated that microglia activated by the Aß peptide, which is deposited in AD, will kill neurones (Meda *et al.* 1995), but the significance of these acute *in vitro* studies is debatable. In the prion diseases it has been stated widely that there is no inflammatory response accompanying the pathology. Recent evidence shows otherwise. Not only is there intense microglial activation in the terminal stage, but there is also a T-lymphocyte and macrophage response early in the disease prior to neuronal degeneration (Betmouni *et al.* 1996). Thus the microglia are well placed to play a role in precipitating or exacerbating the neuronal degeneration. The period during which the microglia are activated is associated with behavioural disturbances in the activity and memory function of the mice suggesting that the microglia either contribute to or indicate some underlying neuronal dysfunction (Betmouni *et al.* 1999). The microenvironment of the CNS, and, in particular, the interaction of neurones with glia, has been considered to down-regulate the glial activity. It has been shown that microglia become less ramified and more 'active' in the ageing brain. Microglia in the brains of aged rats (24 months old) express MHC class II,

CD4, and ED1, which are down-regulated or absent from microglia in 3–6 month-old rats (Perry *et al.* 1993). *In vitro*, neurones tonically inhibit glial activities including their responses to LPS. When the neurones are allowed to die in aged mixed cultures, the responsiveness of glia to LPS is restored. The different phenotype of the microglia in the aged brain may represent a 'primed' state that gives rise to a faster and more pronounced inflammatory response. Traumatic injuries to the CNS of aged rats (36 months) are associated with increased glial activation and increased expression of proinflammatory cytokines compared to equivalent challenges in 3-month-old rats (Kyrkanides *et al.* 2001). Furthermore, serum TNFα levels are higher in aged rats compared to young rats following the intracerebroventricular injection of LPS (Kalehua *et al.* 2000).

1.10 Conclusion

While leucocyte traffic into the normal brain takes place as part of normal physiology, it is clear that the brain has evolved mechanisms to restrict the acute inflammatory response. The mature phenotype of the inflammatory response to injury in the CNS is developmentally acquired, as all the signals necessary to support typical leucocyte recruitment are present in the brain in juvenile animals. The brain becomes able to restrict leucocyte immigration during subsequent postnatal development. It is now becoming more apparent that response to CNS injury and disease cannot be considered in isolation and that there is a peripheral response to focal inflammation in the CNS, which is likely to contribute to outcome. In ageing animals, the phenotype of microglia changes. It is unclear whether the change in phenotype has any functional significance, but the microglia generated a heightened response to proinflammatory challenges. Thus the 'primed' microglia may give rise to increased bystander damage on activation in elderly patients.

References

Akassoglou, K., Bauer, J., Kassiotis, G., Pasparakis, M., Lassmann, H., Kollias, G., and Probert, L. (1998). *Am J Pathol*, 153, 801–13.

Allavena, P., Giardina, G., Bianchi, G., and Mantovani, A. (1997). *J Leukoc Biol*, 61, 729–35.

Anderson, D. C., Hughes, B. J., and Smith, C. W. (1981). *J Clin Invest*, 68, 863–74.

Andersson, P. B., Perry, V. H., and Gordon, S. (1991). *Immunol Lett*, 30, 177–182.

Andersson, P. B., Perry, V. H., and Gordon, S. (1992). *J Exp Med*, 176, 255–9.

Andjelkovic, A. V., Spencer, D. D., and Pachter, J. S. (1999). *J Cell Biol*, 145, 403–12.

Anthony, D., Dempster, R., Fearn, S., Clements, J., Wells, G., Perry, V. H., and Walker, K. (1998). *Curr Biol*, 8, 923–6.

Anthony, D. C., Bolton, S. J., Fearn, S., and Perry, V. H. (1997). *Brain*, 120, 435–44.

Anthony, D. C. and Perry, V. H. (1998). *Curr Biol*, 8, R274–R277.

Bakker, J. M., Kavelaars, A., Kamphuis, P. J., Cobelens, P. M., van Vugt, H. H., van Bel, F., and Heijnen, C. J. (2000). *J Immunol*, 165, 5932–7.

Bell, M. D. and Perry, V. H. (1995). *J Neurocytol*, 24, 695–710.

Bell, M. D., Taub, D. D., and Perry, V. H. (1996). *Neuroscience*, 74, 283–92.

Benigni, F., Faggioni, R., Sironi, M., Fantuzzi, G., Vandenabeele, P., Takahashi, N., et al. (1996). *J Immunol*, 157, 5563–8.

Bernardes-Silva, M., Anthony, D. C., Issekutz, A. C., and Perry, V. H. (2001). *J Cereb Blood Flow Metab*, 21, 1115–24.

Betmouni, S., Perry, V. H., and Gordon, J. L. (1996). *Neuroscience*, 74, 1–5.

Blackwell, T. S., Lancaster, L. H., Blackwell, T. R., Venkatakrishnan, A., and Christman, J. W. (1999). *Am J Respir Crit Care Med*, **159**, 1644–52.

Bokoch, G. M. (1995). *Blood*, **86**, 1649–60.

Bolton, S. J., Anthony, D. A., and Perry, V. H. (1998). *Neuroscience*, **86**, 1245–57.

Bolton, S. J. and Perry, V. H. (1998). *Exp Neurol*, **154**, 231–40.

Breder, C. D., Dinarello, C. A., and Saper, C. B. (1988). *Science*, **240**, 321–4.

Breitner, J. C., Welsh, K. A., Gau, B. A., McDonald, W. M., Steffens, D. C., Saunders, A. M., *et al.* (1995). *Arch Neurol*, **52**, 763–71.

Brown, H., Kozlowski, R., and Perry, H. (1998). *Glia*, **22**, 94–7.

Call, D. R., Nemzek, J. A., Ebong, S. J., Bolgos, G. L., Newcomb, D. E., and Remick, D. G. (2001). *Am J Pathol*, **158**, 715–21.

Chen, Z. L. and Strickland, S. (1997). *Cell*, **91**, 917–25.

Clark, R. S. B., Schiding, J. K., Kaczorowski, S. L., Marion, D. W., and Kochanek, P. M. (1994). *J Neurotrauma*, **11**, 499–506.

Cunningham, E. T., Jr. and De Souza, E. B. (1993). *Immunol Today*, **14**, 171–6.

Cunningham, E. T., Jr., Wada, E., Carter, D. B., Tracey, D. E., Battey, J. F., and De Souza, E. B. (1992). *J Neurosci*, **12**, 1101–14.

Daniel, P. M., Lam, D. K., and Pratt, O. E. (1983). *J Neurol Sci*, **60**, 367–76.

dos Santos, W. L., Rahman, J., Klein, N., and Male, D. K. (1996). *J Neuroimmunol*, **66**, 125–34.

Ericsson, A., Liu, C., Hart, R. P., and Sawchenko, P. E. (1995). *J Comp Neurol*, **361**, 681–98.

Fan, L., Young, P. R., Barone, F. C., Feuerstein, G. Z., Smith, D. H., and McIntosh, T. K. (1995). *Brain Res Mol Brain Res*, **30**, 125–30.

Feuerstein, G. Z., Liu, T., and Barone, F. C. (1994). *Cerebrovasc Brain Metab Rev*, **6**, 341–60.

Flugel, A., Bradl, M., Kreutzberg, G. W., and Graeber, M. B. (2001). *J Neurosci Res*, **66**, 74–82.

Ford, A. L., Foulcher, E., Lemckert, F. A., and Sedgwick, J. D. (1996). *J Exp Med*, **184**, 1737–45.

Fuentes, M. E., Durham, S. K., Swerdel, M. R., Lewin, A. C., Barton, D. S., Megill, J. R., *et al.* (1995). *J Immunol*, **155**, 5769–76.

Gahmberg, C. G., Tolvanen, M., and Kotovuori, P. (1997). *Eur J Biochem*, **245**, 215–32.

Gahmberg, C. G., Valmu, L., Fagerholm, S., Kotovuori, P., Ihanus, E., Tian, L., and Pessa-Morikawa, T. (1998). *Cell Mol Life Sci*, **54**, 549–55.

Gehrmann, J., Mies, G., Bonne-koh, P., Banati, R., Iijima, T., Kreutzberg, G. W., and Hossmann, K.-A. (1993). *Brain Path*, **3**, 11–17.

Graeber, M. B., Lopez-Redondo, F., Ikoma, E., Ishikawa, M., Imai, Y., Nakajima, K., *et al.* (1998). *Brain Res*, **813**, 241–53.

Higgins, G. A. and Olschowka, J. A. (1991). *Brain Res Mol Brain Res*, **9**, 143–8.

Howard, O. M., Oppenheim, J. J., and Wang, J. M. (1999). *J Clin Immunol*, **19**, 280–92.

Huseby, E. S., Sather, B., Huseby, P. G., and Goverman, J. (2001). *Immunity*, **14**, 471–81.

Issekutz, A. C. and Issekutz, T. B. (1993). *Clin Immunol Immunopathol*, **67**, 257–63.

Jiang, N., Moyle, M., Soule, H. R., Rote, W. E., and Chopp, M. (1995). *Ann Neurol*, **38**, 935–42.

Kalehua, A. N., Taub, D. D., Baskar, P. V., Hengemihle, J., Munoz, J., Trambadia, M., *et al.* (2000). *Gerontology*, **46**, 115–28.

Kettenmann, H., Hoppe, D., Gottmann, K., Banati, R., and Kreutzberg, G. (1990). *J Neuroscience Research*, **26**, 278–87.

Kikawa, Y., Shigematsu, Y., and Sudo, M. (1986). *Pediatr Res*, **20**, 402–6.

Konsman, J. P., Blond, D., and Vigues, S. (2000). *Eur Cytokine Netw*, **11**, 699–702.

Kyrkanides, S., O'Banion, M. K., Whiteley, P. E., Daeschner, J. C., and Olschowka, J. A. (2001). *J Neuroimmunol*, **119**, 269–77.

Lawson, L. J., Frost, L., Risbridger, J., Fearn, S., and Perry, V. H. (1994). *J Neurocytol*, **23**, 729–44.

Lawson, L. J. and Perry, V. H. (1995). *Eur J Neurosci*, **7**, 1584–95.

Lawson, L. J., Perry, V. H., Dri, P., and Gordon, S. (1990). *Neuroscience*, **39**, 151–70.

Lawson, L. J., Perry, V. H., and Gordon, S. (1992). *Neuroscience*, **48**, 405–15.

Lawson, L. J., Perry, V. H., and Gordon, S. (1993). *Neuroscience*, 56, 929–38.

Laye, S., Goujon, E., Combe, C., VanHoy, R., Kelley, K. W., Parnet, P., and Dantzer, R. (1996). *J Neuroimmunol*, 68, 61–6.

Liu, T., Clark, R. K., McDonnell, P. C., Young, P. R., White, R. F., Barone, F. C., *et al.* (1994). *Stroke*, 25, 1481–8.

Lucas, R., Lou, J. N., Juillard, P., Moore, M., Bluethmann, H., and Grau, G. E. (1997). *J Neuroimmunol*, 72, 143–8.

Majeed, S. K. (1994). *Arzneimittelforschung*, 44, 1170–3.

Markowitz, S., Saito, K., and Moskowitz, M. A. (1987). *J Neurosci*, 7, 4129–36.

Matsuo, Y., Onodera, H., Shiga, Y., Nakamura, M., Ninomiya, M., Kihara, T., and Kogure, K. (1994). *Stroke*, 25, 1469–75.

Matyszak, M. K. and Perry, V. H. (1996). *Neuropathol Appl Neurobiol*, 22, 44–53.

Matyszak, M. K. and Perry, V. H. (1997). In *Dendritic Cells in Fundamental and Clinical Immunology* (ed., Ricciardi-Castagnoli) Plenum Press, New York, pp. 295–9.

Meda, L., Cassatella, M. A., Szendrei, G. I., Otvos, L., Jr., Baron, P., Villalba, M., *et al.* (1995). *Nature*, 374, 647–50.

Miller, M. D. and Krangel, M. S. (1992). *Crit Rev Immunol*, 12, 17–46.

Parnet, P., Amindari, S., Wu, C., Brunke-Reese, D., Goujon, E., Weyhenmeyer, J. A., Dantzer, R., and Kelley, K. W. (1994). *Brain Res Mol Brain Res*, 27, 63–70.

Perry, V. H., Bolton, S. J., Anthony, D. C., and Betmouni, S. (1998). *Res Immunol*, 149, 721–5.

Perry, V. H., Matyszak, M. K., and Fearn, S. (1993). *Glia*, 7, 60–7.

Perry, V. H., Tsao, J. W., Fearn, S., and Brown, M. C. (1995). *Eur J Neurosci*, 7, 271–80.

Phillips, L. M., Simon, P. J., and Lampson, L. A. (1999). *J Comp Neurol*, 405, 322–33.

Quan, N., Sundar, S. K., and Weiss, J. M. (1994). *J Neuroimmunol*, 49, 125–34.

Schnell, L., Fearn, S., Klassen, H., Schwab, M. E., and Perry, V. H. (1999*a*) *Eur J Neurosci*, 11, 3648–58.

Schnell, L., Fearn, S., Schwab, M. E., Perry, V. H., and Anthony, D. C. (1999*b*) *J Neuropathol Exp Neurol*, 58, 245–54.

Schwartz, M., Lazarov-Spiegler, O., Rapalino, O., Agranov, I., Velan, G., and Hadani, M. (1999). *Neurosurgery*, 44, 1041–5; discussion 1045–6.

Sharples, P. M., Matthews, P. S. F., and Eyre, J. A. (1995). *Journal of Neurology Neurosurgery and Psychiatry*, 58, 153–9.

Tani, M., Fuentes, M. E., Peterson, J. W., Trapp, B. D., Durham, S. K., Loy, J. K., *et al.* (1996). *J Clin Invest*, 98, 529–39.

Tsirka, S. E., Gualandris, A., Amaral, D. G., and Strickland, S. (1995). *Nature*, 377, 2831–41.

Vestweber, D. and Blanks, J. E. (1999). *Physiol Rev*, 79, 181–213.

Webb, L. M., Ehrengruber, M. U., Clark-Lewis, I., Baggiolini, M., and Rot, A. (1993). *Proc Natl Acad Sci USA*, 90, 7158–62.

Wedmore, C. V. and Williams, T. J. (1981). *Nature*, 289, 646–50.

Woodroofe, M. N., Sarna, G. S., Wadhwa, M., Hayes, G. M., Loughlin, A. J., Tinker, A., and Cuzner, M. L. (1991). *J Neuroimmunol*, 33, 227–36.

Yabuuchi, K., Minami, M., Katsumata, S., and Satoh, M. (1994*a*) *Brain Res Mol Brain Res*, 27, 27–36.

Yabuuchi, K., Minami, M., Katsumata, S., Yamazaki, A., and Satoh, M. (1994*b*) *Brain Res Mol Brain Res*, 26, 135–42.

Zhang, Z. G., Chopp, M., Tang, W. X., Jiang, N., and Zhang, R. L. (1995). *Brain Res*, 698, 79–85.

Zielasek, J. and Hartung, H. P. (1996). *Adv Neuroimmunol*, 6, 191–22.

Chapter 2

Imaging inflammation in the brain

Richard B. Banati

2.1 **Introduction**

Brain inflammation is characterized by a number of distinct, pathophysiologically relevant phenomena, including

- regional increases in blood flow
- changes in blood–brain barrier (BBB) permeability
- recruitment of peripheral inflammatory cells and
- regional hypermetabolism by the metabolically active inflammatory cells.

These basic observations have been the foundation for the development of various *in vivo* imaging techniques. For example, regional increases in blood flow can be measured and visualized using the Tc-99m-labelled blood flow tracer hexamethylpropylene amine oxime (99mTc-HMPAO) and single photon emission tomography (SPECT). Likewise, injection of oxygen-15 labelled water and positron emission tomography (PET) can delineate areas of hyperperfusion. BBB permeability is routinely assessed with magnetic resonance imaging (MRI) by detecting the leakage of gadolinium, a paramagnetic contrast agent that does not normally enter the brain. *In vivo* measurements of the recruitment of inflammatory cells can be performed using peripheral leucocytes labelled with 99mTc-HMPAO or other radio-isotopes, though its application in inflammatory brain diseases remains to be developed (Peters 1998). [^{18}F]fluorodeoxyglucose (FDG) and PET has been employed to measure increased metabolism due to the presence of inflammatory cells. Extensive reviews are available covering these clinical *in vivo* imaging techniques (Peters 1998; Rovaris and Fillipi 2000; Filippi and Inglese 2001).

Many of the currently available clinical *in vivo* imaging techniques have important limitations that mainly reflect the relative lack of cellular specificity of the *in vivo* signal. While variations in the diverse spin-echo sequences in MRI may allow measurements of an almost unlimited number of local signal perturbations in the brain structures affected by disease, this high sensitivity is not necessarily accompanied by clear cellular specificity. Thus, histopathologically very different tissue, such as neuronal vacuolation or dense astrogliosis can produce indistinguishable MR signal intensities (Chung *et al.* 1999). A complementary approach is MR spectroscopy (MRS). It allows the highly specific detection of spectra from various brain metabolites. MRS, too, averages the signals from several cellular subpopulations of different physiological and pathological significance. However, it is to a certain extent possible to identify within the averaged spectra, MR signals that are characteristic for one or the other cellular subpopulation, a property that is, for example, used to detect pathology in 'normal-appearing' white matter (Rovaris and Fillipi 2000). Currently, however, the sensitivity and with it the spatial resolution of MRS is relatively poor and remains to be improved.

Brain imaging approaches using specific radioisotopes and PET, also have significant limitations. They are based mostly on the known distribution of a neuroreceptor or metabolic pathway in the CNS of normal individuals, for example, the normal signal pattern of [^{18}F] FDG (2-fluoro-2deoxy-D-glucose) in the healthy cortex. Against this normal standard, the pathological abnormalities in patients with brain disease are usually defined as deficits, that is, relative losses of regional signal. There are some notable exceptions, such as in tumours, where the relevant information of the image lies in an increase of the regional signal. In neurodegenerative diseases, however, current neuroimaging with radiotracers mainly provides 'deficit-images' that are more or less closely correlated to a clinically observed deficit in brain function, raising the occasional question as to what their added value for the understanding of the disease process might be. The number of *in vivo* probes that would allow us to detect and measure the *de novo* expression of molecules specifically associated with those cellular changes that characterize a neuropathological tissue reaction, that is, the 'positive phenomenology' of the disease, is still very limited.

This chapter briefly outlines the rationale for employing [^{11}C](R)-PK11195 PET to detect activated microglia *in vivo* and use their presence as a generic marker of active disease. Putative binding sites of PK11195 and their possible functions have been reviewed elsewhere (Gavish 1999).

2.2 The PK11195 binding site

The isoquinoline PK11195, originally discovered as a compound that partially displaces certain benzodiazepines, such as diazepam, binds to a site that is structurally and functionally unrelated to the central benzodiazepine receptor associated with gamma-aminobutyric acid (GABA)-regulated channels. Particularly abundant in peripheral organs and haematogenous cells but barely present in the normal CNS, the binding site for PK11195 was named 'peripheral benzodiazepine binding site' (PBBS) (for a review see Hertz 1993). The PBBS was found to co-precipitate with the outer membrane of mitochondria (Anholt 1986)—hence its other name, 'mitochondrial benzodiazepine receptor' (MBR). However, PK11195-binding is also present in non-mitochondrial fractions of brain extracts, and mitochondria-free erythrocytes (Hertz 1993; Olson *et al.* 1988) while immunocytochemical staining hints to the possible presence of PBBS in cell nuclei (Hardwick *et al.* 1999). Amongst others, the PBBS plays an important role in steroid synthesis and regulates immunological responses in mononuclear phagocytes. The numerous other putative functions of the PBBS, that still have to merge into a coherent theory of its biological role, have recently been reviewed by Gavish *et al.* (1999).

2.3 The cellular source of PK11195 binding in the CNS

In vitro, astrocytes are found to have high binding of PK11195 (Hertz 1993; Itzhak *et al.* 1993). However, observations made in a number of experimental lesion models and in diseases with BBB damage suggested that focally increased PK11195 binding is due to infiltrating haematogenous cells (Benavides *et al.* 1988; Dubois *et al.* 1988; Price *et al.* 1990).

Subsequent *in vivo* studies found that the distribution pattern of increased PBBS expression matches more closely the distribution of activated microglia rather than that of reactive astrocytes (Dubois *et al.* 1988; Myers *et al.* 1991*a,b*; Stephenson *et al.* 1995; Conway *et al.* 1998, Rao *et al.* 2000). More direct observations using axotomy models demonstrated (Banati *et al.* 1997) that activated microglia are the main source of PK11195 binding *in vivo* (Fig. 2.1). In support of these findings, high-resolution microautoradiography with [^{3}H](R)-PK11195 combined with immunohistochemical cell identification performed on the same tissue section in inflammatory disease, that is, multiple sclerosis and experimental allergic encephalomyelitis, has shown that increased binding of [^{3}H](R)-PK11195 is found on infiltrating blood-borne cells but also on activated microglia (Banati *et al.* 2000). The latter appear to become the dominant source of binding in areas without any obvious histopathology and remote from the primary pathological focus. Some discrepancy, how-ever, still remains: in neurotoxic lesion model, immunoreactivity primarily in and around the nucleus of reactive hippocampal astrocytes was detected by a polyclonal antibody against the peripheral benzodiazepine receptor (Kuhlmann and Guilarte 2000). The failure to find a complete match of the reported immunocytochemical stain for the peripheral benzodi-azepine receptor with the cellular distribution of the microautoradiographic PK11195-label may either have technical reasons, such as sensitivity and specificity of the various detection methods, or indicate that the immunocytochemically detected PBBS is not completely identical with the autoradiographically detected PK11195 binding sites. At present, it may thus be advisable not to view (R)-PK112195 binding as synonymous with the PBBS.

With respect to the above microautoradiographic double-labelling data (Banati *et al.* 2000), it is important that the relative cellular selectivity for activated microglia has been established using the R-enantiomer of PK11195, which has a higher affinity for the PK11195-binding site, rather than the commonly used racemate (Shah *et al.* 1994). The lack of significantly increased [^{11}C](R)-PK11195 binding in astrocyte-rich tissue, such as in patients with hippocampal sclerosis (Banati *et al.* 1999) further supports the view that microglia are the dominant site of (R)-PK11195 binding. Importantly, these patients had a low seizure frequency, as one might expect frequent seizures to induce pathological changes with activation of microglia and consequently increase in PK11195-binding sites. Likewise, long-established lesions identified as hypointense areas in the MRI and known to be sur-rounded by reactive astrogliosis do not show an increased [^{11}C](R)-PK11195 PET signal (Banati *et al.* 2000).

2.4 [^{11}C](R)-PK11195 PET Imaging and the concept of 'Neuroinflammation'

While the exact function of the PBBS has remained elusive, a potentially useful clinical application exists for its specific ligand, PK11195, based on three observations: (1) normal brain shows only minimal binding of PK11195 (2) in CNS pathology, *in vivo* PK11195 binding is predominantly found on activated microglia, and (3) when labelled with carbon-11, PK11195 can be used as a ligand for PET (Benavides *et al.* 1988; Junck *et al.* 1989; Cremer *et al.* 1992; Ramsay *et al.* 1992; Sette *et al.* 1993; Myers *et al.* 1991*a,b*; Myers *et al.* 1999; Banati *et al.* 1999). The use of [^{11}C](R)-PK11195 PET to study the acute and chronic evolution of brain disease introduces the concept of 'neuroinflammation' or 'glial inflam-mation' (Graeber 2001). It is based on the consistently made observation of activated microglia in primarily non-inflammatory, neurodegenerative diseases, such as Alzheimer's

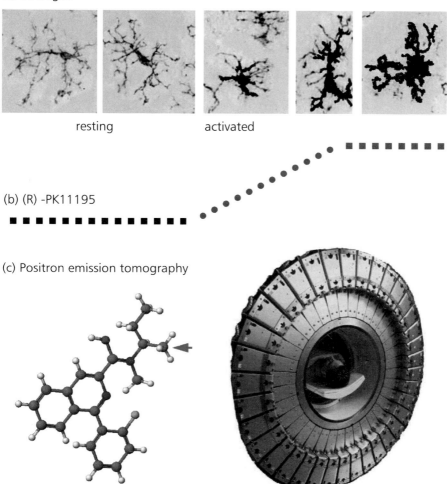

(a) Microglia

resting   activated

(b) (R) -PK11195

(c) Positron emission tomography

Fig. 2.1 Molecular imaging of activated microglia in the living human brain. (a) Microglia respond to a wide variety of pathological stimuli by changing their morphology, proliferation and the expression of numerous biomolecules. (b) Binding of (R)-PK11195 is found to increase in activated microglia. This increase in binding does not require the full transformation of microglia into macrophages. Thus associated with early or subtle activation of microglia, increased (R)-PK11195 binding can be found in tissue with otherwise few signs of active tissue pathology (Banati et al. 1997; Banati et al. 2000). (c) The (R)- PK11195 molecule can be tagged (radiolabelled) with a positron-emitting carbon-11 atom (shown in green). After injection into the blood stream, the radiolabelled molecule enters the brain and binds to activated microglia. The carbon-11 atoms of the marker molecules, bound to microglia, emit positrons that are detected by a ring of crystal detectors placed around the subject's head. This technique is called *positron emission tomography* (PET). Since the marker molecule PK11195 only binds to activated microglia, which themselves are only found in areas of ongoing disease processes, PET-imaging with PK11195 gives a measure of disease distribution and progression. This information can be combined with other markers of brain function, e.g. regional metabolism or the expression of neurotransmitter receptors by specific populations of nerve cells.

disease, Parkinson's disease and others. It has been well established experimentally that neuronal injury *per se* in the absence of any other contributing pathology, such as damage to blood vessels, evokes a rapid, highly localized activation of microglia, the brain's intrinsic macrophages, around the somata of the injured neurones and in anatomical projection areas (Kreutzberg 1996). This neuronally triggered process of microglial activation is associated with the increased expression of immune molecules, such as MHCII. Since, however, lymphocytes, infiltrating macrophages and co-stimulatory are absent its immunological significance is likely to be distinct from that seen in classic inflammation (Graeber 2001).

Peripheral nerve transection experiments demonstrate that 'neuroinflammatory' responses are projected bi-directionally along neural fibre tracts. For example, facial nerve transection leads to a retrograde neuronal reaction and rapid induction of microglial PK11195-binding sites around the somata of lesioned motoneurones facial nucleus, while after sciatic nerve transection, an anterograde response with similar time course occurs in the gracile nucleus in the brain stem, a projection area that contains synaptic terminals from long, ipsilaterally ascending nerve fibres (Kreutzberg 1996; Banati *et al.* 1997). This principle can be observed in stroke patients in whom the cortical injury induces—via the damaged cortico-thalamic connections—a remote microglial response in the ipsilateral thalamus (Myers *et al.* 1991*b*; Sorensen *et al.* 1996) and thus an increased signal of [^{11}C](R)-PK11195 (Pappata *et al.* 2000). Similarly, in individuals with hippocampal damage in the wake of herpes simplex enceph-alitis, [^{11}C](R)-PK11195 PET shows that the distribution pattern of increased [^{11}C](R)-PK11195 binding follows projecting axonal pathways, such as the large association bundles interconnecting mesocortical areas, subicular allocortices and subcortical amygdaloid nuclei (Cagnin *et al.* 2001*c*). It demonstrates how focal damage can lead to widespread microglial activation along almost an entire affected neuronal system, in this case the limbic and associated structures. It has also been possible to predict from this glial activation pattern subsequent anatomical pattern of atrophy as shown by MR-difference imaging (Cagnin, *et al.* 2001*b*; Cagnin *et al.* 2001*c*) (Fig. 2.2).

These findings illustrate that the pattern of microglial activation, as a surrogate marker of neuronal damage, helps to delineate the extent to which a focal lesion impacts on distributed neural connectivities not obvious by standard structural imaging techniques. It should in future, also help to understand so far unexplained differences in the cognitive deficits in patients with apparently similar brain lesions (Eslinger *et al.* 1993). There is already evidence from comparative studies of the functional deficits caused by different types of experimental lesions to the hippocampus or adjacent regions, that indicates so far unaccounted damage leading to a reappraisal of the role of the hippocampus in various aspects of memory (Murray *et al.* 1998; Goulet *et al.* 1998). A closer investigation of the distribution pattern of activated microglia should improve the histopathological description of the effects of neurotoxic lesions as compared to focal structural lesions with respect to the observed variations in the functional outcome.

2.5 What is the significance of a persistent 'neuroinflammatory' response?

Studies with [^{11}C](R)-PK11195 PET in herpes simplex encephalitis patients show that [^{11}C](R)-PK11195 signals can remain elevated for many months if not years and continue to spread along the initially affected neural pathways (Cagnin *et al.* 2001*c*). However, a per-sistent inflammatory tissue response does not necessarily imply continued activity of viral

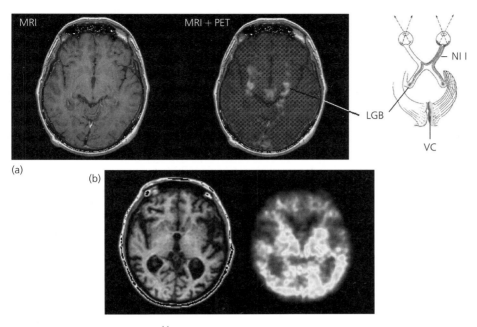

Fig. 2.2 Clinical application of [^{11}C](R)-PK11195 PET. (a) Inflammation of the optic nerve (NII) is a frequent clinical feature of multiple sclerosis. Lesions of the optic nerve lead to the concommittant glial response in those areas to which the optic nerve projects, such as the lateral geniculate body (LGB), which is part of the visual pathway ending in the visual cortex (VC). Using [^{11}C](R)-PK11195 PET, these secondarily involved areas can be visualized. (b) In Alzheimer's disease the gradual loss of nerve cells is accompanied by the activation of glial cells. Typically, the brain areas important for memory functions, such as the temporo-parietal cortex, are most severely affected. In those affected brain areas, the PET scan with [^{11}C](R)-PK11195 indicates a significant involvement of microglia in the disease process (Cagnin *et al.* 2001*a*; Cagnin *et al.* 2001*b*).

products. Detection of viral DNA may establish the latency of the virus in the central nervous system, but the virus usually appears to be inactive (Sobel *et al.* 1986; Esiri *et al.* 1995). This might suggest that such late [^{11}C](R)-PK11195 signals are primarily the consequence of Wallerian-type degeneration of axons and synaptic terminals of the initially damaged neurones. Another experimental observation in mice is that neuronal death alone without BBB damage can lead to the recruitment of peripheral T-lymphocytes and to the appearance of a classical inflammatory reaction despite the absence any infectious agents (Raivich *et al.* 1998).

Some neuropathological evidence suggests that even years after a single toxic event, such as in MPTP-induced parkinsonism (Langston *et al.* 1999), activated microglia are present in selective areas, indicating continuing or secondary neurodegenerative processes. This raises the question of whether the apparent spread of tissue pathology beyond the primarily affected neural pathways represents merely the delayed, full emergence of the initially sustained damage or instead is evidence of more dynamic, trans-synaptic 'knock-on' effects on other not directly injured neural networks, as have been reported for lesions in the visual system and in experimental lesion models of Huntington's disease (Cowey *et al.* 1999; Topper *et al.* 1993). Functionally important, late trans-synaptic microstructural changes are also found in the thalamus of limb-amputated primates where they may occur without significant neuronal cell death and are thought to underlie, at least in part, the cortical plasticity induced by the injury (Jones 2000). Using $[^{11}C](R)$-PK11195 PET, it has recently been possible to show long-term trans-synaptic glial responses in the human thalamus after peripheral nerve injury (Banati *et al.* 2001). Hypothetically, the persistence of activated glia may suggest that even in the chronic stages of the recovery process following brain damage, structural plasticity continues to occur theoretically, allowing for functional plasticity even in the post-acute stages of disease (Knecht *et al.* 1998; Schallert *et al.* 2000).

2.6 Potential role of microglia and the 'peripheral benzodiazepine binding site' (PBBS) in neuronal regeneration

Following activation, microglia change their morphology, proliferate, synthesize numerous bioactive proteins, such as cytokines, and may release neurotoxic metabolites (Giulian and Corpuz 1993; Banati *et al.* 1993). The latter observation in particular, has led to the hypothesis that the activation of microglia is an important pathway in inflammatory as well as neurodegenerative brain diseases, which may result in the loss of neurones through prolonged microglia-mediated damage leading to further progression of disease (McGeer and McGeer 1995; Banati *et al.* 1993). More recently, activated microglia have also been attributed a role in regenerative tissue remodelling (Banati and Graeber 1994). In the context of the present study, it is an intriguing observation that CNS injury causes an increase in the synthesis of neurosteroids with a time course similar to that of the injury-induced up-regulation of the PBBS, that is, the sites to which PK11195 binds. PBBS are known to regulate the synthesis of neurosteroids and through this pathway may influence neuronal functioning and a possible direct participation in CNS regeneration has been suggested (di Michele *et al.* 2000; Lacor *et al.* 1999).

Given these important roles in neuronal re- and degeneration, *in vivo* imaging of activated microglia may be a potentially useful measure of the scope of possible functional rehabilitation and therapeutic efficacy in patients with brain injury. The particular value of $[^{11}C](R)$-PK11195 PET lies in its ability to bind to brain macrophages/microglia as sensors of neuronal injury. In addition to structural neuroimaging it provides a cell biological measure of active disease, the resulting neuronal disconnection, and the protracted large-scale re-organization of the brain following damage to specific regions or pathways. Its application in a variety of brain diseases, such as stroke, multiple sclerosis, autoimmune encephalitis, vasculitis, Parkinson's disease, and atypical Parkinsonism demonstrates the generic value of imaging cellular pathology *in vivo*. Future work will involve the development of improved or new ligands suitable for an '*in vivo* neuropathology', appropriate biomathematical modelling and signal quantification, aspects that were not covered in this outline of the basic concept.

References

Anholt, R. R., Pedersen, P. L., DeSouza, E. B., and Snyder, S. H. (1986). The peripheral-type benzodiazepine receptor. Localisation to the mitochondrial outer membrane. *J Biol Chem*, 261, 776–83.

Banati, R. B., Cagnin, A., Brooks, D. J., Gunn, R. N., Myers, R., Jones, T., *et al.* (2001). Long-term trans-synaptic glial responses in the human thalamus after peripheral nerve injury. *Neuroreport*, 12, 3439–42.

Banati, R. B., Gehrman, J., Schubert, P., and Kreutzberg, G. W. (1993). Cytotoxicity of microglia. *Glia*, 7, 111–18.

Banati, R. B. and Graeber, M. B. (1994). Surveillance, intervention and cytotoxicity: is there a protective role of microglia? *Dev Neurosci*, 16, 114–27.

Banati, R. B., Myers, R., and Kreutzberg, G. W. (1997). PK ('peripheral benzodiazepine')-binding sites in the CNS indicate early and discrete brain lesions: microautoradiographic detection of [3H] PK11195 binding to activated microglia. *J Neurocytol*, 26, 77–82.

Banati, R. B., Goerres, G. W., Myers, R., Gunn, R. N., Turkheimer, F. E., and Kreutzberg, G. W., *et al.* (1999). [11C](R)-PK11195 PET—imaging of activated microglia in vivo in Rasmussen's encephalitis. *Neurology*, 53, 2199–203.

Banati, R. B., Newcombe, J., Gunn, R. N., Cagnin, A., Turkheimer, F., Heppner, F., *et al.* (2000). The peripheral benzodiazepine binding site in the brain in multiple sclerosis: quantitative *in vivo* imaging of microglia as a measure of disease activity. *Brain*, 123, 2321–37.

Benavides, J., Cornu, P., Dennis, T., Dubois, A., Hauw, J.-J., MacKenzie, E. T., *et al.* (1988). Imaging of human brain lesions with an w3 site radioligand. *Ann Neurol*, 24, 708–12.

Cagnin, A., Myers, R., Gunn, R. N., Turkheimer, F. E., Cunningham, V. J., Brooks, D. J., *et al.* (2001a). Imaging activated microglia in the ageing human brain. In *Physiological imaging of the brain with PET* (eds A. Gjedde, S. B. Hansen, G. M. Knudsen and O. B. Paulson, Academic Press, San Diego, pp 361–7.

Cagnin, A., Brooks, D. J., Kennedy, A. M., Gunn, R. N., Myers, R., Turkheimer, F. E., *et al.* (2001b). *In vivo* measurement of activated microglia in dementia. *The Lancet*, 358, 461–7.

Cagnin, A., Myers, R., Gunn, R. N., Lawrence, A. D., Stevens, T., Kreutzberg, G. W., *et al.* (2001c). *In vivo* visualization of activated glia by [11C] (R)-PK11195-PET following herpes encephalitis reveals projected neuronal damage beyond the primary focal lesion. *Brain*, 124, 2014–27.

Chung, Y. L., Williams, A., Ritchie, D., Williams, S. C., Changani, K. K., Hope, J., and Bell, J. D. (1999). Conflicting MRI signals from gliosis and neuronal vacuolation in prion diseases. *Neuroreport*, 10, 3471–7.

Conway, E. L., Gundlach, A. L., and Craven, J. A. (1998). Temporal changes in glial fibrillary acidic protein messenger RNA and [3H] PK11195 binding in relation to imidazoline-I2-receptor and alpha 2-adrenoceptor binding in the hippocampus following transient global forebrain ischaemia in the rat. *Neuroscience*, 82, 805–17.

Cowey, A., Stoerig, P., and Williams, C. (1999). Variance in transneuronal retrograde ganglion cell degeneration in monkeys after removal of striate cortex: effect of size of the cortical lesion. *Vision Res*, 39, 3642–52.

Cremer, J. E., Hume, S. P., Cullen, B. M., Myers, R., Manjil, L. G., Turton, D. R., *et al.* (1992). The distribution of radioactivity in brains of rats given [N-methyl-11C]PK 11195 *in vivo* after induction of a cortical ischaemic lesion. *Int J Radiat Appl Instr B*, 19, 159–66.

di Michele, F., Lekieffre, D., Pasini, A., Bernardi, G., Benavides, J., and Romeo, E. (2000). Increased neurosteroids synthesis after brain and spinal cord injury in rats. *Neurosci Lett*, 284, 65–8.

Dubois, A., Benavides, J., Peny, B., Duverger, D., Fage, D., Gotti, B., *et al.* (1988). Imaging primary and secondary ischaemic and excitotoxic brain lesions. An autoradiographic study of peripheral type benzodiazepine binding sites in the rat and cat. *Brain Res*, 445, 77–90.

Esiri, M. M., Drummond, C. W., and Morris, C. S. (1995). Macrophages and microglia in HSV 1 infected mouse brain. *J Neuroimmunol*, 62, 201–5.

Eslinger, P. J., Damasio, H., Damasio, A. R., and Butters, N. (1993). Non verbal amnesia and asymmetric cerebral lesions following encephalitis. *Brain Cogn*, 21, 140–52.

Fillipi, M. and Inglese, M. (2001). Overview of diffusion-weighted magnetic resonance studies in multiple sclerosis. *J Neurol Sci*, 186(1), S37–43.

Gavish, M., Bachman, I., Shoukrun, R., Katz, Y., Veenman, L., Weisinger, G., and Weizman, A. (1999). Enigma of the peripheral benzodiazepine receptor. *Pharmacol Rev*, 51, 629–50.

Giulian, D. and Corpuz, M. (1993). Microglial secretion products and their impact on the nervous system. *Adv Neurol*, 59, 315–20.

Goulet, S., Dore, F. Y., and Murray, E. A. (1998). Aspiration lesions of the amygdala disrupt the rhinal corticothalamic projection system in rhesus monkeys. *Exp Brain Res*, 119, 131–40.

Graeber, M. B. (2001). Glial inflammation in neurodegenerative diseases. *Immunology*, 101(1), 52.

Hardwick, M., Fertikh, D., Culty, M., Li, H., Vidic, B., and Papadopoulos, V. (1999). Peripheral-type benzodiazepine receptor (PBR) in human breast tissue: correlation of breast cancer cell aggressive phenotype with PBR expression, nuclear localization and PBR-mediated cell proliferation and nuclear transport of cholesterol. *Cancer Res*, 59, 831–42.

Hertz, L. (1993). Binding characteristics of the receptor and coupling to transport proteins. In *Peripheral Benzodiazepine Receptors* (ed. E. Giessen-Crouse) pp. 27–51. Academic Press, London.

Itzhak, Y., Baker, L., and Norenberg, M. D. (1993). Characterization of the peripheral-type benzodiazepine receptors in cultured astrocytes: evidence for multiplicity. *Glia*, 9, 211–18.

Jones, E. G. (2000). Cortical and subcortical contributions to activity-dependent plasticity in primate somatosensory cortex. *Annu Rev Neurosci*, 23, 1–37.

Junck, L., Olson, J. M., Ciliax, B. J., Koeppe, R. A., Watkins, G. L., Jewett, D. M., *et al.* (1989). PET imaging of human gliomas with ligands for the peripheral benzodiazepine binding site. *Ann Neurol*, 26, 752–58.

Knecht, S., Henningsen, H., Hohling, C., Elbert, T., Flor, H., Pantev. C., and Taub, E. (1998). Plasticity of plasticity? Changes in the pattern of perceptual correlates of reorganization after amputation. *Brain*, 121, 717–24.

Kreutzberg, G. W. (1996). Microglia: a sensor for pathological events in the CNS. *Trends Neurosci*, 19, 312–18.

Kuhlmann, A. C. and Guilarte, T. R. (2000). Cellular and subcellular localization of peripheral benzodiazepine receptors after trimethyltin Neurotoxicity. *J Neurochem*, 4, 1694–704.

Lacor, P., Gandolfo, P., Tonon, M. C., Brault, E., Dalibert, I., Schumacher, M., Benavides, J., and Ferzaz, B. (1999). Regulation of the expression of peripheral benzodiazepine receptors and their endogenous ligands during rat sciatic nerve degeneration and regeneration: a role for PBR in neurosteroidogenesis. *Brain Res*, 815, 70–80.

Langston, J. W., Forno, L. S., Tetrud, J., Reeves, A. G., Kaplan, J. A., and Karluk, D. (1999). Evidence of active nerve cell degeneration in the substantia nigra of humans years after 1-methyl-4-phenyl-1,2,3,6-tetrahydropyridine exposure. *Ann Neurol*, 46, 598–605.

McGeer, P. L. and McGeer, E. G. (1995). The inflammatory response system of brain: implications for therapy of Alzheimer and other neurodegenerative diseases. *Brain Res Brain Res Rev*, 21, 195–218.

Murray, E. A., Barker, M. G., and Gaffan, D. (1998). Monkeys with rhinal cortex damage or neurotoxic hippocampal lesions are impaired on spatial scene learning and object reversals. *Behav Neurosci*, 112, 1291–303.

Myers, R., Manjil, L. G., Cullen, B. M., Price, G. W., Frackowiak, R. S. J., and Cremer, J. E. (1991a). Macrophage and astrocyte populations in relation to [3H] PK11195 binding in rat cerebral cortex following a local ischaemic lesion. *J Cereb Blood Flow Metab*, 11, 314–22.

Myers, R., Manjil, L. G., Cullen, B. M., Price, G. W., Frackowiak, R. S. J., and Cremer, J. E. (1991b). (3H) PK 11195 and the localisation of secondary thalamic lesions following focal ischemia in rat motor cortex. *Neurosci Lett*, 133, 20–4.

Myers, R., Gunn, R. N., Cunningham, V. J., Banati, R. B., and Jones, T. (1999). Cluster analysis and the reference tissue model in the analysis of clinical [11C](R)-PK11195 PET. *J Cereb Blood Flow Metab*, 19 Supplement, 789.

Olson, J. M., Ciliax, B. J., Mancini, W. R., and Young, A. B. (1988). Presence of peripheral-type benzodiazepine binding sites on human erythrocyte membranes. *Eur J Pharmacol*, 152, 47–53.

Pappata, S., Levasseur, M., Gunn, R. N., Myers, R., Crouzel, C., Syrota, A., *et al.* (2000). Thalamic microglial activation in ischemic stroke detected *in vivo* by PET and [11C] PK11195. *Neurology*, 55, 1052–4.

Peters, A. M. (1998). The use of nuclear medicine in infections. *Br J Radiol*, 71, 252–61.

Price, G. W., Ahier, R. G., Hume, S. P., Myers, R., Manjil, L. G., Cremer, J. E., *et al.* (1990). *In vivo* binding to peripheral benzodiazepine binding sites in lesioned rat brain: comparison between [3H] PK 11195 and (^{18}F) PK 14105 as markers for neuronal damage. *J Neurochem*, 55, 175–85.

Raivich, G., Jones, L. L., Kloss, C. U. A., Werner, A., Neumann, H., and Kreutzberg, G. W. (1998). Immune surveillance in the injured nervous system: T-lymphocytes invade the axotomized mouse facial motor nucleus and aggregate around sites of neuronal degeneration. *J Neurosci*, 18, 5804–16.

Ramsay, S. C., Weiller, C., Myers, R., Cremer, J. E., Luthra, S. K., Lammertsma, A. A., and Frackowiak, R. S. J. (1992). Monitoring by PET of macrophage accumulation in brain after ischaemic stroke. *The Lancet*, 339, 1054–5.

Raghavendra Rao, V. L., Dogan, A., Bowen, K. K., and Dempsey, R. J. (2000). Traumatic Brain Injury Leads to Increased Expression of Peripheral-Type Benzodiazepine Receptors, Neuronal Death, and Activation of Astrocytes and Microglia in Rat Thalamus. *Exp Neurol*, 16, 102–14.

Rovaris, M. and Fillipi, M. (2000). Contrast enhancement and the acute lesion in multiple sclerosis. *Neuroimaging Clinics of North America*, 10, 705–16.

Schallert, T., Leasure, J. L., and Kolb, B. (2000). Experience-associated structural events, subependymal cellular proliferative activity, and functional recovery after injury to the central nervous system. *J Cereb Blood Flow Metab*, 20, 1513–28.

Sette, G., Baron, J. C., Young, A. R., Miyazawa, H., Tillet, I., Barre, L., *et al.* (1993). *In vivo* mapping of brain benzodiazepine receptor changes by positron emission tomography after focal ischemia in the anesthetized baboon. *Stroke*, 24, 2046–57.

Shah, F., Pike, V. W., Ashworth, S., and McDermott, J. (1994). Synthesis of the enantiomer of [N-methyl-11C]PK11195 and comparison of their behaviours as PK (peripheral benzodiazepine) binding site radioligands in rats. *Nucl Med and Biol*, 21, 573–81.

Sobel, R. A., Collins, A. B., Colvin, R. B., and Bhan, A. K. (1986). The *in situ* cellular immune response in acute herpes simplex encephalitis. *Am J Pathol*, 125, 332–8.

Sorensen, J. C., Dalmau, I., Zimmer, J., and Finsen, B. (1996). Microglial reactions to retrograde degeneration of racer-identified thalamic neurones after frontal sensorimotor cortex lesions in adult rats. *Exp Brain Res*, 11, 203–12.

Stephenson, D. T., Schober, D. A., Smalstig, E. B., Mincy, R. C., Gehlert, D. R., and Clemens, J. A. (1995). Peripheral benzodiazepine receptors are colocalized with activated microglia following transient global forebrain ischemia in the rat. *J Neurosci*, 15, 5263–74.

Topper, R., Gehrmann, J., Schwarz, M., Block, F., Noth, J., and Kreutzberg, G. W. (1993). Remote microglial activation in the quinolinic acid model of Huntington's disease. *Exp Neurol*, 123, 271–83.

Chapter 3

Astrocytic networks and brain injury

A. Verkhratsky and O. T. Jones

3.1 Introduction

Brain function is executed by a continuous interaction of two cellular circuits, neuronal and astroglial. Cellular networks integrated by intercellular communication pathways represent both circuits. Neuronal networks rely on fast (10–100 m s^{-1}) electrical signal propagation and chemical synapses, whereas astrocytes communicate by relatively slow (20–40 μm s^{-1}) propagating intercellular calcium waves. These waves, which can be regarded as a substrate for glial excitability, are produced by intracellular routes, employing intracellular organelles, specifically, the endoplasmic reticulum and the mitochondria. While astrocytic networks are equipped with an extended complement of receptors allowing them to sense neuronal activity, astrocytes can send signals to neurones by releasing neurotransmitters such as glutamate or ATP. Astrocytes are heavily involved in responses to brain injury, and various pathological signals may travel through astrocytic networks. In the present chapter we give an overview of recent advances in identifying the role of astroglia in brain pathology.

3.2 Astrocyte communication

3.2.1 Endoplasmic reticulum-dependent calcium signalling in glial cells

Once regarded as purely supportive elements of the nervous system, astroglia have recently emerged as an important part of information processing in the brain. It appears that astrocytes can respond to a variety of neurotransmitters, can release neurotransmitters by themselves and are endowed with a means for long-range intercellular communication (Kim *et al.* 1994; Deitmer *et al.* 1998; Giaume and Venance 1998; Verkhratsky *et al.* 1998; Araque *et al.* 1999). There is, however, a fundamental difference between neurones and glia with respect to the mechanisms of signal propagation. Neuronal excitability arises from the plasmalemma, where voltage-gated ion channels, which give birth to propagating action potentials, reside. The action potentials can spread along the nerve fibres at a high speed approaching 10–100 m s^{-1}. The excitability of astrocytes is different as it stems from a tubulovesicular structure, the endoplasmic reticulum (ER), which extends throughout the cytoplasm (Presley *et al.* 1997) and which contains a specific complement of inositol-(1,4,5) tri-phosphate (InsP$_3$)/Ca^{2+}gated Ca^{2+} release channels. Interestingly, there is evidence for some spatial heterogeneity in the astrocytic ER with respect to the sites of calcium release (Golovina and Blaustein 1997) and for amplification of the Ca^{2+} waves in astrocytes

(Simpson *et al.* 1998). These latter sites are identifiable by accumulations of calreticulin, type 2 InsP$_3$ receptors, and by the presence of mitochondria, which may regulate Ca^{2+} release.

The initiation of Ca^{2+} signals in astrocytes depends primarily upon the activation of plasmalemmal metabotropic receptors coupled via G-proteins to the activation of phospholipase C, which in turn generates InsP$_3$. The latter interacts with InsP$_3$-receptors resident in the ER membrane, triggering Ca^{2+} release. The membrane of the ER can convey signals in space by generating a wave of Ca^{2+}-dependent recruitment of Ca^{2+} release channels, therefore producing a propagating cytosolic Ca^{2+} signal. This propagating signal is not confined within the astrocytic boundary, as it is able to spread without decrement to adjacent astrocytes and, thus, through astrocytic networks. This transcellular Ca^{2+} wave forms a substrate for long-range signalling within the astrocytic syncytium, which propagates at a rate of about 10–40 m s^{-1}. Such long distance Ca^{2+} waves were initially described in cultured astrocytes (Cornell Bell *et al.* 1990; Charles *et al.* 1991; Cornell Bell and Finkbeiner 1991), and subsequently were detected in retinal preparations and cultured hippocampal slices *in situ* (Newman and Zahs 1997; Harris-White *et al.* 1998).

The mechanisms of transcellular Ca^{2+} signalling are not yet completely understood, but almost certainly involve two important routes: (i) their direct spread through the gap junctions and/or (ii) release of neurotransmitters which support the wave. The first hypothesis to emerge postulated that the Ca^{2+} wave is a result of diffusion of InsP$_3$ through gap junctions (see Section 3.2.2). Indeed, the artificial expression of gap junctions in C6 glioma cells, where they are normally largely absent, resulted in the appearance of propagating Ca^{2+} waves, which otherwise could not be generated (Charles *et al.* 1992). The gap-junction-mediated diffusion theory, however, did not explain the mechanisms for InsP$_3$ regeneration along the wave path. Thus, an alternative theory has been proposed that invokes the involvement of an extracellular messenger (most likely ATP or glutamate), which is released from the astrocytes and supports wave propagation (Enkvist and McCarthy 1992; Hassinger *et al.* 1997). In all likelihood, both pathways probably coexist, and are modulated by each other (Cotrina *et al.* 1998*b*; Cotrina *et al.* 2000), so that it is their coordinated activity that underlies long-range astrocyte signalling.

3.2.2 Gap junctions and the astrocytic syncytium

In contrast to neurone-to-neurone connections, where the continuity of the network is interrupted by chemical synapses, and intercellular signalling employs an extracellular neurotransmitter messenger, astrocyte–astrocyte communication seems to be integrated into a much tighter network. Numerous experiments deploying morphological, electrophysiological, and dye-transfer techniques have demonstrated that astrocytes in the grey matter are tightly coupled to form a functional syncytium (see Rash *et al.* 1997; Dermietzel 1998*a,b*; Nagy and Rash 2000 for reviews) whose molecular substrate is the gap junctions. The latter are comprised of channels that have an extraordinarily high permeability to diverse molecules ranging in size up to 1 kDa. Each gap junction is a hemi-channel formed through the co-assembly of six transmembrane spanning subunits known as connexins (Bennett *et al.* 1991; Dermietzel and Spray 1993). The apposition of two such hemi-channels, one each contributed by the adjoining cell, allows for the formation of a functional gap junction channel. Molecular cloning studies have identified at least 15 different connexins (abbreviated as 'Cx' followed by molecular weight designation) with each belonging to one of three distinct gene families (Willecke *et al.* 1991; Nagy and Rash 2000). At least 10 types of connexin have been identified in the brain, with each showing a differential pattern of expression between distinct cell types (neurones vs. oligodendrocytes vs. astrocytes) and between brain regions. The specificity of gap junction formation between adjacent cell types is determined by the extracellular domains of specific connexins, and thus, reflects the appropriate complementarity in their patterns of gene expression in adjacent cells. Astrocytes *in vivo* express mostly Cx43 and Cx30 (Nagy *et al.* 1997; Nagy and Rash 2000). However, the expression of Cx46 in astroglial cells in culture (Dermietzel 1998*b*) or alternate forms in Cx43 knockout mice (Scemes *et al.* 1998) suggests their expression is plastic and tailored to the specific cell or tissue milieu.

Astrocytic gap junctions are quite abundant, so, together with their ability to access the cytoplasm of each apposed cell, readily afford a means for integrating the astrocytes into a functional syncytium. These direct intercellular pathways contribute to important functions of astrocytic networks, notably the spatial buffering of K^+ via the rapid redistribution of excess K^+ ions between adjacent cells (Newman 1986*a,b*, 1996)—a process that parallels water transport. Astrocytic gap junctions are also readily permeable to glucose and its derivatives, serving, thus, as an important pathway for the distribution of energy metabolites in the grey matter (Tabernero *et al.* 1996; Giaume *et al.* 1997). Significantly, the permeability of gap junctions is regulated by various factors, such as pH, neurotransmitters, neuro-modulators, and eicosanoids, thereby providing a mechanism for the specific regulation of intercellular communication within astrocytic networks. Furthermore, various agents released by neurones influence coupling between astrocytes, thereby, linking neuronal activity to signalling within the astroglial network. Such neurone-dependent regulation of astrocyte gap junctions has been observed in both culture and preparations *in situ*. For example, noradrenaline decreases (Giaume *et al.* 1991), and K^+ ions and glutamate increase (Enkvist and McCarthy 1994) coupling in cultured astrocytes. Similarly, stimulation of optic nerve increased coupling in adjacent astrocytic networks (Marrero and Orkand 1996). Other agents, which may also be released by nerve cells, namely ATP, endothelin-1, nitric oxide, arachidonic acid, were reported to decrease coupling between astrocytes (see Nagy and Rash 2000 for review). Although the intracellular pathways that regulate the permeability of gap junctions remain to be clarified, it has been demonstrated that Cx43 is regulated by phosphorylation (Nagy *et al.* 1992). The observation that such phosphorylation occurs in response to nerve activity, neural injury and mediators of inflammation like interleukin (IL)-1β (John *et al.* 1999), strongly argues that it is likely to be a relevant pathway for connexin regulation *in vivo* (Nagy and Rash 2000). Another possible mechanism for regulating gap junction permeability may involve the heteromeric assembly of Cx43/Cx30 subunits. Heteromultimerization is reported to affect, significantly, both the conductance and even the ionic selectivity of the gap junction (Veenstra 1996).

3.2.3 Astrocyte–neuronal communication

Astrocytes release neurotransmitters

Astrocytes express another feature that always was believed to be a prerogative of neurones—specifically, they are able to secrete classical neurotransmitters. Furthermore, the release of such neurotransmitters occurs in response to Ca^{2+} waves, and it very likely involves the vesicular release of transmitter via the exocytotic pathway. Several ligands, triggering Ca^{2+} signals in cultured astrocytes, produce significant release of the excitatory amino acids glutamate and aspartate (Parpura *et al.* 1994; Bezzi *et al.* 1998). Similarly, astrocytic calcium waves evoke spreading waves of extracellular ATP, as visualized by luciferin–luciferase chemiluminescent assays (Guthrie *et al.* 1999). Finally, glutamate release from astrocytes has been detected in brain slices treated with tetanus toxin to inhibit neuronal (synaptic) pathways (Bezzi *et al.* 1998). The ability of astrocyte-released neurotransmitters to activate receptors, evoking electrical or Ca^{2+} responses in adjacent neurones, (Pasti *et al.* 1997; Araque *et al.* 1998, 2000, 2001; Pasti *et al.* 2001) suggests they may have important consequences for nerve function.

Direct coupling between astrocytes and neurones

Another, quite intriguing, pathway for astrocyte–neuronal communication has emerged recently that is mediated by direct gap-junction contacts. The initial suggestion that Ca^{2+} signals may spread directly from astrocytes to neurones using gap-junction contacts was made by Nedergaard (1994), although for quite a while this was believed to be a culture artefact. Extensive ultrastructural studies on diverse brain regions have failed to find any evidence for nerve–astrocyte gap junctions (Rash *et al.* 1997). Nevertheless, recent findings by Alvarez-Maubecin *et al.* (2000) now provide compelling functional and microscopic evidence that gap junctions can couple neurones and astroglia in the locus coeruleus. Although the functional significance of this phenomenon remains to be established, at least in certain brain regions, astrocytes and neurones may form continuous networks.

3.3 Astrocyte networks during brain injury

3.3.1 Ischaemia induced astrocyte reactions

Generally, astrocytes are deemed to be considerably less vulnerable to ischaemia than neurones (Ransom and Fern 1996). Likewise astrocytes are less susceptible to glutamatergic excitotoxicity (Choi and Rothman 1990). Moreover, astrocytes may assume a neuroprotective role, reducing nerve cell death. Most likely the neuroprotective action of astrocytes is achieved by their ability to support a 'chemical homeostasis' of the interstitial fluid by removing excess potassium ions and glutamate. Nonetheless, in certain conditions astrocytes may exacerbate neuronal damage by either extensive swelling (Siesjö 1985) or by releasing glutamate through a reversal of the Na^+/glutamate transporter (Billups and Attwell 1996).

Short periods of hypoxia–hypoglycemia (3.3–7.5 min) have been shown to trigger an elevation of $[Ca^{2+}]_i$ in astrocytes in hippocampal slices (Duffy and MacVicar 1996) as a result of both Ca^{2+} release from internal stores and Ca^{2+} entry through voltage-gated Ca^{2+} channels. Nonetheless, the elevation of $[Ca^{2+}]_i$ in astrocytes was found to be much smaller than that in neurones from the same preparation. Furthermore, while short periods of hypoxia–hypoglycemia caused an irreversible and fatal elevation of $[Ca^{2+}]_i$ elevation in neurones, this did not occur for astrocytes. In contrast, in neonatal astrocytes from the optic nerve, ischaemia triggered a substantial Ca^{2+} influx through both the L- and T- types of Ca^{2+} channels which was associated with large $[Ca^{2+}]_i$ increases and subsequent cell death.

Ischaemic insults also affect cytoplasmic Na^+ in astroglial cells. Thus, 45 min of combined hypoxia–hypoglycemia has been found to increase the cytoplasmic concentration to 140 mM in cultured rat cortical astrocytes (Rose *et al.* 1998). However, these changes in $[Na^+]_i$ may vary significantly between astrocytes derived from different brain regions. Simulated ischaemia, through metabolic inhibition, results in only a modest elevation in $[Na^+]_i$ in mouse astroglial cells (Silver *et al.* 1997). Similarly, cultured spinal cord astrocytes maintain low intracellular sodium (20 mM) even after 60 min of energy metabolism inhibition (Rose *et al.* 1998). Energy metabolism inhibition renders the Na^+/K^+ pump completely inefficient, via ATP depletion, and its effects on $[Na^+]_i$ can be mimicked by ouabain, a Na^+/K^+ pump inhibitor (Rose *et al.* 1998). Therefore, these data indicate that Na^+ influx through the astroglial plasmalemma is normally very low and a very steep inward sodium gradient exists across the astrocyte plasmalemma. This gradient is very important for the normal functioning of the astrocytic Na^+/glutamate transporter, whose ability to clear glutamate from the extracellular space contributes to the neuroprotective role of astroglial cells. Nevertheless, prolonged episodes of ischaemia may eventually result in overloading the astrocytes with Na^+ with a consequent reversal of the Na^+/glutamate and other transporters leading to an additional release of glutamate, H^+ and K^+ into the extracellular space (Billups and Attwell 1996; Rose *et al.* 1998).

3.3.2 Death signal propagates through astrocyte networks?

The development of ischaemic damage to brain tissue has a complicated kinetics. The cessation of, or a considerable decrease in, cerebellar blood flow triggers the onset of infarction. At this stage, cells located within the core of the ischaemic region undergo an anoxic depolarization and rapidly lose their ability to maintain transmembrane ion gradients (Siesjö 1992). This results in a considerable Na^+ and Ca^{2+} influx into the cells accompanied by a substantial K^+ efflux, so that very soon (within minutes) the extracellular ion concentration deteriorates severely: for example in the grey matter $[K^+]_o$ rises to 40–60 mM, whereas $[Na^+]_o$ and $[Ca^{2+}]_o$ decline to 60 mM and 0.2–0.5 mM respectively (Sykova *et al.* 1994; Kraig *et al.* 1995). Simultaneously, the extracellular pH drops to 6.5 and extracellular levels of glutamate increase markedly. These events amost immediately kill the neurones and most likely, the glial cells, too. A much slower process of expansion of the infarction zone follows this initial formation of infarction core, in a process that is accomplished several hours or even days later (Ginsberg 1995). This slow progression of cell death implicates specific signalling processes propagating from the infarction core towards surrounding tissue. Neuronal signalling pathways can be excluded, as their activity is fully abolished with even a mild reduction of cerebral blood flow (Hossmann 1994). On this basis it has been proposed (Cotrina *et al.* 1998*a*) that astrocytic networks may provide a pathway for the propagation of 'death signals' (Lin *et al.* 1998) which contribute to the expansion of the injury.

Indeed, excessive glutamate released from damaged neurones may initiate aberrant $[Ca^{2+}]_i$ waves in an astrocytic syncytium, which may in turn evoke the distant release of glutamate from astrocytes beyond the ischaemic focus. Thus, a propagating wave of glutamate release from the astrocytes can contribute to the extension of infarction. Although astrocytes are endowed with a defence mechanism, because excessive long-lasting increases in $[Ca^{2+}]_i$ decrease the gap junction permeability, coupling is sufficiently persistent (Cotrina *et al.* 1998*a*) to afford a pathway for various chemical substance to migrate through the astrocyte network. Compelling evidence for the importance of a gap-junction-mediated spread of 'cell death' signals has come from recent experiments showing that transfection of normal and Bcl-2 enriched ischaemia-resistant C6 glioma cells with connexins dramatically increases the vulnerability of the latter to Ca^{2+} ionophores or metabolic insults (Lin *et al.* 1998).

3.4 **ER as a signalling organelle—another source of death signal?**

The initiation and maintenance of glial calcium signals, which act as a communication vehicle within glial networks, is intimately associated with the storage of calcium by the ER. It seems, however, that the importance of calcium dynamics in the ER may be much broader than originally anticipated and may be associated with a variety of novel signals relevant to both physiological and pathological conditions.

Calcium homeostasis in the ER is severely impaired by acute brain insults. Thus, a profound disruption of ER Ca^{2+} homeostasis has been observed in hippocampal neurones undergoing ischaemic insult (Kirino 1982) and depletion of ER calcium stores has been observed under conditions of oxygen–glucose deprivation as well as after global cerebral ischaemia (Pisani *et al.* 2000).

A link between ER calcium homeostasis and neuropathology has also been suggested by studies on various intracellular components involved in neurodegenerative diseases. For example, alteration of ER Ca^{2+} handling by ionophores results in expression of amyloid-beta (Aβ) peptide (Querfurth and Selkoe 1994), a protein involved in the pathogenesis of Alzheimer's disease. The latter may enter the stage in two forms, a relatively benign A (1–40) and a highly toxic Aβ (1–42), a process controlled by another set of ER-resident peptides, presenilins. The formation of Aβ proteins in turn appears to amplify the disruption of ER calcium homeostasis since these peptides have ionophore-like properties (Engstrom *et al.* 1995), thus forming an additional route for Ca^{2+} leakage from the store. A direct influence of Aβ proteins on Ca^{2+} content of the ER has been directly demonstrated in cultured cortical neurones, where they inhibit carbachol-induced Ca^{2+} release (Kelly *et al.* 1996).

Some of the most important evidence for a mechanistic link between ER Ca^{2+} content and cell injury stems from numerous experiments (Tsukamoto and Kaneko 1993; Kaneko and Tsukamoto 1994; Takei and Endo 1994; Bian *et al.* 1997; Nath *et al.* 1997; Zhou *et al.* 1998; see also (Paschen 2001) for review), which have demonstrated that severe and irreversible depletion of ER calcium stores by thapsigargin trigger cell death via either apoptotic or necrotic (Silverstein and Nelson 1992; Paschen 2001) pathways. Unfortunately, while the precise basis for such phenomena has been elusive, evidence is now emerging to suggest that changes in intra-ER free Ca^{2+}, and Ca^{2+} efflux from the ER may trigger powerful stress responses via transcriptional activation. These mechanisms are now discussed.

Besides being an indispensable source for cytoplasmic calcium signalling, the ER plays a fundamental role in cellular biochemistry and trafficking events. The folding and assembly of newly synthesized proteins takes place within the ER lumen in a series of steps catalyzed by numerous enzymatic cascades which require high levels of free Ca^{2+} for correct functioning (Lodish and Kong 1990; Kuznetsov *et al.* 1992; Lodish *et al.* 1992; Paschen 2001). High intraluminal Ca^{2+} concentrations are extremely important for maintaining normal protein synthesis. Consequently, large changes in calcium can trigger bursts of protein misfolding and accumulation of unfolded proteins within the ER lumen. In various cell types such accumulations are now known to trigger specific stress responses that are manifest as two distinct types of pathological cascades: (i) the ER overload response (EOR—(Pahl and Baeuerle 1997)) and (ii) the unfolded protein response (UPR—(Pahl 1999; Patil and Walter, 2001)). The EOR is characterized by an activation of the transcription factor NF-κB, which in turn upregulates the transcription of genes responsible for pro-inflammatory proteins

(Glazner *et al.* 2000). In contrast, the UPR is characterized by an induction in the synthesis of ER-resident stress proteins and the suppression of global protein synthesis.

Not surprisingly, the outcome of the ER stress responses is multifaceted, bearing both protective and pathological functions. For example, the activation of the UPR, upregulates the expression of glucose-regulated protein, grp78 a protein whose overexpression reduces the susceptibility of neurones to oxidative stress and excitotoxicity (Yu *et al.* 1999). In contrast, the downregulation of grp78 has been reported to augment apoptotic neuronal demise (Lee *et al.* 1999). The pathological face of the ER stress response is revealed most prominently in the EOR, which results in activation of NF-κB with subsequent cell death. The latter is also linked to ER Ca^{2+} content, as treatment of cultured neurones with specific inhibitor of InsP$_3$ receptors, Xestospongin C, eliminates NF-κB activation (Glazner *et al.* 2001). Moreover, it seems that protein components of the ER stress response and intra-ER calcium homeostasis are intimately linked. For example, the observation that grp78 over-expression in neurones reduces the amplitude of glutamate-triggered $[Ca^{2+}]_i$ elevations while antisense depletion of grp78 significantly increases glutamate-induced cytosolic Ca^{2+} loads (Yu *et al.* 1999) argues that at least one function of the UPR may be to protect the ER by stabilizing Ca^{2+} homeostasis.

Further support for an interplay between ER stress responses and calcium homeostasis comes from studies showing that depletion of ER calcium in neurones undergoing ischaemic insults coincides with an increase of mRNA encoding ER-stress proteins, such as grp78, grp94 (Wang *et al.* 1993; Lowenstein *et al.* 1994) or transcription factor gadd 153 (Paschen *et al.* 1998). This upregulation of ER-stress proteins is not affected by chelation of cytosolic Ca^{2+}, thus highlighting the importance of lumenal Ca^{2+} exhaustion (Linden *et al.* 1998). In accord with this assumption, inhibition of Ca^{2+} release from the ER by dantrolene or TMB-8, has been found to have a neuroprotective effect, rescuing cells from damage induced by ischaemia or seizures (Mody and MacDonald 1995; Malcolm *et al.* 1996).

Overall it is clear that the ER is a highly important signalling organelle, with the potential for integrating rapid signalling, (Ca^{2+} release) with long-lasting cellular plasticity. Any disruption in ER Ca^{2+} homeostasis, therefore, has the demonstrated potential to trigger various pathological reactions, ultimately resulting in cell injury and death. Unfortunately, the ER stress responses in astrocytes remain largely unexplored, although it seems reasonable to suggest, that they may play an important role in the response of glial networks to brain injury. For example, in diseases such as cerebral ischaemia, aberrant calcium waves produced by indices of ischaemia/infarction in grey matter may cause a severe depletion of astrocytic ER calcium leading to a stress response that can be indirectly propagated throughout the astrocyte syncytium away from the infarct core, thus, further contributing in development of the ischaemic damage.

3.5 **Conclusion**

In this review we have discussed the potential and established roles of astroglial networks in healthy and diseased nervous tissue. Much of our focus has been on the cellular and intercellular mechanisms involved in signal propagation. Thus, we suggest a new view of the ER where it acts as a signalling organelle capable of providing a direct link between environmental stimulation and the generation of transcriptional signals, in particular those mediating stress responses. By playing a key role in long-range intercellular communication, we suggest that astrocytes propagate not only beneficial but also deleterious signals, and equally important *signalling responses*, throughout healthy and diseased brain tissues.

References

Alvarez-Maubecin, V., Garcia-Hernandez, F., Williams, J. T., and Van Bockstaele, E. J. (2000). Functional coupling between neurons and glia. *J Neurosci*, **20**, 4091–8.

Araque, A., Carmignoto, G., and Haydon, P. G. (2001). Dynamic signaling between astrocytes and neurons. *Annu Rev Physiol*, **63**, 795–813.

Araque, A., Sanzgiri, R. P., Parpura, V., and Haydon, P. G. (1998). Calcium elevation in astrocytes causes an NMDA receptor-dependent increase in the frequency of miniature synaptic currents in cultured hippocampal neurons. *J Neurosci*, **18**, 6822–9.

Araque, A., Parpura, V., Sanzgiri, R. P., and Haydon, P. G. (1999). Tripartite synapses: glia, the unacknowledged partner. *Trends Neurosci*, **22**, 208–15.

Araque, A., Li, N., Doyle, R. T., and Haydon P. G. (2000). SNARE protein-dependent glutamate release from astrocytes. *J Neurosci*, **20**, 666–73.

Bennett, M. V., Barrio, L. C., Bargiello, T. A., Spray, D. C., Hertzberg, E., and Saez, J. C. (1991). Gap junctions: new tools, new answers, new questions. *Neuron*, **6**, 305–20.

Bezzi, P., Carmignoto, G., Pasti, L., Vesce, S., Rossi, D., and Rizzini, B. L., *et al.* (1998). Prostaglandins stimulate calcium-dependent glutamate release in astrocytes. *Nature*, **391**, 281–5.

Bian, X., Hughes, F. M., Jr., Huang, Y., Cidlowski, J. A., and Putney, J. W., Jr. (1997). Roles of cytoplasmic Ca^{2+} and intracellular Ca^{2+} stores in induction and suppression of apoptosis in S49 cells. *Am J Physiol*, **272**, C1241–9.

Billups, B., Attwell, D. (1996). Modulation of non-vesicular glutamate release by pH. *Nature*, **379**, 171–4.

Charles, A. C., Merrill, J. E., Dirksen, E. R., and Sanderson, M. J. (1991). Intercellular signaling in glial cells: calcium waves and oscillations in response to mechanical stimulation and glutamate. *Neuron*, **6**, 983–92.

Charles, A. C., Naus, C. C., Zhu, D., Kidder, G. M., Dirksen, E. R., and Sanderson, M. J. (1992). Intercellular calcium signaling via gap junctions in glioma cells. *J Cell Biol*, **118**, 195–201.

Choi, D. W. and Rothman, S. M. (1990). The role of glutamate neurotoxicity in hypoxic-ischemic neuronal death. *Annu Rev Neurosci*, **13**, 171–82.

Cornell Bell, A. H. and Finkbeiner, S. M. (1991). Ca^{2+} waves in astrocytes. *Cell Calcium* **12**, 185–204.

Cornell Bell, A. H., Finkbeiner, S. M., Cooper, M. S., and Smith, S. J. (1990). Glutamate induces calcium waves in cultured astrocytes: long-range glial signaling. *Science*, **247**, 470–3.

Cotrina, M. L., Lin, J. H., Lopez-Garcia, J. C., Naus, C. C., and Nedergaard, M. (2000). ATP-mediated glia signaling. *J Neurosci*, **20**, 2835–44.

Cotrina, M. L., Kang, J., Lin, J. H., Bueno, E., Hansen, T. W., He, L., *et al.* (1998a). Astrocytic gap junctions remain open during ischemic conditions. *J Neurosci*, **18**, 2520–37.

Cotrina, M. L., Lin, J. H., Alves-Rodrigues, A., Liu, S., Li, J., Azmi-Ghadimi, H., *et al.* (1998b). Connexins regulate calcium signaling by controlling ATP release. *Proc Natl Acad Sci USA*, **95**, 15735–40.

Deitmer, J. W., Verkhratsky, A. J., Lohr, C. (1998). Calcium signalling in glial cells. *Cell Calcium*, **24**, 405–16.

Dermietzel, R. (1998a). Diversification of gap junction proteins (connexins) in the central nervous system and the concept of functional compartments. *Cell Biol Int*, **22**, 719–30.

Dermietzel, R. (1998b). Gap junction wiring: a 'new' principle in cell-to-cell communication in the nervous system? *Brain Res Brain Res Rev*, **26**, 176–83.

Dermietzel, R. and Spray, D. C. (1993). Gap junctions in the brain: where, what type, how many and why? *Trends Neurosci*, **16**, 186–92.

Duffy, S. and MacVicar, B. A. (1996). *In vitro* ischemia promotes calcium influx and intracellular calcium release in hippocampal astrocytes. *J Neurosci*, 16, 71–81.

Engstrom, I., Ronquist, G., Pettersson, L., and Waldenstrom, A. (1995). Alzheimer amyloid beta-peptides exhibit ionophore-like properties in human erythrocytes. *Eur J Clin Invest*, 25, 471–6.

Enkvist, M. O. and McCarthy, K. D. (1994). Astroglial gap junction communication is increased by treatment with either glutamate or high K^+ concentration. *J Neurochem* 62, 489–95.

Enkvist, M. O. K. and McCarthy, K. D. (1992). Activation of protein kinase C blocks astroglial gap junction communication and inhibits the spread of calcium waves. *J Neurochem*, 59, 519–26.

Giaume, C. and Venance, L. (1998). Intercellular calcium signaling and gap junctional communication in astrocytes. *Glia*, 24, 50–64.

Giaume, C., Tabernero, A., and Medina, J. M. (1997). Metabolic trafficking through astrocytic gap junctions. *Glia*, 21, 114–23.

Giaume, C., Marin, P., Cordier, J., Glowinski, J., and Premont, J. (1991). Adrenergic regulation of intercellular communications between cultured striatal astrocytes from the mouse. *Proc Natl Acad Sci USA*, 88, 5577–81.

Ginsberg, M. (1995). Neuroprotection in brain ischemia: an update. *The Neuroscientist*, 1, 95–103.

Glazner, G. W., Camandola, S., and Mattson, M. P. (2000). Nuclear factor-kappaB mediates the cell survival-promoting action of activity-dependent neurotrophic factor peptide-9. *J Neurochem*, 75, 101–8.

Glazner, G. W., Camandola, S., Geiger, J. D., and Mattson, M. P. (2001). Endoplasmic reticulum D-myo-inositol 1,4,5-trisphosphate-sensitive stores regulate nuclear factor-kappaB binding activity in a calcium-independent manner. *J Biol Chem*, 276, 22 461–7.

Golovina, V. A. and Blaustein, M. P. (1997). Spatially and functionally distinct Ca^{2+} stores in sarcoplasmic and endoplasmic reticulum. *Science*, 275, 1643–8.

Guthrie, P. B., Knappenberger, J., Segal, M., Bennett, M. V., Charles, A. C., and Kater, S. B. (1999). ATP released from astrocytes mediates glial calcium waves. *J Neurosci*, 19, 520–8.

Harris-White, M. E., Zanotti, S. A., Frautschy, S. A., and Charles, A. C. (1998). Spiral intercellular calcium waves in hippocampal slice cultures. *J Neurophysiol*, 79, 1045–52.

Hassinger, T. D., Guthrie, P. B., Atkinson, P. B., Bennett, M. V. L., and Kater, S. B. (1997). An extracellular signaling component in propagation of astrocytic calcium waves. *Proc Natl Acad Sci USA*, 93, 13 268–73.

Hossmann, K. A. (1994). Viability thresholds and the penumbra of focal ischemia. *Ann Neurol*, 36, 557–65.

John, G. R., Scemes, E., Suadicani, S. O., Liu, J. S., Charles, P. C., Lee, S. C., *et al.* (1999). IL-1beta differentially regulates calcium wave propagation between primary human fetal astrocytes via pathways involving P2 receptors and gap junction channels. *Proc Natl Acad Sci USA*, 96, 11 613–18.

Kaneko, Y. and Tsukamoto, A. (1994). Thapsigargin-induced persistent intracellular calcium pool depletion and apoptosis in human hepatoma cells. *Cancer Lett*, 79, 147–55.

Kelly, J. F., Furukawa, K., Barger, S. W., Rengen, M. R., Mark, R. J., Blanc, E. M., *et al.* (1996). Amyloid beta-peptide disrupts carbachol-induced muscarinic cholinergic signal transduction in cortical neurons. *Proc Natl Acad Sci USA*, 93, 6753–8.

Kim, W. T., Rioult, M. G., and Cornell Bell, A. H. (1994). Glutamate-induced calcium signaling in astrocytes. *Glia*, 11, 173–84.

Kirino, T. (1982). Delayed neuronal death in the gerbil hippocampus following ischemia. *Brain Res* 239, 57–69.

Kraig, R. P., Lascola, C. D., and Caggiano, A. (1995). Glial response to brain ischemia. In: *Neuroglia* (ed. H. Kettenmann and B. R. Ransom) OUP, New York, pp. 964–76.

Kuznetsov, G., Brostrom, M. A., and Brostrom, C. O. (1992). Demonstration of a calcium requirement for secretory protein processing and export. Differential effects of calcium and dithiothreitol. *J Biol Chem*, 267, 3932–9.

Lee, J., Bruce-Keller, A. J., Kruman, Y., Chan, S. L., and Mattson, M. P. (1999). 2-Deoxy-D-glucose protects hippocampal neurons against excitotoxic and oxidative injury: evidence for the involvement of stress proteins. *J Neurosci Res*, 57, 48–61.

Lin, J. H., Weigel, H., Cotrina, M. L., Liu, S., Bueno, E., Hansen, A. J., *et al.* (1998). Gap-junction-mediated propagation and amplification of cell injury. *Nat Neurosci*, 1, 494–500.

Linden, T., Doutheil, J., and Paschen, W. (1998). Role of calcium in the activation of erp72 and heme oxygenase-1 expression on depletion of endoplasmic reticulum calcium stores in rat neuronal cell culture. *Neurosci Lett*, 247, 103–6.

Lodish, H. F., Kong, N. (1990). Perturbation of cellular calcium blocks exit of secretory proteins from the rough endoplasmic reticulum. *J Biol Chem*, 265, 10 893–9.

Lodish, H. F., Kong, N., and Wikstrom, L. (1992). Calcium is required for folding of newly made subunits of the asialoglycoprotein receptor within the endoplasmic reticulum. *J Biol Chem*, 267, 12 753–60.

Lowenstein, D. H., Gwinn, R. P., Seren, M. S., Simon, R. P., and McIntosh, T. K. (1994). Increased expression of mRNA encoding calbindin-D28K, the glucose-regulated proteins, or the 72 kDa heat-shock protein in three models of acute CNS injury. *Brain Res Mol Brain Res*, 22, 299–308.

Malcolm, C. S., Ritchie, L., Grieve, A., and Griffiths, R. (1996). A prototypic intracellular calcium antagonist, TMB-8, protects cultured cerebellar granule cells against the delayed, calcium-dependent component of glutamate neurotoxicity. *J Neurochem*, 66, 2350–60.

Marrero, H. and Orkand, R. K. (1996). Nerve impulses increase glial intercellular permeability. *Glia*, 16, 285–9.

Mody, I. and MacDonald, J. F. (1995). NMDA receptor-dependent excitotoxicity: the role of intracellular Ca^{2+} release. *Trends Pharmacol Sci*, 16, 356–9.

Nagy, J. I. and Rash, J. E. (2000). Connexins and gap junctions of astrocytes and oligodendrocytes in the CNS. *Brain Res Brain Res Rev*, 32, 29–44.

Nagy, J. I., Ochalski, P. A., Li, J., and Hertzberg, E. L. (1997). Evidence for the co-localization of another connexin with connexin-43 at astrocytic gap junctions in rat brain. *Neuroscience*, 78, 533–48.

Nagy, J. I., Yamamoto, T., Sawchuk, M. A., Nance, D. M., and Hertzberg, E. L. (1992). Quantitative immunohistochemical and biochemical correlates of connexin43 localization in rat brain. *Glia*, 5, 1–9.

Nath, R., Raser, K. J., Hajimohammadreza, I., and Wang, K. K. (1997). Thapsigargin induces apoptosis in SH-SY5Y neuroblastoma cells and cerebrocortical cultures. *Biochem Mol Biol Int*, 43, 197–205.

Nedergaard, M. (1994). Direct signaling from astrocytes to neurons in cultures of mammalian brain cells. *Science*, 263, 1768–71.

Newman, E. A. (1986*a*). High potassium conductance in astrocyte endfeet. *Science* 233, 453–4.

Newman, E. A. (1986*b*). Regional specialization of the membrane of retinal glial cells and its importance to K^+ spatial buffering. *Ann N Y Acad Sci*, 481, 273–86.

Newman, E. A. (1996). Acid efflux from retinal glial cells generated by sodium bicarbonate cotransport. *J Neurosci* 16, 159–68.

Newman, E. A. and Zahs, K. R. (1997). Calcium waves in retinal glial cells. *Science*, 275, 844–7.

Pahl, H. L. (1999). Signal transduction from the endoplasmic reticulum to the cell nucleus. *Physiol Rev* 79, 683–701.

Pahl, H.L. and Baeuerle, P. A. (1997). The ER-overload response: activation of NF-kappa B. *Trends Biochem Sci*, 22, 63–7.

Parpura, V., Basarsky, T. A., Liu, F., Jeftinija, K., Jeftinija, S., and Haydon, P. G. (1994). Glutamate-mediated astrocyte-neuron signalling. *Nature*, 369, 744–7.

Paschen, W. (2001). Dependence of vital cell function on endoplasmic reticulum calcium levels: implications for the mechanisms underlying neuronal cell injury in different pathological states. *Cell Calcium*, 29, 1–11.

Paschen, W., Gissel, C., Linden, T., Althausen, S., and Doutheil, J. (1998). Activation of gadd153 expression through transient cerebral ischemia: evidence that ischemia causes endoplasmic reticulum dysfunction. *Brain Res Mol Brain Res*, 60, 115–22.

Pasti, L., Volterra, A., Pozzan, T., and Carmignoto, G. (1997). Intracellular calcium oscillations in astrocytes: a highly plastic, bidirectional form of communication between neurons and astrocytes in situ. *J Neurosci* 17, 7817–30.

Pasti, L., Zonta, M., Pozzan, T., Vicini, S., and Carmignoto, G. (2001). Cytosolic calcium oscillations in astrocytes may regulate exocytotic release of glutamate. *J Neurosci*, 21, 477–84.

Patil, C. and Walter, P. (2001). Intracellular signaling from the endoplasmic reticulum to the nucleus: the unfolded protein response in yeast and mammals. *Curr Opin Cell Biol*, 13, 349–55.

Pisani, A., Bonsi, P., Centonze, D., Giacomini, P., and Calabresi, P. (2000). Involvement of intracellular calcium stores during oxygen/glucose deprivation in striatal large aspiny interneurons. *J Cereb Blood Flow Metab*, 20, 839–46.

Presley, J. F., Cole, N. B., Schroer, T. A., Hirschberg, K., Zaal, K. J., and Lippincott-Schwartz, J. (1997). ER-to-Golgi transport visualized in living cells. *Nature* 389, 81–5.

Querfurth, H. W. and Selkoe, D. J. (1994). Calcium ionophore increases amyloid beta peptide production by cultured cells. *Biochemistry* 33, 4550–61.

Ransom, B. R. and Fern, R. (1996). Anoxic-ischemic glial cells injury: mechanisms and consequences. In: *Tissue oxygen deprivation* (ed. G. G. Haddad and G. Lister), Dekker, New York, pp. 617–52.

Rash, J. E., Duffy, H. S., Dudek, F. E., Bilhartz, B. L., Whalen, L. R., and Yasumura, T. (1997). Grid-mapped freeze-fracture analysis of gap junctions in gray and white matter of adult rat central nervous system, with evidence for a 'panglial syncytium' that is not coupled to neurons. *J Comp Neurol* 388, 265–92.

Rose, C. R., Waxman, S. G., and Ransom, B. R. (1998). Effects of glucose deprivation, chemical hypoxia, and simulated ischemia on Na^+ homeostasis in rat spinal cord astrocytes. *J Neurosci*, 18, 3554–62.

Scemes, E., Dermietzel, R., and Spray, D. C. (1998). Calcium waves between astrocytes from Cx43 knockout mice. *Glia*, 24, 65–73.

Siesjö, B. K. (1985). Membrane events leading to glial swelling and brain edema. In: *Brain edema* (ed. Inaba Y), Springer, Berlin, pp. 200–9.

Siesjö, B. K. (1992). **Pathophysiology and treatment of focal cerebral ischemia. Part II: Mechanisms of damage and treatment.** *J Neurosurg*, 77, 337–54.

Silver, I. A., Deas, J., and Erecinska, M. (1997). Ion homeostasis in brain cells: differences in intracellular ion responses to energy limitation between cultured neurons and glial cells. *Neuroscience*, 78, 589–601.

Silverstein, F. S. and Nelson, C. (1992). The microsomal calcium-ATPase inhibitor thapsigargin is a neurotoxin in perinatal rodent brain. *Neurosci Lett* 145, 157–60.

Simpson, P. B., Mehotra, S., Langley, D., Sheppard, C. A., and Russell, J. T. (1998). Specialized distributions of mitochondria and endoplasmic reticulum proteins define Ca^{2+} wave amplification sites in cultured astrocytes. *J Neurosci Res* 52, 672–83.

Sykova, E., Svoboda, J., Polak, J., and Chvatal, A. (1994). Extracellular volume fraction and diffusion characteristics during progressive ischemia and terminal anoxia in the spinal cord of the rat. *J Cereb Blood Flow Metab*, 14, 301–11.

Tabernero, A., Giaume, C., and Medina, J. M. (1996). Endothelin-1 regulates glucose utilization in cultured astrocytes by controlling intercellular communication through gap junctions. *Glia*, 16, 187–95.

Takei, N., and Endo, Y. (1994). Ca^{2+} ionophore-induced apoptosis on cultured embryonic rat cortical neurons. *Brain Res*, 652, 65–70.

Tsukamoto, A., and Kaneko, Y. (1993). Thapsigargin, a Ca^{2+}-ATPase inhibitor, depletes the intracellular Ca^{2+} pool and induces apoptosis in human hepatoma cells. *Cell Biol Int*, 17, 969–70.

Veenstra, R. D. (1996). Size and selectivity of gap junction channels formed from different connexins. *J Bioenerg Biomembr*, **28**, 327–37.

Verkhratsky, A., Orkand, R. K., and Kettenmann, H. (1998). Glial calcium: homeostasis and signaling function. *Physiol Rev* **78**, 99–141.

Wang, S., Longo, F. M., Chen, J., Butman, M., Graham, S. H., Haglid, K. G., and Sharp, F. R. (1993). Induction of glucose regulated protein (grp78) and inducible heat shock protein (hsp70) mRNAs in rat brain after kainic acid seizures and focal ischemia. *Neurochem Int*, **23**, 575–82.

Willecke, K., Hennemann, H., Dahl, E., Jungbluth, S., and Heynkes, R. (1991). The diversity of connexin genes encoding gap junctional proteins. *Eur J Cell Biol*, **56**, 1–7.

Yu, Z., Luo, H., Fu, W., and Mattson, M. P. (1999). The endoplasmic reticulum stress-responsive protein GRP78 protects neurons against excitotoxicity and apoptosis: suppression of oxidative stress and stabilization of calcium homeostasis. *Exp Neurol*, **155**, 302–14.

Zhou, Y. P., Teng, D., Dralyuk, F., Ostrega, D., Roe, M. W., Philipson, L., and Polonsky, K. S. (1998). Apoptosis in insulin-secreting cells. Evidence for the role of intracellular Ca^{2+} stores and arachidonic acid metabolism. *J Clin Invest*, **101**, 1623–32.

Chapter 4

Blood–brain barrier and perivascular cells

Barbro B. Johansson

4.1 Introduction

The blood–brain barrier (BBB) is a dynamic interface between blood and brain that restricts the entry of plasma constitutents that could interfere negatively with brain function while allowing substances that are essential for brain metabolism and function to enter the brain via complex carrier and receptor-mediated transport mechanisms, which also regulate the brain to blood efflux of metabolites and neuromodulaters. In addition, perivascular astrocytes and other perivascular cells influence the induction, maintenance, and modulation of the BBB.

4.1.1 Structural basis for the blood–brain barrier

The brain endothelial cells contain few pinocytotic vesicles and are sealed together by continuous and complex tight junctions, zonula occludens (Brightman and Tao-Cheng 1993). A schematic illustration of the BBB interface is shown in Fig. 4.1. Tight junctions are composed of transmembrane and cytoplasmatic proteins linked to an actin-based cytoskeleton that allow the junctions to form a seal while remaining capable of rapid modulation and regulation (Lapierre 2000; Kniesel and Wolburg 2000; Huber *et al.* 2001). Most studies on the molecular structure and regulation of tight junctions have been performed on epithelial tight junctions. Transmembrane tight junction proteins include claudin, occludin, and junction adhesion molecules (JAM), members of the immunoglobulin superfamily. The permeability of tight junctions varies with the function of the tissue forming the barrier (Lapierre 2000). In the mouse, the heterogeneity of endothelial junctions is reflected by different expression and specific subcellular localization of three JAM molecules with the highest vascular expression of JAM-1 found in the adult brain (Aurrand-Lions *et al.* 2001). In addition tight junctions are made up of accessory proteins that are necessary for structural support such as zonula occludens proteins ZO1, ZO2, ZO3 and 7H6 antigen. The primary cytosketal protein actin has binding sites to all ZO proteins, to claudin and occluding and actin filaments have structural and dynamic functions. Signalling molecules regulating tight junction permeability include protein kinase C, cAMP, G-protein coupled events, and calcium (Huber *et al.* 2001). Cytokines and growth factors can modulate tight junctions *in vitro* and *in vivo* (Walsh *et al.* 2000).

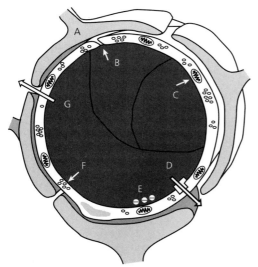

Fig. 4.1 Schematic representation of a cerebral capillary. (A = astrocytic end feet, B = tight junction, C = mitochondria, D = transport mechanism for, for example, glucose and amino acids, E = endothelial cell negative charge, F = enzymes in brain capillaries, G = receptor-mediated peptide transport).

4.1.2 Polarity of brain endothelial cells

The brain endothelial cells share many characteristics with tight and polarized epithelial cells. They have a high electrical resistance and the abluminal and luminal plasma membranes differ. Na^+–K^+-ATPase and 5-nucleotidase are predominantly found on the abluminal side, whereas gamma-glutamyltranspeptidase (GGT), that is not present in any detectable amounts in other capillary beds, is found predominantly on the luminal side. The distribution within the brain differs indicating regional heterogeneity in brain microvessels (Wolff *et al.* 1992). The polarity provides the basis for transcellular transport. The Na^+–K^+-ATPase on the abluminal side removes potassium from the brain extracellular fluid and transport sodium in the opposite direction, an important function for maintaining homeostasis of the neuronal environment. The complex ion transport over the BBB is reviewed by Keep *et al.* (1998).

4.1.3 Carrier-mediated transport of nutrients

Because of the tight junctions, the passage of solutes is mainly transcellular and essentially determined by the lipid solubility of the substances. Exceptions to this rule are substances that have access to specific carrier mechanisms in the endothelial cells.

A high content of mitochondria reflects the metabolic activity needed to maintain ion differentials between blood plasma and brain extracellular fluid and to maintain the unique functions of the brain endothelial cells (Oldendorf *et al.* 1977). A large number of carrier-mediated transport systems have been identified in the brain endothelial cells, (Bradbury 1992; Keep *et al.* 1998; Pardridge 1998, 1999; Cornford and Hyman 1999; Begley *et al.* 2000). Major transport systems for metabolic substrates are carriers for hexosis, monocarboxylic acids, and amino acids. The main energy source for the brain, D-glucose, enters the brain via a saturable and stereospecific facilitated transport using the GLUT-1 transporter (Kalaria *et al.* 1988; Gjedde 1992). During the neonatal period, the main substances for the brain are pyruvate, lactate, and beta-hydroxy-butyrate, substrates that use a monocarboxylic acid transporter that has a high capacity in the post-natal period and then declines. The decline seems to be regulated by diet and linked to weaning. During starvation, the monocarboxylic carrier can again increase its capacity allowing ketone bodies to substitute glucose as main energy substrate for the brain. Studies in man implies that the influx of ketone bodies into the brain is largely determined by the amount of ketones present in the blood and that any condition in which ketonaemia occurs will lead to an increased ketone influx (Hasselbalch *et al.* 1995).

The presence of three amino acid transport mechanisms were demonstrated more than thirty years ago, and recent studies have demonstrated several more (Smith and Stoll 1998). Most of the plasma neutral amino acids are transported by a stereospecific, bi-directional sodium/energy independent transporter. Because the transporter is heavily saturated at normal plasma concentrations, it is sensitive to competition. Another stereospecific, sodium/ energy independent and bi-directional carrier system mediates the brain uptake of three cationic amino acids: arginine, lysine, and ornithine. A further system is a sodium dependent amino acid transport system with affinity for neutral amino acids. Because most *in vivo* studies have shown little evidence for transport of these amino acids into brain it was proposed, and later confirmed that the transporter was confined to the capillary abluminal membrane. It may have an important role in removal of amino acids from the brain extracellular fluid. Amino acids with transmitter functions within the brain, GABA, glutamate, glycine, and aspartate, have little access to the brain in *in vivo* studies, and a low activity transporter for glutamate and aspartate may function to pump anionic amino acids out of the brain.

In general, protein and peptides have difficulty in passing the BBB. Some peptides, for example, insulin, insulin-like growth factor and transferrin enter the brain by a receptor-mediated transcytosis, and other peptide can be coupled to such vectors to get access to the brain (Pardridge 1998, 1999; Begley *et al.* 2000; Bickel *et al.* 2001). However, to what extent various peptides including cytokines enter the brain is controversial (Banks and Kastin 1996) and there might be species differences. Thus, human interleukin-1 (IL-1) alpha is transported across the murine but not the rat BBB (Plotkin *et al.* 2000). It has been suggested that transporters associated with smaller peptides such as enkephalin and vasopressin may function in a similar manner to the carriers associated with amino acid transport (Begley 1996). Numerous receptors for peptides are present on cerebral capillary endothelial cells and peptides probably can interact with the blood–brain interface without actually entering the brain. Some examples for cytokines are given in Section 4.7 of this review. As discussed in the following section, an efflux transporter can deliver peptides from brain to blood (King *et al.* 2001).

4.1.4 Efflux transport systems

P-glycoprotein, a multidrug resistance gene product, is an ATP-dependent transport protein that functions as an active efflux pump in any cells, including brain endothelial cells (Schinkel 1999). Disruption of the mdr P-glycoprotein gene in the mouse significantly enhances the uptake of many drugs including cyclosporin A, vinblanstin, quinidine, verapamin, actinomycin D (Schinkel *et al.* 1995). Efflux can be inhibited by competition (Jette *et al.* 1995), and potent P-glykoprotein inhibitors increase the acute toxicity to cyclosporin A (Diedier and Loor 1995). A P-glycoprotein mediated efflux of phenytoin, has recently been observed in the rat brain (Potschka and Loscher 2001). Bilirubin is an endogenous substance that may be prevented from brain entry by this mechanism (Watchko *et al.* 1998). P-glycoprotein is present at the abluminal surface of the endothelial cells on neighbouring astrocyte foot processes (Golden and Pardridge 2000), and is expressed in rat astrocyte cultures although at lower levels than in endothelial cell cultures (Declèves *et al.* 2000).

The functional implication of P-glycoprotein on systemic bioavailability of xenobiotics and anticancer drugs remains to be defined in humans. P-glycoprotein inhibition leads to enhanced disruptive effects by anti-microtubule cytostatics at the BBB *in vitro* (van der Sandt *et al.* 2001). Several inhibitors of P-glycoprotein are currently on the clinical trial stage and natural inhibitors of P-glycoprotein have been discovered. Polymorphism, noted in animals and malignant cells, may if present in humans, be critically important for pharmacotherapy (Liu and Hu 2000).

Studies have so far been directed toward the capacity of the efflux system to prevent substances from entering the brain. However, as indicated in a recent report on transport of opiods from the brain to the blood by P-glycoprotein (King *et al.* 2001), an important physiological function may be to pump active neuromodulators from the brain to the periphery. A second efflux transport protein subfamily is the multidrug resistance protein (MRP) family that has been less studied in the brain (Lee *et al.* 2001). In contrast to P-glycoprotein, higher levels of MRP1 have been observed in primary astrocytes than in brain endothelial cells (Declèves *et al.* 2000).

4.1.5 Enzymatic barriers

Enzymes in the brain endothelial cells can degrade substances that are not impeded by the luminal endothelial membrane (Hardebo and Owman 1990). Degrading enzymes present in brain endothelial cells include aromatic L-amino acid decarboxylase, monoamine oxidase, angiotensin converting enzyme, aminopeptidase A-degrading angiotensin II and enkephalin degrading aminopeptidase. The precursors of dopamine and serotonin, L-dopa and tryptophan, enter the brain by facilitated transport and are then decarboxylated to dopamine and serotonin, substances that are metabolized by monoaminoxidase and catechol-O-methyltransferase (COMT). However, these enzymes have a limited capacity and if given in high doses, L-dopa can enter the brain parenchyma. By combining L-dopa with a peripheral decarboxylase inhibitor, the dose and side effects can be reduced and the clinical response improved.

High activities of enzymes primarily involved in the metabolism of lipophilic xenobiotics in the liver, for example, cytochrome P-450-linked monooxygenase, epoxidehydrolase, NADP-cytochrome P-450-reductase and 1-naphtol-UDP-glycuronyl-transferase are present in rat brain microvessels and are likely to reduce the brain toxicity of lipophilic xenobiotics (Ghersi-Egea *et al.* 1994; el-Bacha and Minn 1999). Enzymatic drug metabolism by cerebral endothelial cells can thus provide protection to the brain against blood-born toxic molecules but have also been proposed to synthesize toxic substances from exogenous and endogenous sources, thereby generating reactive metabolites responsible for some brain dysfunctions and neurodegenerative disorders.

4.1.6 Endothelial charge

Glycocalyx, a negatively charged layer of a fibrous chain of macromolecules mainly glycoproteins cover the luminal surface of endothelial cells. It is a dynamic structure presenting a barrier to movement of macromolecules from plasma to the endothelial surface. Anionic sites are also present in the plasmolemma and the basement membrane of brain endothelial cells. The pattern of glycocalyx and endothelial cell anionic sites in the brain differs from those in other capillary beds (Johansson 2001), and a comparison of brain endothelial cells *in vitro* and *in vivo* have indicated differences in anion composition and distribution (Dos Santos *et al.* 1995). One possible explanation could be the absence of astrocytes in the culture. An astrocyte-derived protein factor promotes proteoglycan synthesis in endothelial cells resulting in increased charge selectivity of the BBB during development (Yamagata *et al.* 1997), which is consistent with an earlier shown sequential appearance of anionic domains in the developing BBB (Vorbrodt *et al.* 1990). Because of the glycocalyx and endothelial negative charge, anionic molecules enter the brain less readily than uncharged or cationic molecules of equal size. Cationization of serum albumin, immunoglobulin G, and anti-bodies significantly increases their passage into the brain (Triguero *et al.* 1989). Intracarotid infusion of polycations rapidly and transiently increase the passage of plasma constituents into the brain (see Johansson 2001).

4.2 **Astrocytes and the blood–brain barrier**

Astrocytic foot processes cover more than 90 per cent of the brain capillary circumference. Astrocytes stimulate tight junction strand formation and enhance the barrier function of brain capillary endothelial cells *in vitro* (Janzer and Raff 1987; Wolburg *et al.* 1994; Hayashi *et al.* 1997). Tight junctions are formed early in rat fetus and the BBB to albumin is estab-lished at that time. In contrast, the barrier to sucrose and inulin tightens markedly between the fourth and ninth day after birth and reaches adult degree by 2–3 weeks (Ferguson and Woodbury 1969), a time corresponding to the maturation of the glial foot processes sur-rounding the larger part of the endothelial cell surface and the capillary basement membrane. Endothelial cells in culture lose the BBB characteristics after a few passages *in vitro*. Co-culture with astrocytes help the endothelial cells to retain their BBB characteristics in culture, and tight junctions can be induced in endothelial cells of non-neuronal origin by astrocytes or a soluble astrocyte-derived factor (Janzer and Raff 1987). Astrocytes may participate in maintenance of ionic homeostasis by regulating Na-K-Cl co-transporter function at the BBB (Sun *et al.* 1997). By induction of manganese superoxide dismutase, a free radical scavenger, they protect in the endothelial cells (Schroeter *et al.* 2001). Soluble factors produced by glial cells help restrict development of inflammation within the CNS under basal culture conditions (Prat *et al.* 2001). However, when activated in response to signals generated within the brain or the immune system, they produce inflammatory molecules that increase permeability and promote lymphocyte passage.

Endothelial cells have recently been reported to induce astrocyte differentiation which sup-porting a bi-directional interaction (Mi *et al.* 2001). Astrocytes and endothelial cells respond to a variety of stimuli with an increase in intracellular free calcium, and fast-acting calcium signals can be communicated to adjacent cells through an intracellular/gap junctional pathway and an extracellular purinergic pathway (Leybaert *et al.* 1998; Braet *et al.* 2001).

4.3 **Perivascular cells**

4.3.1 **Pericytes**

Pericytes are perivascular cells enclosed within the basal membrane of microvessels in both fenestrated and continuous endothelial cells, and extend long cytoplastic processes over the surface of the endothelial cell. Communicating gap junctions, tight junctions, and adhesion plaques are present at points of contact. (Allt and Lawrenson 2001). Pericytes show structural and functional heterogeneity and have multifunctional activities. Interactions between pericytes and endothelial cells are thought to be important for the maturation, remodelling, and maintenance of the vascular system. In the brain, pericytes are involved in the transport across the BBB and regulation of vascular permeability. They contain BBB specific enzymes including high amounts of GGT, possibly relevant in amino acid transport (Frey *et al.* 1991; Risau *et al.* 1992). The presence of aminopeptidase N suggests that cerebral pericytes are involved in amino acid and peptide catabolism and that they may constitute part of the enzymatic BBB (Krause *et al.* 1993). The pericytes in the pre- and post-capillary regions contain actin filaments, which have been suggested to be able to modify brain microcirculation and tight junctions. Several agents have been shown to regulate contraction of vascular pericytes (Rucker *et al.* 2000). In the view of Thomas (1999), pericytes in the brain possess the full macrophage functions and behave similar to other tissue macrophages. Others do not ascribe them any phagocytotic activity (Kida *et al.* 1993; Angelov *et al.* 1998; Bechmann *et al.* 2001). Pericytes in other organs have been shown to give rise to various mesodermal cell types including smooth muscle cells, fibroblasts, osteoblasts, and chondroblasts. Thomas (1999) has suggested that also brain pericytes may be multipotent and serve as precursors for a variety of other cell types including microglia. According to him, some pericytes or pericytes-similar cells can be observed outside the basal membrane and share many characteristics with microglia. The same opinion has been proposed based on an electron microscopic study (Monteiro *et al.* 1996).

4.3.2 Perivascular macrophages and microglia

Although much progress has been made on understanding the origin and function of perivascular cells, some controversies remain as to their origin and whether or not they can migrate into the brain (Hickey *et al.* 1992; Graeber 1993; Kida *et al.* 1993; Thomas 1999; Rucker *et al.* 2000; Bechmann *et al.* 2001; Allt and Lawrenson 2001; Williams *et al.* 2001). Some investigators distinguish phagocytic perivascular cells, pericytes, and perivascular microglia based on their location in relation to the three basement membranes between endothelium and glia limitans, others restrict the term perivascular cells to those present in the Virchow–Robin space, an extension of the subpial space that surrounds arteries entering and veins emerging from the cerebral cortex. At the capillary level the vascular and glial basement membranes fuse together, obliterating the fluid-filled space. The Virchow–Robin space contains macrophages which may be distinguished from pericytes and microglia by their anatomical location, size, relatively small number under normal conditions, and by the absence of actin. As mentioned in the previous section, others do not draw a sharp line between pericytes, microglia, and macrophages (Monteiro *et al.* 1996; Thomas 1999; Rucker *et al.* 2000).

According to Lassmann *et al.* (1991) processes of parenchymatous microglial cells are incorporated in the layer of astrocytic foot processes of the perivascular glia limitans, proposed to function in presenting p antigen to T-cells that enter the central nervous system (CNS). Gehrmann *et al.* (1995) defined two subsets of macrophages/microglia close to the blood vessels, that is, perivascular cells enclosed within the basal lamina which can undergo replacement with bone marrow-derived cells and juxtavascular microglia which make direct contact with the parenchymatous side of the CNS vascular basal lamina but represent true intraparenchymal resident microglia.

Bone marrow chimeric experiments indicate that a high percentage of the perivascular cells undergo replacement with bone marrow-derived cells (Hickey *et al.* 1992). This has been questioned (Kida *et al.* 1993) but confirmed in a recent study. With a double labeling technique with macrophages injected with 4 weeks interval, the tracers were shown to be taken up within hours and remain stable in perivascular cells for at least 8 weeks. During that time no cells were seen to enter the brain parenchyma (Bechmann *et al.* 2001). The constantly replaced pool of perivascular cells probably represents an entry route by which HIV infected monocytes get access to the brain (Fischer-Smith *et al.* 2001).

With current knowledge of cell differentiation and its interaction with the environment, it seems reasonable to assume that the further fate of monocytes entering the brain may differ depending on factors, such as whether or not they enter the brain, where the blood vessels are surrounded by the fluid filled Virchow–Robin space or at the capillary level. Different terminology used may reflect subpopulations of perivascular cells within different anatomical regions and experimental paradigm, neuropathological conditions and species studied (Williams *et al.* 2001).

4.3.3 Perivascular mast cells

Mast cells are located in the leptomeninges and concentrated in the brain parenchyma along the blood vessels in the thalamus on the brain side of the BBB which recently been shown to enter the brain through intact brain blood vessels (Silverman *et al.* 2000). Their functions are still poorly understood although they are known to increase in activity and number in response to changed physiological conditions.

4.4 Lymphocyte surveillance of the brain

Polynuclear leucocytes are considered not to enter an intact BBB, although systemic lipo-polysaccharide injection has recently been shown to induce an influx of granulocytes into the healthy brain (Bohatschek *et al.* 2001). It is, however, generally accepted that the brain is subjected to limited immunological surveillance, and lymphocytes are normally present in small numbers in the cerebrospinal fluid. Activated T-lymphocyte introduced into the circulation rapidly appear in the CNS reaching a peak between 9 and 12 h and exited within 1–2 days (Hickey *et al.* 1991). Activation of adhesion molecules in the endothelial cells by cytokines will increase the expression of intercellular adhesion molecules and facilitate the entry of lymphocytes (Lassmann 1997; de Vries *et al.* 1997; Eden and Parkos 2000; Starzyk *et al.* 2000; Brown 2001). The passage of lymphocytes over the BBB may differ more in degree than in nature from passage over other endothelial cells (Hickey 2001). After passage the lymphocyte may die by apoptosis or leave the brain via the cerebrospinal fluid (CSF) that drains predominantly via the arachnoid villi on the brain surface or directly to blood over the endothelial cells. An alternative route of possible significance under pathological conditions is the drainage of brain extracellular fluid to the retropharyngeal lymph glands via the cribriform plate in the nasal cavity, a passage that is well documented in animals (Bradbury *et al.* 1981; Widner *et al.* 1987, 1988; Cserr *et al.* 1992) and in man (Löwhagen *et al.* 1994).

4.5 Interaction between endothelium, perivascular cells and environment in response to chronic and acute infection

Resident perivascular cells are well situated to interact with activated T-lymphocytes and they are probably of prime importance in initiating immunological processes in the brain.

The role of resident perivascular cells as compared to invading monocytes and macrophages in response to neuronal injury is debated. The majority of proliferating cells that respond to selective neuronal injury, including macrophages and monocytes, are probably not intrinsic but entering from the blood. The perivascular cell may have a main role as initiating processes allowing monocytes and macrophages to enter from the blood. Monocytes interact with cerebral endothelial cells via adhesion molecules, and activation of adhesion molecules leads to increased production of inflammatory mediators, which in turn can induce reactive oxygen species shown to enhance the migration of cells across the BBB *in vitro* (van der Goes *et al.* 2001). Participation of specific cytokines may vary with the experimental model used. See Section 4.7.

Paracellular permeability is altered during the migration of leucocyte across the apical junctions complex and the apical junction complex plays an important role in the regulation of leukocyte transmigration through the endothelium (Martin-Padura *et al.* 1998; Edens and Parkos 2000). TNF alpha and IFN-gamma have been shown to alter the distribution of junctional molecules and the actin cytoskeleton concurrent with an observed increase in permeability and leucocyte transmigration (Edens and Parkos 2000).

Resident meningeal and perivascular macrophages play a protective role during bacterial meningitis (Polfliet *et al.* 2001). Depletion of those cells reduces the influx of leucocytes and aggravates the symptom despite high production of relevant chemokines.

In addition to cellular elements, the possible role of the perivascular matrix is currently discussed. Matrix metalloproteinases, a family of Zn^{2+} dependent endopeptidases, act as an effector mechanism of tissue remodelling in physiological and pathological conditions and as modulator of inflammation. Current research into their potential influence on the BBB, invasion of blood-derived immune cells, shedding of cytokines and cytokine receptors, and direct damage to the CNS has recently been reviewed. (Leppert *et al.* 2001).

4.6 Alternative ways of blood to brain exchange

4.6.1 The choroid plexus

The choroid plexus in an important interface between the blood and the CSF. Unlike the cerebral capillaries, the capillaries of the choroid plexus are fenestrated and thus permit ultrafiltration of plasma and passage of many water-soluble substances that cannot pass the BBB. The interstitium is surrounded by specialized epithelium of cuboidal cells joined to its neighbour at the apical surface by tight junctions (Brightman and Tao-Cheng 1993) where the CSF is secreted as a result of complex inorganic ion exchanges. The paracellular permeability of the choroidal epithelium is higher than the brain endothellial cells and polar substances that do not pass the BBB can slowly diffuse into the CSF. Tranport mechanisms from brain to CSF include amino acids, vitamins and peptides. A wide range of drugs and endogenous metabolic molecules can be transported from CSF to blood via organic anion transporters and MRP (Strazielle and Ghersi-Egea 1999, 2000; Segal 2001). Enzymes of drug metabolism (see 4.1.5) display higher activities in the choroid plexus and the circumventricular organs than at the BBB and conjugating activities are very high in the choroid plexus (el-Bacha and Minn 1999). Recent studies indicate that the choroid plexus plays an important part in the immunoregulatory functions of the brain (Strazielle and Ghersi-Egea 2000; Engelhart *et al.* 2001).

4.6.2 **The circumventricular organs**

The circumventricular organs (CVO) have fenestrated capillaries and high permeability and provide an important link in the regulation of metabolic and endocrine function (Ferguson and Bains 1996; McKinley *et al.* 1998; Ganong 2000). Whereas septic doses of lipopoly-saccaride (LPS) induce global expression of pro-inflammatory cytokines in the brain, subseptic doses increase IL-beta and TNF alpha mRNA only in the choroids plexus, the CVO, and meninges (Quan *et al.* 1999). They CVO can be separated into two classes according to their neuronal content and proposed roles in the blood–brain communications. The median eminence and area postrema consist primarily of axon terminals and the lack of BBB facilitates diffusion of released hypothalamic peptides from axonal terminal into the blood stream following release. The primary direction of communication is from hypothalamic neurosecretory neurones to the circulation. The subfornical organ, area postrema and organum vasculosum of the lamina terminalis contain large numbers of neuronal cell bodies and high densities of peptidergic receptors for substances like angiotensin, vasopressin, endotheline. They send extensive neuronal efferents to important local autonomic control centres and appear to receive relative sparse neuronal input. The high permeability permits circulating substances that cannot cross the BBB to access neuronal tissue within these structures allowing them to monitor the physiological state of the body. The primary afferent control of these neurones is most likely derived from circulating chemical messengers such as angiotensin, atrial natriuretic peptide, vasopressin, endothelin, cholecystokinin, and nerve growth factor. Functional and/or structural barriers seem to reduce extracellular diffusion of molecules from the CVO into the brain. Substances may, however, reach other parts of the brain by retrograde axonal transport. The extent to which substances acting on receptors or cells in the circumventricular organs and influence other parts of the brain is not clear. Although these structures lack a BBB they have a barrier to the CSF where tanocytes, a modified type of astrocytes, are joined together by tight junctions. Thus, whereas there is no barrier between the brain extracellular space and the CSF in other parts of the brain, substances cannot enter the CVO from the CSF.

4.7 **Brain–immune system interaction at the blood–brain barrier**

The brain blood vessels exhibit both constitutive and induced expression of receptors for TNF alpha, IL-1beta, and IL-6. Stimulating these receptors can extensively modify the endothelial cells as well as have distant actions (Rivest 2001). The temporal and spatial patterns of c-fos mRNA induced by i.v. IL-1 indicate a cascade of non-neuronal cellular activation at the BBB. The first activation pattern, 0.5 h after the injection, was seen in the meninges, blood vessels, and choroids plexus; the second activation, at 3 h, appeared in cells just inside the now quiescent barrier cells. In addition each CVO showed characteristic spatio-temporal labelling patterns. It was proposed that the first wave of activation was elicited by blood-borne immune signals and the second was caused by molecules generated within the first set of activated cells with the signal propagated to neighbouring receptive cells by extracellular diffusion (Herkenham *et al.* 1998).

Depending on the challenges and cytokines involved, the transduction signals in cells of the BBB can orient the neuronal activity in a very specific manner in activating the transcription and production of soluble factors. Systemic injection of IL-1 beta rapidly induces a cyclooxygenase (COX-2) mRNA signal, a gene encoding for the production of pros-taglandins, in brain microvessels (Lacroix and Rivest 1998). It has been proposed that the microvasculature is the source of prostaglandin formation into the brain during systemic inflammatory challenges (LPS, IL-1 and TNF) that trigger the nuclear factor kappa B (NF-kappaB) signalling pathways and COX-2 transcription within the cerebral endothelium (Rivest 2001).

Lipopolysaccaride is thought to exert its action on mononuclear phagocytes via the cell surface receptor CD14. Under basal conditions low levels of CD14 mRNA are found in the leptomeninges, choroids plexus, and the brain microvasculature. Systemic injection of LPS causes a profound increase of gene expression for CD14 within the same structures as well as in the circumventricular organs (Lacroix *et al.* 1998). Furthermore, intravenous injection of LPS, TNF alpha and IL-1beta induces a robust transcription activation of the gene encoding monocyte chemoattractant protein-1 (MCP-1) in brain microvessels (Thibeault *et al.* 2001).

4.8 Concluding remarks

The BBB and its interaction with the endocrine and immune systems is a rapidly expanding field of research. Most studies on the BBB have so far been performed on experimental animals or *in vitro* models, and the results vary with the models, experimental conditions, and species used. However, most basic BBB functions are likely to be similar in rodents and man. The present technological development in microbiology and human brain imaging is likely to lead to new ways to study the human BBB in health and disease.

References

Allt, G. and Lawrenson, J. G. (2001). Pericytes: cell biology and pathology. *Cells Tissues Organs*, 169, 1–11.

Angelov, D. N., Walther, M., Streppel, M., Guntinas-Lichius, O., and Neiss, W. F. (1998). The cerebral perivascular cells. *Adv Anat, Embryol Cell Biol*, 147, 1–87.

Aurrand-Lions, M., Johnson-Leger, C., Wong, C., Du Pasquier, L., and Imhof, B. A. (2001). Heterogeneity of endothelial junctions is reflected by differential expression and specific subcellular localization of the three JAM family members. *Blood*, 98, 3699–707.

Banks, W. A. and Kastin, A. J. (1996). Passage of peptides across the blood-brain barrier: pathophysiological perspectives. *Life Sci*, 59, 1923–43.

Bechmann, I., Kwidzinski, E., Kovac, A. D., *et al.* (2001). Turnover of rat brain perivascular cells. *Exp Neurol*, 168, 242–9.

Begley, D. J., Bradbury, M. W., and Kreuter, J. (eds.) (2000). *The blood-brain barrier and drug delivery to the CNS*. Marcel Dekker, New York.

Begley, D. J. (1996). The blood-brain barrier: principles for targeting peptides and drug to the central nervous system. *J Pharm Pharmacol*, 48, 136–46.

Bickel, U., Yoshikawa, T., and Pardridge, W. M. (2001). Delivery of peptides and proteins through the blood-brain barrier. *Adv Drug Deliv Rev*, 46, 47–79.

Bohatschek, M., Werner, A., and Raivich, G. (2001). Systemic LPS injection leads to granulocyte influx into normal and injured brain: effect of ICAM-1 deficiency. *Exp Neurol*, 172, 137–52.

Bradbury, M. W. B. (ed.) (1992). *Physiology and Pharmacology of the blood-brain barrier. Handbook of experimental pharmacology*, Vol. 103. Springer-Verlag, Heidelberg-New York.

Bradbury, W. B., Cserr, H. F., and Westrop, J. (1981). Drainage of cerebral interstitial fluid into deep cervical lymph of the rabbit. *Amer J Physiol*, 240, F329–36.

Braet, K., Paemeleire, K., D'Herde, K., Sanderson, M. J., and Leybaert, L. (2001). Astrocyte-endothelial cell calcium signals conveyed by two signalling pathways. *Eur J Neurosci*, 3, 79–91.

Brightman, M. W. and Tao-Cheng, J. H. (1993). Tight junctions of brain endothelium and epithelium. In *The Blood–brain barrier*, (ed. W. M. Pardridge) Raven Press, New York, pp. 107–25.

Brown, K. A. (2001). Factors modifying the micration of lymphocytes across the blood-brain *Int Immunopharmacol*, 1, 2043–62.

Cserr, H. F., Harling-Berg, C. J., and Knopf, P. M. (1992). Drainage of brain extracellular fluid into blood and deep cervical lymph and its immunological significance. *Brain Pathol*, 2, 269–76.

Cornford, E. M. and Hyman, S. (1999). Blood–brain barrier permeability to small and large molecules. *Adv Drug Deliv Rev*, 36, 145–63.

Declèves, X., Regina, A., Laplanche, J. L., *et al.* (2000). Functional expression of P-glycoprotein and multidrug resistance-associated protein (Mrp1) in primary cultures of rat astrocytes. *J Neurosci Res*, 60, 594–601.

De Vries, H. E., Kuiper, J., De Boer, A. G., Van Berkel, J. C., and Breimer, D. D. (1997). The blood–brain barrier in neuroinflammatory diseases. *Pharmacol Rev*, 49, 143–55.

Didier, A. D. and Loor, F. (1995). Decreased biotolerability for ivermectin and cyclosporin A in mice exposed to potent P-glycoprotein inhibitors. *Int J Cancer*, 63, 263–7.

dos Santos, W. L. C., Rahman, J., Klein, N., and Male, D. K. (1995). Distribution and analysis of surface charge on brain endothelium in vitro and in situ. *Acta Neuropathol*, 90, 305–11.

Edens, H. A. and Parkos, C. A. (2000). Modulation of epithelial and endothelial paracellular permeability by leukocytes. *Adv Drug Deliv Rev*, 41, 315–28.

el-Bacha, R. S. and Minn, A. (1999). Drug metabolizing enzymes in cerebrovasclular endothelial cells afford a metabolic protection to the brain. *Cell Mol Biol*, 45, 15–23.

Engelhardt, B., Wolburg-Buchholz, K., and Wolburg, H. (2001). Involvement of the choroid plexus in central nervous system inflammation. *Microsc Res Tech*, 52, 112–29.

Ferguson, A. V. and Bains, J. S. (1996). Electrophysiology of the circumventricular organs. *Frontiers Neuroendocrinol*, 17, 440–75.

Ferguson, R. K. and Woodbury, D. M. (1969). Penetration of 14C-inulin and 14C-sucrose into brain, cerebrospinal fluid and skeletal muscle of developing rats. *Exp Brain Res*, 7, 181–94.

Fischer-Smith, T., Croul, S., and Sverstiuk, A. E. (2001). CNS invation by CD14+/CD16+ peripheral blood-derived monocytes in HIV dementia: perivascular accumulation and reservoir of HIV infection. *J Neurovirol*, 7, 528–41.

Frey, A., Meckelein, B., Weiler-Güttler, H., Möckel, B., Flach, R., and Gassen, H. G. (1991). Pericytes of the brain microvasculature express γ-glutamyl transpeptidase. *Eur J Biochem*, 202, 421–9.

Ganong, W. F. (2000). Circumventricular organs: definition and role in the regulation of endocrine and autonomic function. *Clin Exp Pharmacol Physiol*, 27, 422–7.

Gehrmann, J., Matsumoto, Y., and Kreutzberg, G. W. (1995). Microglia: intrinsic immunoeffector cell of the brain. *Brain Res Brain Res*, 20, 269–87.

Ghersi-Egea, J. F., Leininger-Muller, B., Suleman, G., Siest, G., and Minn, A. (1994). Localization of drug-metabolizing enzyme activities to blood-brain interfaces and circumventricular organs. *J Neurochem*, 62, 1089–96.

Ghersi-Egea, J. F. and Strazielle, N. (2001). Brain drug delivery, drug metabolism, and multidrug resistance at the choroid plexus. *Microsc Res Tech*, 52, 83–8.

Gjedde, A. (1992). Blood-brain glucose transfer. In: *Physiology and pharmacology of the blood–brain barrier*. In *Handbook of Experimental Pharmacology*, Vol. 103, (ed. M. B. B. Bradbury) Springer-Verlag, Heidelberg-New York, pp. 65–115.

Golden, P. L. and Pardridge, W. M. (2000). Brain microvascular P-glycoprotein and a revised model of multidrug resistance in brain. *Cell Mol Neurobiol*, 20, 165–81.

Graeber, M. B. (1993). Microglia, macrophages and the blood–brain barrier. *Clin Neuropathol*, 12, 296–7.

Hardebo, J. E. and Owman, C. (1990). Enzymatic barrier mechanisms for neurotransmitter monoamines and their precursors at the blood-brain interface. In *The Pathophysiology of the blood–brain barrier*, Fernström Foundation Series, Vol. 14, (eds. B. B. Johansson, C. Owman, and H. Widner) Elsevier, Amsterdam. pp. 41–55.

Hasselbalch, S. G., Knudsen, G. M., Jakobsen, J., Hageman, L. P., Holm, S., and Paulson, O. B. (1995). Blood–brain barrier permeability of glucose and ketone bodies during short-term starvation in humans. *Amer J Physiol*, **268**, E1161–6.

Hayashi, Y., Nomura, M., Yamagishi, S., Harada, S., Yamashita, J., and Yamamoto, H. (1997). Induction of various blood–brain barrier properties in non-neural endothelial cells by close apposition to co-cultured astrocytes. *Glia*, **19**, 13–26.

Herkenham, M., Lee, H. Y., and Baker, R. A. (1998). Temporal and spatial patterns of c-fos mRNA induced by intravenous interleukin-1: a cascade of non-neuronal cellular activation at the blood–brain barrier. *J Comparat Neurol*, **400**, 175–96.

Hickey, W. F. (2001). Basic principles of immunological surveillance of the normal central nervous system. *Glia*, **36**, 118–24.

Hickey, W. F., Hsu, B. L., and Kimura, H. (1991). T-lymphocyte entry into the central nervous system. *J Neurol Sci Res*, **28**, 254–60.

Hickey, W. F., Vass, K., and Lassmann, H. (1992). Bone marrow-derived elements in the central nervous system: an immunohistochemical and ultrastructural survey of rat chimeras. *J Neuropathol Exp Neurol*, **51**, 246–56.

Huber, J. D., Egleton, R. D., and Davis, T. P. (2001). Molecular physiology and pathophysiology of tight junctions in the blood-brain barrier. *Trends Neurosci*, **24**, 719–25.

Janzer, R. C. and Raff, M. C. (1987). Astrocytes induce blood–brain barrier properties in endothelial cells. *Nature*, **325**, 253–7.

Jetté, L., Murphy, G. H., Leclerc, J. M., and Béliveau, R. (1995). Interaction of drugs with P-glyco-protein in brain capillaries. *Biochem Pharmacol*, **50**, 1701–9.

Johansson, B. B. (2001). Blood–brain barrier: role of brain endothelial surface charge and glycocalyx. In *Ichemic blood flow in the brain* (Y. Fukuuchi, M. Tomita M, A. Koto, eds.). Springer-Verlag, Tokyo, pp. 33–8.

Kalaria, R. N., Gravina, S. A., Schmidley, J. W., Perry, G., and Harik, S. I. (1988). The glucose transporter of the human brain and blood–brain barrier. *Ann Neurol*, **24**, 57–76.

Keep, R., Ennis, S. R., and Betz, A. L. (1998). Blood–brain barier ion transport. In *Introduction to the blood-brain barrier* (ed. M. Pardridge), Cambridge University Press, Cambridge, UK pp. 207–13.

Kida, S., Steart, P. V., Zhang, E.-T., and Weller, R. O. (1993). Perivascular cells act as scavengers in the cerebral perivascular spaces and remain distinct from pericytes, microglia and macrophages. *Acta Neuropathol*, **85**, 646–52.

King, M., Su, W., Chang, A., Zuckerman, A., and Pasternak, G. W. (2001). Transport of opioids from the brain to the periphery by P-glycoprotein: peripheral actions of central drugs. *Nature Neurosci*, **4**, 268–74.

Kniesel, U. and Wolburg, H. (2000). Tight junctions of the blood–brain barrier. *Cell Mol Neurobiol*, **20**, 57–76.

Krause, D., Kunz, J., and Dermietzel, R. (1993). Cerebral pericytes—a second line of defense in controlling blood–brain barrier peptide metabolism. *Adv Exp Med Biol*, **331**, 149–52.

Lacroix, S., Feinstein, D., and Rivest, S. (1998). The bacterial endotoxin lipopolysaccharide has the ability to target the brain in upregulating its membrane CD14 receptor within specific cellular populations. *Brain Pathol*, **8**, 625–40.

Lacroix, S. and Rivest, S. (1998). Effect of acute systemic inflammatory response and cytokines on the transcription of the genes encoding cyclooxygenase enzymes (COX-1 and COX-2) in the rat brain. *J Neurochem*, **70**, 452–66.

Lapierre, L. A. (2000). The molecular structure of the tight junction. *Adv Drug Deliv Rev*, **41**, 255–64.

Lassmann, H. (1997). Basic mechanisms of brain inflammation. *J Neural Transmission Suppl*, **50**, 183–99.

Lassmann, H., Zimprich, F., Vass, K., and Hickey, W. F. (1991). Microglial cells are a component of the perivascular glia limitans. *J Neurol Sci Res*, 28, 236–43.

Lee, G., Dallas, S., Hong, M., and Bendayan, R. (2001). Drug transporters in the central nervous system: brain barriers and brain parenchyma considerations. *Pharmacol Rev*, 53, 569–96.

Leppert, D., Lindberg, R. L., Kappos, L., and Leib, S. L. (2001). Matric metalloproteinases: multifunctional effectors of inflammation in multiple sclerosis and bacterial meningitis. *Brain Res, Brain Res Rev*, 36, 249–57.

Leybaert, L., Paemeleire, K., Strahonja, A., and Sanderson, M. J. (1998). Inositol-trisphosphate-dependent intercellular calcium signaling in and between astrocytes and endothelial cells. *Glia*, 24, 398–407.

Liu, Y. and Hu, M. (2000). P-glycoprotein and bioavailability—implication of pylymorphism. *Clin Chem Lab Med*, 38, 877–81.

Löwhagen, P., Johansson, B. B., and Nordborg, C. (1994). The nasal route of cerebrospinal fluid drainage in man. A light-microscope study. *Neuropathol Appl Neurobiol*, 20, 543–50.

Martin-Padura, I., Lostaglio, S., Schneemann, M., et al. (1998). Junctional adhesion molecule, a novel member of the immunoglobulin superfamily that distributes at intercellular junction and modulates monocyte transmigration. *J Cell Biol*, 142, 117–27.

McKinley, M. J., Allen, A. M., Burn, P., Colvill, L. M., and Oldfield, B. J. (1998). Interaction of circulating hormones with the brain: the roles of the subfornical organ and the organum vasculosum of the lamina terminalis. *Clin Exp Pharmacol Physiol*, Supplement 25, S61–7.

Mi, H., Haeberle, H., and Barres, B. A. (2001). Induction of astrocyte differentiation of endothelial cells. *J Neurosci*, 21, 1538–47.

Monteiro, R. A., Rocha, E., and Marini-Abreu, M. M. (1996). Do microglia arise from pericytes? An ultrastructural and distribution study in the rat cerebellar cortex. *J Submicrosc Cytol Pathol*, 28, 457–69.

Oldendorf, W. H., Cornform, M. E., and Brown, W. J. (1977). The large apparent work capability of the blood–brain barrier: a study of the mitochondrial content of capillary endothelial cells in brain and other tissues of the rat. *Ann Neurol*, 1, 409–17.

Pardridge, W. M., ed. (1998). *Introduction to the blood–brain barrier. Methodology, biology and pathology*. Cambridge University Press, Cambridge, UK.

Pardridge, W. M. (1999). Blood-brain barrier biology and methodology. *J Neurovirol*, 5, 556–69.

Plotkin, S. R., Banks, W. A., Maness, L. M., and Kastin, A. J. (2000). Differential transport of rat and human interleukin-1alpha across the blood–brain barrier and blood–testis barrier in rats. *Brain Res*, 881, 57–61.

Polfliet, M. M., Zwijnenburg, P. J., and van Furth, A. M. (2001). Meningeal and perivascular macrophages of the central nervous system play a protective role during bacterial meningitis. *J Immunol*, 167, 4644–50.

Potschka, H. and Loscher, W. (2001). *In vivo* evidence of P-glycoprotein-mediated transport of phenytoin at the blood–brain barrier of rats. *Epilepsia*, 42, 1231–40.

Prat, A., Biernacki, K., Wosik, K., and Antel, J. P. (2001). Glial cell influence on the human blood–brain barrier. *Glia*, 36, 145–55.

Quan, N., Stern, E. L., Whiteside, M. B., and Herkenham, M. (1999). Induction of pro-inflammatory cytokine mRNA in the brain after peripheral injection of subseptic doses of lipopolysaccharide in the rat. *J Neuroimmunol*, 93, 72–80.

Risau, W., Dingler, A., Albrecht, U., Dehouck, M.-P., and Cecchelli, R. (1992). Blood–brain barrier pericytes are the main source of g-glutamyltranspeptidase activity in brain capillaries. *J Neurochem*, 58, 667–72.

Rivest, S. (2001). How circulating cytokines trigger the neural circuits that control the hyothalami-pituitary-adrenal axis. *Psychoneuroendocrinology*, 26, 761–88.

Rucker, H. K., Wynder, H. J., and Thomas, W. E. (2000). Cellular mechanisms of CNS pericytes. *Brain Res Bull*, 51, 363–9.

Schinkel, A. H. (1999). P-glucoprotein, a gatekeeper in the blood–brain barrier. *Adv Drug Deliv Rev*, **36**, 179–94.

Schinkel, A. H., Wagenaar, E., Ven Deemter, L., Mol, C. A. A. M., and Borst, P. (1995). Absence of the mdr 1a P-glycoprotein in mice affect tissue distribution and pharmacokinetics of dexamethasone, digoxin and cyclosporin A. *J Clini Invest*, **96**, 1698–705.

Schroeter, M. L., Muller, S., Linenau, J., *et al.* (2001). Astrocytes induce mangenese superoxide dismutase in brain capillary endothelial cells. *Neuroreport*, **12**, 2513–7.

Segal, M. B. (2001). Transport of nutrients across the choroid plexus. *Microsc Res Tech*, **52**, 38–48.

Silverman, A. J., Sutherland, A. K., Wilhelm, M., and Silver, R. (2000). Mast cells migrate from blood brain. *J Neurosci*, **20**, 401–8.

Smith, Q. R. and Stoll, J. (1998). In *Introduction to the blood–brain barrier*, (ed. M. Pardridge) Cambridge University Press, Cambridge, UK, pp. 188–97.

Starzyk, R. M., Rosenow, C., Frye, J., *et al.* (2000). Cerebral cell adhesion molecule: a novel leukocyte adhesion determinant on blood–brain barrier capillary endothelium, *J Infecti Dis*, **181**, 181–7.

Strazielle, N. and Ghersi-Egea, J. F. (1999). Demonstration of a coupled metabolism-efflux process at the choroid plexus as a mechanism of brain protection towards xenobiotics. *J Neurosci*, **19**, 6275–89.

Strazielle, N. and Ghersi-Egea, J. F. (2000). Choroid plexus in the cental nervous system; biology and Physiopathology. *J Neuropathol Exp Neurol*, **59**, 561–74.

Sun, D., Lytle, C., and O'Donnell, M. E. (1997). IL-6 secreted by astroglial cells regulate NA-K-Cl cotransport in brain microvessel rndothelial cells. *Amer J Physiol*, **272**, C1829–35.

Thomas, W. E. (1999). Brain macrophages: on the role of pericytes and perivascular cells. *Brain Res Rev*, **31**, 42–57.

Thibeault, I., Laflamme, N., and Rivest, S. (2001). Regulation of the gene encoding the monocyte chemoattractant protein 1 (MCP-1) in the rat brain in response to circulating LPS and proinflammatory cytokines. *J Comparat Neurol*, **434**, 461–77.

Triguero, D., Buciak, J. B., Yang, J., and Pardridge, W. M. (1989). Blood–brain barrier transport of cationized immunoglobulin G: Enhanced delivery compared to native protein. *Proc Nat Acad Sci USA*, **86**, 4761–5.

van der Goes, A., Wouters, D., van der Pol, S. M., *et al.* (2001). Reactive oxygen species enhance the migration of monocytes across the blood-brain barrier *in vitro*. *FASEB J*, **15**, 1852–64.

van der Sandt, I. C., Gaillard, P. J., Voorwinden, H. H., de Boer, A. G., and Breimer, D. D. (2001). P-glygoprotein inhibition leads to enhanced disruptive effects by anti-microtubule cytostatics at the *in vitro* blood–brain barrier. *Pharmacol Res*, **18**, 587–92.

Vorbrodt, A. W., Lossinsky, A. S., Dobrogowska, D. H., and Wisniewski, H. M. (1990). Sequential appearance of anionic domains in the developing blood–brain barrier. *Brain Res Develop Brain Res*, **52**, 31–7.

Walsh, S. V., Hopkins, A. M., and Nusrat, A. (2000). Modulation of tight junction structure and function by cyrokines. *Adv Drug Deliv Rev*, **4**, 303–13.

Watchko, J. F., Daood, M. J., and Hansen, T. W. (1998). Brain bilirubin content is increased in P-glycoprotein-deficient transgenic null mutant mice. *Pediatr Res*, **44**, 763–6.

Widner, H., Jönsson, B.-A., Hallstadius, L., Wingårdh, K., Strand, S.-E., and Johansson, B. B. (1987). Scintigraphic method to quantify the passage from brain parenchyma to the deep cervical lymph nodes in rats. *Eur J Nucl Med*, **13**, 456–61.

Widner, H., Möller, G., and Johansson, B. B. (1988). Immune response in deep cervical lymph nodes and spleen in the mouse after antigen deposition in different intracerebral sites. *Scand J Immunol*, **28**, 563–71.

Williams, K., Alvarez, X., and Lackner, A. A. (2001). Central nervous system perivascular cells are immunoregulatory cells that connect the CNS with the peripheral immune system. *Glia*, **36**, 156–64.

Wolburg, H., Neuhaus, J., Kniesel, U., *et al.* (1994). Modulation of tight junction structure in blood–brain barrier endothelial cells. Effects of tissue culture, second messengers and cocultured astrocytes. *J Cell Sci*, **107**, 1347–57.

Wolff, J. E. A., Belloni-Olivi, L., Bressler, J. P., and Goldstein, G. W. (1992). γ-glutamyl transpeptidase activity in brain microvessels exhibits regional heterogeneity. *J Neurochem*, **58**, 909–15.

Yamagata, K., Tagami, M., Nara, Y., *et al.* (1997). Astrocyte-conditioned medium induces blood–brain barrier properties in endothelial cells. *Clin Exp Pharmacol Physiol*, **24**, 710–3.

Chapter 5

CNS responses to peripheral insults

Jan Pieter Konsman and Giamal N. Luheshi

5.1 Introduction

Peripheral tissue injury, trauma, or infection, triggers a complex series of reactions mounted by the host to prevent further damage, isolate and destroy infectious organisms and initiate repair processes. These responses are collectively known as the acute phase response (APR) which refers to a set of specific defence mechanisms that are rapidly activated following peripheral insults (Baumann and Gauldie 1994).

The APR is initiated by mast cell degranulation or microbial products which activate tissue macrophages to produce certain inflammatory mediators. The best known of these belong to a family of pro-inflammatory cytokines, and include interleukin-1β (IL-1β), interleukin-6 (IL-6) and tumor necrosis factor α (TNFα), which are probably the most important cytokines involved in this type of response. The activity of these immune messengers appears to be compartmentalized and can be divided into local, systemic and central nervous components depending on the site of action.

Peripheral tissue injury or infection is often accompanied by elevations in body temperature, behavioural changes such as loss of appetite as well as loss of interest in usual activities and activation of the pituitary–adrenal axis resulting in the release of adrenocorticotropin and glucocorticoid hormones all of which are controlled by the central nervous system (CNS). In this chapter we will focus on the importance of the central nervous components of the APR for the host as well as the CNS structures and immune-to-brain signalling pathways involved in mediating these responses.

5.2 Central nervous components of the APR are important to host survival

Of all the CNS mediated responses comprising APR, fever is probably the best studied. The fever response was historically considered to be beneficial to the host, but this idea was not tested scientifically until the last quarter of the twentieth century. Clinical studies demonstrated that patients developing a moderate fever survive bacterial peritonitis and bacteraemia to a greater extent than those who fail to develop fever (Mackowiak et al. 1997). These observations were confirmed with experimental evidence which showed that administration of antipyretics in animals increases mortality and duration of illness after viral or bacterial infection (Husseini et al. 1982; Vaughn et al. 1980). Enhanced migration of phagocytic leucocytes to the site of infection (Roberts 1991) and increased delivery of lympohocytes to lymph nodes (Evans et al. 2001) at febrile temperatures are mechanisms that may explain the beneficial effect of fever on host survival after infection. Mounting a febrile response is, however, metabolically demanding requiring the mobilization of energy stores originating from adipose tissue, muscle protein, and liver glycogen as a consequence of the activation of the sympathetic nervous system (Jepson *et al.* 1988) and the release of glucocorticoids by the adrenal (Schöbitz *et al.* 1994).

Besides the energy needed to raise body temperature, the maintenance of a febrile temperature of up to 2°C above normal levels for hours or days during sickness also requires an increase in energy consumption (>20 per cent). However, metabolic rate is often not actually raised. It is, therefore, not surprising that fever is almost always accompanied by behavioural responses that contribute to conserving energy. These include reduced loco-motor activity and sleep which are critical components of APR. The reduction of behav-ioural activity and adoption of body posture to limit the exposed body surface contribute to limiting heat loss and thus to the maintenance of an elevated body temperature. The reduction of behavioural activity in response to deep tissue injury, (which may or may not be accompanied by haemorrhage) is also adaptive, as it prevents further tissue damage and blood loss. Therefore, although the reduction of behavioural activity in response to per-ipheral insults have often been neglected, it is in fact an integral part of the host's response to overcome tissue infection or injury.

The reduction in food intake typically seen during the APR can be construed as a direct result of loss of function, which counteracts the action of the mobilization of energy supplies to increase body temperature. Indeed, when fat reserves are mobilized to produce heat during cold exposure, hyperphagia normally follows resulting in the replenishment of energy stocks (Bing *et al.* 1998). It can however be argued that these behavioural symptoms of sickness can also be adaptive responses to acute infection. Despite the fact that anorexia during disease induces a negative energy balance, it is important to host survival. For example, food deprivation preceding experimental bacterial infection of mice increases survival rate (Wing and Young 1980). Conversely, force-feeding mice infected with Listeria to ensure normal energy intake increases mortality rate (Murray and Murray 1979). The mechanisms by which anorexia contributes to survival of the host during infection are not yet fully understood, but seem to be related to prevention of feeding-induced rises in plasma iron levels (Murray *et al.* 1978). Indeed, low plasma iron concentrations together with increased temperature inhibit bacterial growth (Kluger and Rothenburg 1979). It is clear that the CNS controlled events constitute a major component of the APR, so a great deal of research has focused on the brain mechanisms underlying these responses.

5.3 CNS structures activated by peripheral insults

Given the adaptive nature of the central nervous components of the APR, one would expect specific brain structures to be activated in response to specific peripheral insults. Validation of the immediate-early gene c-fos as a cellular activity marker has provided a means to study activation of CNS cell groups in response to a wide variety of stimuli (Kovács 1998). C-fos induction is related closely to rises in extracellular calcium and is a marker of cellular/trans-synaptic activations that exceed a certain threshold (Kovács 1998). Interestingly, some of the hypothalamic structures that are activated by peripheral insults can be related to the hor-monal and metabolic central nervous components of the APR. Immune stimuli consisting of peripheral injections of bacterial lipopolysaccharide (LPS), cell wall components of gram negative bacteria or pro-inflammatory cytokines such as IL-1β for instance, induce c-fos in corticotropin-releasing hormone (CRH) containing neurones of the paraventricular nucleus of the hypothalamus (PVH), (Ericsson *et al.* 1994; Rivest and Laflamme 1995), which control the activity of hypothalamus–pituitary–adrenal (HPA) axis. Interruption of the ascending catecholaminergic input from the brainstem attenuates IL-1β induced Fos immuno-reactivity and increases in CRH mRNA in the PVH (Ericsson *et al.* 1994). Moreover, peripheral administration of LPS or IL-1β in rats induces c-fos expression in catecholaminergic neurones of the nucleus of the solitary tract (NTS) and the ventrolateral medulla (VLM) (Ericsson *et al.* 1994; Sagar *et al.* 1995). Finally, lesions of the VLM including the A1 catecholaminergic cell group prevent intravenous IL-1β-induced activation of the PVH (Buller *et al.* 2001). Haemorrhage is a potential consequence of peripheral insults, and a loss in blood volume results in Fos expression in neurones of the NTS and the VLM that project to the PVH of rats (Krukoff *et al.* 1995). Together, these findings indicate that catecholaminergic brainstem projections to the PVH are responsible for activation of the HPA-axis in response to peripheral insults.

The PVH also plays a role in fever, as lesions of this structure prevent the rise in body temperature normally induced by peripheral administration of LPS (Horn *et al.* 1994; Lu *et al.* 2001). Lesions of the preoptic hypothalamus, at the level of the organum vasculosum of the laminae terminalis (OVLT), also attenuate fevers induced by peripheral administration of LPS (Blatteis *et al.* 1983; Caldwell *et al.* 1998), indicating that neuronal projections from the preoptic area to the PVH are involved in fever. Neurones in the ventromedial preoptic area (VMPO) and the median preoptic nucleus express c-fos after peripheral administration of bacterial LPS and project to the PVH. They may, therefore, constitute a neuronal substrate underlying the fever response (Elmquist and Saper 1996). The role of the PVH in the fever response is not necessarily related to activation of CRH neurones controlling the HPA-axis, as peripheral LPS administration also induces c-fos in PVH neurones that project to the level of the spinal cord innervating brown adipose tissue, an important source of energy in rats (Zhang *et al.* 2000).

Another hypothalamic structure showing c-fos expression after peripheral LPS or IL-1β administration is the arcuate nucleus (Reyes and Sawchenko 2000; Sagar *et al.* 1995). Neurones in the arcuate nucleus of the hypothalamus express receptors for hormones reflecting energy status, such as insulin and leptin, and are thus thought to act as first order neurones in the regulation of energy homeostasis and food intake (Schwartz *et al.* 2000). One of the neuronal populations in the arcuate nucleus expresses α-melanocyte stimulating hormone (α-MSH), which is known to inhibit food intake (Schwartz *et al.* 2000). Interestingly, intracerebroventricular (icv) administration of a melanocortin antagonist prevents the reduction in food intake in response to peripheral injection of bacterial LPS in rats (Huang *et al.* 1999). In view of this observation, one can speculate that activation of the α-MSH neurones in the arcuate nucleus plays a role in mediating anorexia during the APR. However, lesions of the arcuate nucleus do not affect anorexia induced by peripheral administration of IL-1β (Reyes and Sawchenko 2000). Instead, these lesions result in increased fever responses (Martin *et al.* 1990; Opp *et al.* 1990). Arcuate α-MSH neurones might be responsible for this latter effect, as exogenous icv administration of this peptide inhibits fever in response to peripheral IL-1 (Deeter *et al.* 1988; Lipton *et al.* 1994). Moreover, icv administration of a melanocortin antagonist or a neutralizing antiserum to α-MSH augments fever induced by peripheral LPS- or IL-1β (Huang *et al.* 1999; Shih *et al.* 1986). Collectively, these results suggest that arcuate α-MSH neurones are part of antipyretic brain circuitry, whereas α-MSH neurones outside the arcuate nucleus seem to be involved in mediating anorexia during the APR. Besides hypothalamic structures, peripheral administration of IL-1β also induces c-fos expression in enkephalinergic neurones of the dorsolateral bed nucleus of the stria terminalis and the lateral part of the central amygdala (CEA) (Day *et al.* 1999), and in neurones of the lateral parabrachial nuclei. Although it is tempting to speculate that activation of these brainstem and limbic structures play a role in the behavioural central nervous components of the APR, such as behavioural depression, this remains to be established.

Despite the fact that the same brain structures seem to be activated in response to insults as different as peripheral infection, sterile tissue injury and haemorrhage, the inducing stimuli may differ. The stimulus responsible for c-fos induction in response to peripheral insults resulting in haemorrhage may be hypotension, which induces the same pattern of c-fos expression (Graham *et al.* 1995; Li and Dampney 1994). Hypotension is also one of the symptoms of septic shock and of intravenous administration of high doses of LPS or IL-1β (Tkacs *et al.* 1997). It is, therefore, possible that the c-fos pattern obtained in response to these stimuli is due to hypotension. However, intravenous administration of LPS at a dose that provokes fever, but not hypotension, readily induces c-fos expression in the medial preoptic area (MPO), PVH, and in limbic structures (Tkacs *et al.* 1997). This demonstrates that hypotension is not necessarily the stimulus responsible for c-fos induction in the brain in response to peripheral administration of bacterial LPS. Since intravenous administration of low doses of IL-1β, in contrast to other pro-inflammatory cytokines, mimics the pattern of c-fos expression in the brain observed after administration of LPS, IL-1β may be the stimulus responsible for activation of CNS structures during infectious and inflammatory conditions.

In addition to mimicking LPS-induced c-fos pattern in the brain, peripheral administration of IL-1β also provokes all central nervous components of the APR in rodents, including fever, activation of the HPA-axis, and reduced food intake, as well as behavioural activity (Berkenbosch *et al.* 1987; Crestani *et al.* 1991; Dascombe *et al.* 1989; Kent *et al.* 1992). Moreover, peripheral administration of the naturally occurring interleukin-1 receptor antagonist (IL-1ra) attenuates fever, HPA-axis activation, and the reduction in behavioural activity and food intake caused by bacterial LPS or induction of sterile inflammation and tissue injury by intramuscular turpentine injection (Bluthé *et al.* 1992; Ebisui *et al.* 1994; Luheshi *et al.* 1996, 1997; Schotanus *et al.* 1993; Swiergiel *et al.* 1997). However, IL-1β is a hydrophilic peptide that cannot cross the blood–brain barrier (BBB) passively, giving rise to the question as to how IL-1β signals the nervous system.

5.4 **Humoural immune-to-brain signalling**

One hypothesis to explain the activation of brain structures and central nervous components of the APR proposes that circulating IL-1β induces the synthesis of prostaglandins (PGs) at the BBB (Elmquist *et al.* 1997; Rivest 1999). These small and lipophilic mediators easily cross biological membranes (O'Neill 1994) and PGs of the E family have long been known to increase body temperature (Milton and Wendlandt 1970). Moreover, PGE levels are increased in the cerebrospinal fluid (CSF) and the preoptic area of the hypothalamus (Dey *et al.* 1974; Philipp-Dormston and Siegert 1974; Sehic *et al.* 1996), an important structure in the control of body temperature (Boulant 1981). The observation that peripheral administration of IL-1β, bacterial LPS or turpentine all induce the PG-synthesizing enzyme cyclooxygenase-2 (COX-2) in BBB-related cells (Cao *et al.* 1995; Elmquist *et al.* 1997;

Lacroix and Rivest 1998) provided a mechanism. Prostaglandins are thus thought to cross the BBB and act on their receptors in brain parenchyma to induce the central nervous components of the APR (Elmquist *et al.* 1997; Rivest 1999). Finally, the observation that IL-1β-induced c-fos expression colocalizes to a certain extent with prostaglandin PGE receptor mRNA in the preoptic hypothalamus and VLM (Ek *et al.* 2000; Oka *et al.* 2000) is in accordance with the hypothesis that PGs synthesized at the BBB act on their receptors in brain parenchyma.

Non-steroidal anti-inflammatory drugs (NSAIDs), such as salicylates and indomethacin inhibit PG synthesis (Flower and Vane 1974) and attenuate central nervous components of the APR (Crestani *et al.* 1991; Hashimoto *et al.* 1988; Morimoto *et al.* 1989; Murakami and Watanabe 1989; Sirko *et al.* 1989; Uehara *et al.* 1989). These findings seem at first sight to provide support for the role of IL-1β-induced PG synthesis at the BBB in immune-to-brain signalling. Conventional NSAIDs, like aspirin and indomethacin, show, however, little selectivity for the cytokine-inducible form of COX, coined COX-2 and also inhibit prostaglandin synthesis by the constitutively, widely expressed COX-1 (O'Neill *et al.* 1995). In addition, salicylates inhibit activation of the NF-kappa-B transcription factor (Yin *et al.* 1998) which is an important factor mediating both the induction and effects of IL-1β (Hiscott *et al.* 1993; O'Neill and Greene 1998). Acute treatment with indomethacin increases plasma levels of corticosterone (Rivier and Vale 1991), which is known to attenuate both IL-1β synthesis and IL-1β-induced responses (Schöbitz *et al.* 1994). This indicates that the alleviating effects of agonists such as aspirin and indomethacin on central nervous components of the APR may be due to inhibition of interleukin-1β synthesis or biological responses induced by this cytokine other than COX-2 induction.

It has been shown that a COX-2 specific inhibitor attenuates fever and the rise in adrenocorticotropin hormone after peripheral administration of IL-1β or bacterial LPS (Cao *et al.* 1997; Parsadaniantz *et al.* 2000), but this does not necessarily mean that these effects are due to inhibition of prostaglandin synthesis by COX-2 at the BBB. Macrophages are a major source of PG during inflammation, and inhibition of COX-2 in stimulated peritoneal macrophages results in decreased IL-6 synthesis (Hinson *et al.* 1996; Williams and Shacter 1997). Furthermore, NSAIDs attenuate IL-1β-induced activation of the vagus nerve (Ek *et al.* 1998; Niijima 1996). This indicates that peripheral administration of NSAIDs will not only inhibit COX-2 activity in BBB-related cells, but also activation of the vagus nerve and the synthesis of IL-6 by macrophages. Interestingly, both circulating IL-6 and IL-1β action on the vagus nerve have recently been shown to be part of alternative immune-to-brain signalling pathways. This, together with emerging evidence indicating that IL-1β-induced PG synthesis at the BBB, cannot account for the initiation of central nervous components of the APR (Blatteis *et al.* 2000) has led to a more complex view of immune-to-brain signalling involving several mediators and mechanisms.

An important review article by Kluger (1991) set out criteria describing the properties that define a circulating pyrogen. IL-1 satisfies most of these criteria, since injection of IL-1β into experimental animals or humans induces fever (Dascombe *et al.* 1989; Tewari *et al.* 1990) and inhibiting the action of this cytokine by its receptor antagonist IL-1ra attenuates the fever in response to peripheral administration of bacterial LPS (Long *et al.* 1990; Luheshi *et al.* 1996). However, plasma levels of IL-1β are not detectable at fever onset in animals or humans (Cannon *et al.* 1990; Kluger 1991) suggesting that this cytokine cannot act as a circulating pyrogen. Recently it was shown that subcutaneous injection of LPS into an air pouch resulted in a significant increase in IL-1β levels in the air pouch, while circulating levels of this cytokine were undetectable (Cartmell *et al.* 2000; Miller *et al.* 1997). These and other evidence suggest that instead of acting at the level of the circulation, IL-1 action is limited to the site of infection or inflammation, and that a different mediator acts as the circulating pyrogen.

Several lines of evidence now indicate that, IL-6 is an important circulating mediator involved in the febrile response to localized LPS injections. Plasma IL-6 levels rise dramatically, and precede fever onset in response to local LPS administration or sterile tissue inflammation in rats (Cartmell *et al.* 2000; Luheshi *et al.* 1996, 1997; Ross *et al.* 2000). Furthermore, immunoneutralization of circulating IL-6 attenuates the febrile response to subcutaneous LPS administration (Cartmell *et al.* 2000). Circulating, IL-6 does not induce the prostaglandin-synthesizing enzyme COX-2 at the BBB (Lacroix and Rivest 1998), but probably acts in the CNS, since icv administration of a neutralizing antiserum inhibits the fever response to intraperitoneal LPS injection (Rothwell *et al.* 1991). In accordance with this observation, icv administration of recombinant IL-6 induces fever, but not behavioural depression (Lenczowski *et al.* 1999), suggesting that circulating IL-6 action in the CNS during peripheral infection or inflammation is limited specifically to the fever response. Interleukin-6, in contrast to other pro-inflammatory cytokines, can act directly within the CNS, since its receptors are found in circumventricular organs (Vallières and Rivest 1997), small midline brain structures where the BBB is non-functional (Gross 1992). In accordance with this, intravenous administration of IL-6 induces the cellular activation marker c-fos found in these brain circumventricular organs.

Interestingly, local injection of IL-1ra at sites of peripheral inflammation/infection attenuates the fever response and rises in plasma IL-6 levels induced by intraperitoneal or subcutaneous LPS administration or sterile tissue inflammation (Luheshi *et al.* 1996, 1997; Miller *et al.* 1997) suggesting that local tissue, and not circulating, levels of IL-1β are important to the fever response, possibly through its induction of circulating IL-6. Given the overwhelming evidence supporting a role of IL-6 as a circulating signal in fever, systemic administration of this cytokine should induce a febrile response. Surprisingly this is not to be the case. Intraperitoneal injection of rat recombinant IL-6, at concentrations several hundred fold higher than that detected in the plasma at the peak of the fever response after LPS, has no effect on body temperature (Cartmell *et al.* 2000). This may be a result of the relatively short half-life of this cytokine in circulation (a few minutes), or activity could be curtailed by failure of the protein to interact with its soluble receptor in the absence of other stimuli such as LPS or IL-1. The existence of a synergistic mechanism that ensures the activity of IL-6 in fever was demonstrated by Cartmell *et al.* (2000), where the same dose of IL-6 which previously failed to induce fever, was shown to be a very potent pyrogen when co-administered with a non-pyrogenic dose of IL-1β in rats.

It seems obvious from these and other data that IL-6 is an essential component for relaying the signal from the periphery to CNS structures to activate the fever response during sickness. It seems however that this is not the only route of communication. Evidence from numerous research groups have also supported a role for neural afferents as the main route between the periphery and the brain.

5.5 Neural immune-to-brain signalling

An alternative mechanism by which local tissue concentrations of IL-1β may play a role in immune-to-brain signalling is via its action on neural afferents (Dantzer 1994; Kent *et al.* 1992). Infection often occurs through a break in the protective barrier formed by the skin. The injection of bacterial LPS into a previously formed subcutaneous pouch filled with sterile air is an experimental approach to mimic these types of infection. Using this approach one study has tested the involvement of neural afferents at the level of the site of infection or inflammation by using local anesthetics to disrupt the firing of nerve fibres. This study demonstrated that local anesthetics can indeed attenuate, but not abolish the fever response induced by LPS, but only at relatively low concentrations of the stimulus (10 µg/kg) (Ross *et al.* 2000). Similarly, C-fibre deafferentiation attenuates the early fever response induced by intramuscular turpentine injection in rats (Cooper and Rothwell 1991). These findings suggest that local subcutaneous, and deeper tissue afferent nerves play a role in CNS afferent signals induced by low doses of bacterial LPS and sterile tissue injury. Most of the recent investigations in this area have, however, focused on the role of subdiaphragmatic vagal afferents, which innervate the stomach, liver, and small intestine.

The gastrointestinal tract contains the organism's largest external surface and, in contrast to the skin, has to absorb valuable nutrients while preventing bacteria and viruses from infecting the organism. Intestinal and peritoneal macrophages represent a first line of defence against infecting micro-organisms (Hau 1990). These macrophages express the LPS binding, Toll-like receptor 4 (Akashi *et al.* 2000) and produce IL-1β in response to intra-peritoneally derived LPS (Takai *et al.* 1997). The first experimental evidence in favour of IL-1β action on peripheral nerves was obtained by Niijima, who showed that intraportal infusion of IL-1β increased discharge activity of the hepatic branch of the vagus nerve in the anesthetized rat (Niijima 1996). After intraperitoneal injection of LPS in rats, IL-1β is found in macrophages and dendritic cells associated with vagal branches innervating the peritoneal cavity before it appears in the circulation (Goehler *et al.* 1999). In addition, IL-1 receptors are expressed by vagal neurones (Ek *et al.* 1998) indicating that vagal afferents can indeed present a target for locally released IL-1.

To address the role of vagal afferents in immune-to-brain signalling in response to intraperitoneal LPS administration, several groups have studied the impact of subdiaphragmatic vagotomy on APR responses to LPS or IL-1β. At this anatomic level the vagus nerve consists of more than 70 per cent of afferent fibres (Berthoud and Neuhuber 2000), so this procedure affects mostly afferent vagal signalling. Subdiaphragmatic vagotomy sometimes attenuates, but never completely prevents, intraperitoneal IL-1β or LPS-induced fever (Hansen *et al.* 2000, 2001; Kapás *et al.* 1998). In contrast, it either prevents or attenuates adrenocorticotropin release as well as the reduction in behavioural activity and food-motivated behaviour depending on the dose of intraperitoneal LPS or IL-1β (Bluthé *et al.* 1996, 1994; Bret-Dibat *et al.* 1995; Gaykema *et al.* 1995; Kapcala *et al.* 1996; Konsman *et al.* 2000). Moreover, we found that the febrile response to intraperitoneal injection of a dose of LPS or IL-1β was not altered by subdiaphragmatic vagotomy which did prevent LPS-induced behavioural depression (Konsman *et al.* 2000; Luheshi *et al.* 2000). This suggests that vagal fibres play a more important role in immune-to-brain signalling underlying behavioural depression as compared to fever in response to intraperitoneal LPS administration.

Vagus-dependent and -independent activation of CNS structures is probably best illu-strated by quantifying the number of c-fos containing cells in different brain nuclei of vagotomized and sham-operated animals after peripheral LPS injection. We demonstrated, for example, that LPS-induced c-fos expression in the OVLT of the preoptic area was not affected by subdiaphragmatic vagotomy (Konsman *et al.* 2000). This, together with the observed translocation of the IL-6 inducible Stat3 transcription factor in the OVLT, suggests that circulating IL-6 acts on this structure, lacking a BBB, to induce fever (Konsman *et al.* 2000). However, subdiaphragmatic vagotomy prevents c-fos induction in the NTS, on to which vagal afferents project as well as in the neuroendocrine PVH and limbic structures, which receive projections from the NTS, 2 h after intraperitoneal LPS administration (Konsman *et al.* 2000) (see Fig. 5.1). These findings illustrate that subdiaphragmatic afferents are responsible for rapid immune-to-brain signalling underlying activation of limbic structures and the neuroendocrine hypothalamus.

When infection persists and spreads from the peritoneal cavity or skin, infectious microorganisms may gain access to the circulation. Hepatic Kupffer cells make up the largest population of tissue macrophages and form a line of defence once micro-organisms have gained access to the circulation (Ruiter *et al.* 1981). Although it hardly represents the kinetics of a natural infection, intravenous or intra-arterial bolus injection of bacterial LPS can be used to mimic situations in which bacteria have caused the general condition. In this

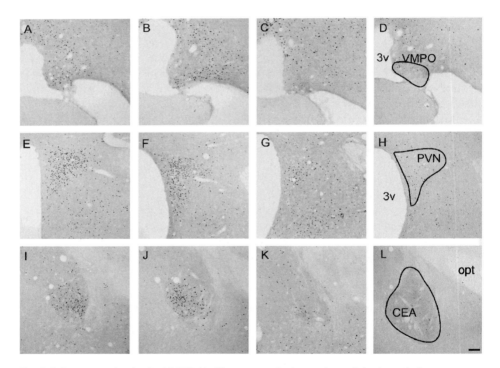

Fig. 5.1 Fos expression in the VMPO (A–D), paraventricular nucleus of the hypothalamus (PVH; E–H) and CEA (I–L) 2 h after intraperitoneal injection of saline or bacterial LPS in vagotomized (VGX) and sham-operated rats. The left panel (A, E, I) shows sections of a sham-operated animal injected with 250 μg/kg LPS route? Panels (B, F, J) display sections from an animal injected with LPS, that was judged to be incompletely vagotomized based on the persistence of isolectin binding in the NTS. The pattern of Fos expression after LPS in this animal is similar to that seen in a sham-operated animal. However, LPS-induced Fos expression is almost completely absent in a rat that was completely vagotomized (C, G, K). Panels D, H, L shows a completely vagotomized animal injected with saline. 3v = third ventricle. Scale bar = 100 μm. (Reproduced with permission from Konsman *et al.* 2000)

experimental model, fever and adrenocorticotropin hormone release occur within 30 min of intravenous or intra-arterial administration of low doses of LPS (Givalois *et al.* 1994; Sehic *et al.* 1996), during which no rise in cytokine plasma levels is observed (Givalois *et al.* 1994). Kuppfer cells take up its intravenous by injected LPS and are responsible for these fast responses, as temporal elimination of these cells blocks the fever response to systemic administration of a low dose of LPS (Sehic *et al.* 1998). Moreover, Kuppfer cell elimination prevents the rise in PGE2 seen normally in the preoptic hypothalamus during the first 30 min after systemic LPS administration (Sehic *et al.* 1998). This suggests the release of either a preformed or rapidly generated peripheral messenger. Local prostaglandin PGE2 might constitute such a messenger, as LPS-stimulated macrophages produce this within 30 min, that is, before COX-2 induction becomes detectable (Ribardo *et al.* 2001). Although the underlying mechanism is at present unclear, fast local PGE2 production by Kuppfer cells may signal the brain via the vagus nerve, as its neurones express PG receptors (Ek *et al.* 1998).

In accordance with this hypothesis, subdiaphragmatic vagotomy not only attenuates, but also prevents, the rapid fever responses to systemic administration of low doses of LPS (Romanovsky *et al.* 1997; Sehic and Blatteis 1996). Moreover, subdiaphragmatic vagotomy prevents the rise in PGE2 levels in the preoptic area (Sehic and Blatteis 1996), which is important for fever induction (Sehic *et al.* 1996). Neurones of the solitary tract on which vagal fibres terminate, contain noradrenaline and project to the preoptic area (Saper *et al.* 1983). Interestingly, noradrenaline injected into the preoptic area increases PGE2 production (Sehic *et al.* 1996). The production of PGE2 in neurones of the preoptic area does not require de novo synthesis, as COX-2 is expressed constitutively by neurones in this structure (Breder *et al.* 1995). Collectively, these findings indicate that in response to intravenous administration of low doses of LPS, a mediator, produced by Kuppfer cells, acts rapidly on the vagus nerve, which in turn activates a neuronal circuit resulting in the release of PGE2 in the preoptic area and ultimately fever.

In summary, at least three immune-to-brain signalling pathways other than cytokine-induced PG synthesis at the BBB seem to be involved in the initiation of central nervous components of the APR namely action of circulating IL-6 in the CNS as well as IL-1β-dependent and independent activation of peripheral nerves (see Fig. 5.2). The relative importance of each pathway depends on the site of the insult and the response studied.

5.6 **Cytokine production and action within the CNS**

Given that other immune-to-brain signalling mechanisms are responsible for initiation of central nervous components of the APR, can PG induction at the BBB account for the maintenance of fever, HPA-axis activation and behavioural changes as well as the activation of CNS structures in response to peripheral insults? Our recent observations indicate that the IL-1 type 1 receptor (IL-1R1), the only known signalling receptor for IL-1β, is present in blood vessels of the preoptic area, the supraoptic nucleus of the hypothalamus, the NTS and the VLM (Konsman *et al.* 2000). Furthermore, the PG-synthesising enzyme COX-2 is found around blood vessels of these brain areas after intravenous injection of IL-1β or intraperitoneal administration of LPS, (Konsman, unpublished observations). With these descriptive data in mind, one would expect inhibition of PG synthesis to attenuate activation of these hypothalamic and brainstem structures more than in other brain nuclei displaying c-fos induction in response to peripheral IL-1β or bacterial LPS. Indeed,

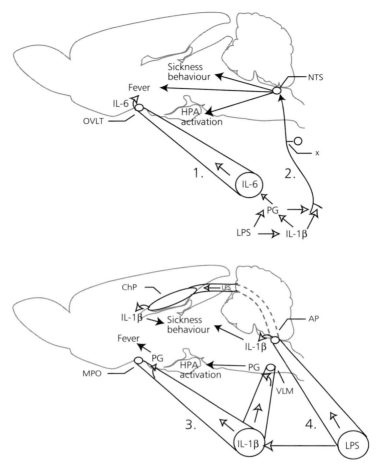

Fig. 5.2 Schematic drawing of a saggital brain section to summarize the role of different immune-to-brain signalling pathways after peripheral infection with bacteria containing LPS fragments. The upper panel shows fast immune-to-brain signalling pathways including (1) action of circulating IL-6 at the level of brain circumventricular organs and (2) local IL-1β or PG action on neural afferents. The lower panel displays slower immune-to-brain signalling mechanisms involving (3) PG synthesis at the BBB or (4) production of IL-1β within brain circumventricular organs and choroid plexus (ChP). (1) Local IL-1β release induces IL-6 production, which enters the blood stream and acts at the level of brain circumventricular organs, such as the OVLT, where the BBB is absent. This hormonal type of action contributes to the fever response. (2) Local IL-1β or PG action on neural afferents of for example the vagus nerve (x) results in activation of neurones of the NTS. NTS neurones, in turn, project to brain structures involved in the fever response, activation of the HPA axis and sickness behaviour. At later time points after local infection bacterial LPS and IL-1β gain access to the blood stream. (3) Circulating IL-1β acts on its receptors present on blood vessels of, amongst others the VLM and the MPO to induce the synthesis of PG. PGs diffuse across the BBB and can act on their receptors in the VLM and MPO to sustain the HPA axis and fever response respectively. (4) Circulating LPS can act on its receptor present in circumventricular organs, such as the area postrema (AP) in the brainstem and ChP to stimulate the production of IL-1β in these brain structures. Diffusion of thus produced IL-1β to IL-1 receptors in the AP or from the ChP to forebrain structures bearing its receptor is thought to underlie the maintenance of sickness behaviour. Open arrows indicate diffusion of inflammatory mediators, while closed arrows refer to the activation of neural pathways.

peripheral administration of drugs known to inhibit prostaglandin synthesis attenuate LPS- or IL-1β-induced c-fos expression in the preoptic area, supraoptic and paraventricular nucleus of the hypothalamus as well as in the VLM (Ericsson *et al.* 1997; Lacroix and Rivest 1997; Wan *et al.* 1994; Zhang and Rivest 2000). However, these treatments did not alter peripheral LPS- or IL-1β-induced c-fos expression in the parabrachial nuclei, the central nucleus of the amygdala, or the bed nucleus of the stria terminalis (Ericsson *et al.* 1997; Lacroix and Rivest 1997; Zhang and Rivest 2000). These findings indicate that PG synthesis accounts only for the maintenance of activation of brainstem and hypothalamic structures associated with the febrile and neuroendocrine responses during the APR (see Fig. 5.2).

Although subdiaphragmatic vagotomy attenuates the reduction in social behaviour induced by intraperitoneally administered IL-1β, it does not affect the same response after intravenous injection of IL-1β (Bluthé *et al.* 1996). This indicates that besides the vagus nerve, other types of IL-1β-to-brain signalling mechanisms are involved in mediating sickness behaviour. Since IL-1 type 1 receptors are present in brain parenchyma (Cunningham *et al.* 1992; Ericsson *et al.* 1995), we addressed the role of parenchymal IL-1 in CNS components of the APR. The naturally occurring antagonist for IL-1 (IL-1ra) was administered either into the lateral cerebral ventricle or into the peritoneal cavity before intraperitoneal injection of IL-1β. Intraperitoneal or icv administration of IL-1ra attenuated the reduction in social interaction and food-motivated behaviour induced by intraperitoneal injection of IL-1β (Kent *et al.* 1992). In contrast, the fever response induced by intraperitoneal injection of IL-1β was abrogated only by administration of IL-1ra via the same route (Kent *et al.* 1992). These observations indicate that peripherally administered interleukin-1β acts on the brain side of the BBB on receptors within the CNS to induce sickness behaviour, but not fever.

An active blood-to-brain transport system exists for IL-1β, but only 0.1 per cent of systemically administered IL-1 enters the brain (Banks *et al.* 1991). Thus, this form of transport of IL-1β across the BBB may come in to play only when plasma concentrations of this cytokine are at levels achieved by a bolus injection, or possibly when infection is severe and widespread. LPS administration induces the secretion of pro-inflammatory cytokines, including IL-1β, in a pattern similar to that seen in natural infection (Chen *et al.* 1992). Bacterial LPS appears in the circulation before any pro-inflammatory cytokine after its intraperitoneal injection (Hansen *et al.* 2000; Lenczowski *et al.* 1997). Circumventricular organs and choroid plexus, which lack a functional BBB (Gross 1992), express the LPS-binding molecules CD14 and Toll-like receptor 4 (Laflamme and Rivest 2001). These observations suggest that circulating LPS can act on these brain structures to induce IL-1β synthesis.

We recently tested the hypothesis that IL-1β is produced in circumventricular organs and choroid plexus (ChP) after peripheral administration of LPS. These studies revealed IL-1β-immunoreactive phagocytic cells in circumventricular organs and ChP as early as 2 h after intraperitoneal injection of bacterial LPS (Konsman *et al.* 1999). However, at this time point brain IL-1β, in contrast to plasma IL-1β, is not yet bioactive as measured by an IL-1 receptor-dependent thymocyte proliferation assay (Quan *et al.* 1994). At later time points, IL-1β-immunoreactive cells are observed in brain parenchyma adjacent to circumventricular organs and over the ventricular surface of the ChP, that is, behind the cellular barrier that separates the ChP from the CSF (Konsman *et al.* 1999). Moreover, bioactive IL-1 can be found in the brain extracellular and ventricular CSF at similar time points (Quan *et al.* 1994). These findings suggest that after peripheral injection of LPS, IL-1β produced in circumventricular organs and ChP spreads throughout the brain extracellular space (Konsman *et al.* 2000). It is probable, therefore, that brain IL-1β plays a role in suppressing behavioural activity and food intake during the APR. Indeed, icv administration of IL-1ra attenuates anorexia and behavioural depression, but not fever or neuroendocrine activation, at time points beyond 4 h after LPS administration (Layé *et al.* 2000; J.P. Konsman, PhD-thesis, Groningen 2000). Earlier studies have, however, reported that icv injection of IL-1ra attenuates ip LPS-induced fever (Luheshi *et al.* 1996), or activation of the HPA-axis (Kakucska *et al.* 1993), using repeated or continuous administration of IL-1ra started at time points when IL-1β in the brain was not yet bioactive. However, since icv administration of cytokines results in higher and longer lasting plasma and liver levels of these cytokines compared to those induced by intravenous injection (Di Santo *et al.* 1999), prevention of circulating IL-1β action cannot be excluded in these earlier studies. Collectively, this indicates that IL-1β production and action within the CNS constitutes a relatively slow way of IL-1β-to-brain signalling involved in maintaining activation of limbic structures and the behavioural components of the APR (see Fig. 5.2).

5.7 Conclusion

The central nervous components of the APR, including fever, HPA-axis activation and reduced behavioural activity and food intake can be considered adaptive to the host faced with a peripheral insult. These responses are the result of activation of hypothalamic and presumably limbic circuits in response to circulating IL-6 as well as to the action of IL-1β, and other, as yet unidentified, mediators on peripheral nerves, and are maintained by PG synthesis at the BBB and cytokine production and action within the CNS. Better understanding of the role of these immune-to-brain signalling mechanisms is important for identifying new target and developing future therapeutic strategies for treatment of diseases in which central nervous components of the APR persist.

References

Akashi, S., Shimazu, R., Ogata, H., Nagai, Y., Takeda, K., Kimoto, M., and Miyake, K. (2000). Cutting edge: cell surface expression and lipopolysaccharide signaling via the toll-like receptor 4-MD-2 complex on mouse peritoneal macrophages. *J Immunol*, **164**, 3471–5.

Banks, W. A., Ortiz, L., Plotkin, S. R., and Kastin, A. J. (1991). Human interleukin (IL) 1 alpha, murine IL-1 alpha and murine IL-1 beta are transported from blood to brain in the mouse by a shared saturable mechanism. *J Pharmacol Exp Ther*, **259**, 988–96.

Baumann, H. and Gauldie, J. (1994). The acute phase response. *Immunology Today*, **15**, 74–80.

Berkenbosch, F., van Oers, J., del Rey, A., Tilders, F., and Besedovsky, H. (1987). Corticotropin-releasing factor-producing neurons in the rat activated by interleukin-1. *Science*, **238**, 524–6.

Berthoud, H. R. and Neuhuber, W. L. (2000). Functional and chemical anatomy of the afferent vagal system. **85**, 1–17.

Bing, C., Frankish, H. M., Pickavance, L., Wang, Q., Hopkins, D. F., Stock, M. J., and Williams, G. (1998). Hyperphagia in cold-exposed rats is accompanied by decreased plasma leptin but unchanged hypothalamic NPY. *Amer J Physiol*, **274**, R62–8.

Blatteis, C. M., Bealer, S. L., Hunter, W. S., Llanos-Q, J., Ahokas, R. A., and Mashburn, T. A. Jr. (1983). Suppression of fever after lesions of the anteroventral third ventricle in guinea pigs. *Brain Res Bull*, **11**, 519–26.

Blatteis, C. M., Sehic, E., and Li, S. (2000). Pyrogen sensing and signaling: old views and new concepts. *Clin Infect Dis*, 31 **Suppl** 5, S168–177.

Bluthé, R. M., Dantzer, R., and Kelley, K. W. (1992). Effects of interleukin-1 receptor antagonist on the behavioral effects of lipopolysaccharide in rat. *Brain Res*, **573**, 318–20.

Bluthé, R. M., Michaud, B., Kelley, K. W., and Dantzer, R. (1996). Vagotomy attenuates behavioural effects of interleukin-1 injected peripherally but not centrally. *Neuroreport*, **7**, 1485–8.

Bluthé, R. M., Michaud, B., Kelley, K. W., and Dantzer, R. (1996). Vagotomy blocks behavioural effects of interleukin-1 injected via the intraperitoneal route but not via other systemic routes. *Neuroreport*, **7**, 2823–7.

Bluthé, R. M., Walter, V., Parnet, P., Layé, S., Lestage, J., Verrier, D., *et al*. (1994). Lipopolysaccharide induces sickness behaviour in rats by a vagal mediated mechanism. *Comptes Rendus De L Academie Des Sciences. Serie Iii, Sciences De La Vie*, **317**, 499–503.

Boulant, J. A. (1981). Hypothalamic mechanisms in thermoregulation. *Federation Proc*, **40**, 2843–50.

Breder, C. D., Dewitt, D., and Kraig, R. P. (1995). Characterization of inducible cyclooxygenase in rat brain. *J Comparat Neurol*, **355**, 296–315.

Bret-Dibat, J. L., Bluthé, R. M., Kent, S., Kelley, K. W., and Dantzer, R. (1995). Lipopolysaccharide and interleukin-1 depress food-motivated behavior in mice by a vagal-mediated mechanism. *Brain, Behav, Immunity*, **9**, 242–6.

Buller, K., Xu, Y., Dayas, C., and Day, T. (2001). Dorsal and ventral medullary catecholamine cell groups contribute differentially to systemic interleukin-1beta-induced hypothalamic pituitary adrenal axis responses. *Neuroendocrinology*, **73**, 129–38.

Caldwell, F. T., Graves, D. B., and Wallace, B. H. (1998). Studies on the mechanism of fever after intravenous administration of endotoxin. *J Trauma*, **44**, 304–12.

Cannon, J. G., Tompkins, R. G., Gelfand, J. A., Michie, H. R., Stanford, G. G., van der Meer, J. W., *et al*. (1990). Circulating interleukin-1 and tumor necrosis factor in septic shock and experimental endotoxin fever. *J Infect Dis*, **161**, 79–84.

Cao, C., Matsumura, K., Yamagata, K., and Watanabe, Y. (1995). Induction by lipopolysaccharide of cyclooxygenase-2 mRNA in rat brain; its possible role in the febrile response. *Brain Res*, **697**, 187–96.

Cao, C., Matsumura, K., Yamagata, K., and Watanabe, Y. (1997). Involvement of cyclooxygenase-2 in LPS-induced fever and regulation of its mRNA by LPS in the rat brain. *Amer J Physiol*, **272**, R1712–25.

Cartmell, T., Poole, S., Turnbull, A. V., Rothwell, N. J., and Luheshi, G. N. (2000). Circulating interleukin-6 mediates the febrile response to localised inflammation in rats. *J Physiol*, **526**, 653–61.

Chen, T. Y., Lei, M. G., Suzuki, T., and Morrison, D. C. (1992). Lipopolysaccharide receptors and signal transduction pathways in mononuclear phagocytes. *Curr Topics Microbiol Immunol*, **181**, 169–88.

Cooper, A. L. and Rothwell, N. J. (1991). Mechanisms of early and late hypermetabolism and fever after localized tissue injury in rats. *Amer J Physiol*, **261**, E698–705.

Crestani, F., Seguy, F., and Dantzer, R. (1991). Behavioural effects of peripherally injected interleukin-1: role of prostaglandins. *Brain Res*, **542**, 330–5.

Cunningham, E. T. J., Wada, E., Carter, D. B., Tracey, D. E., Battey, J. F., and De Souza, E. B. (1992). *In situ* histochemical localization of type I interleukin-1 receptor messenger RNA in the central nervous system, pituitary, and adrenal gland of the mouse. *J Neurosci*, **12**, 1101–14.

Dantzer, R. (1994). How do cytokines say hello to the brain? Neural versus humoral mediation. *Eur Cytokine Network*, **5**, 271–3.

Dascombe, M. J., Rothwell, N. J., Sagay, B. O., and Stock, M. J. (1989). Pyrogenic and thermogenic effects of interleukin 1 beta in the rat. *Amer J Physiol*, **256**, E7–11.

Day, H. E., Curran, E. J., Watson, S. J., and Akil, H. (1999). Distinct neurochemical poulations in the rat central nucleus and bed nucleus of the stria terminalis: evidence for their selective activation by interleukin-1beta. *J Comparat Neurol*, **413**, 113–28.

Deeter, L. B., Martin, L. W., and Lipton, J. M. (1988). Antipyretic properties of centrally administered alpha-MSH fragments in the rabbit. *Peptides*, **9**, 1285–8.

Dey, P. K., Feldberg, W., Gupta, K. P., Milton, A. S., and Wendlandt, S. (1974). Further studies on the role of prostaglandin in fever. *J Physiol*, **241**, 629–46.

Di Santo, E., Benigni, F., Agnello, D., Sipe, J. D., and Ghezzi, P. (1999). Peripheral effects of centrally administered interleukin-1beta in mice in relation to its clearance from the brain into the blood and tissue distribution. *Neuroimmunomodulation*, **6**, 300–4.

Ebisui, O., Fukata, J., Murakami, N., Kobayashi, H., Segawa, H., Muro, S., *et al.* (1994). Effect of IL-1 receptor antagonist and antiserum to TNF-alpha on LPS-induced plasma ACTH and corticosterone rise in rats. *Amer J Physiol*, **266**, E986–92.

Ek, M., Arias, C., Swachenko, P. E., and Ericsson-Dahlstrandt, A. (2000). Distribution of the EP3 prostaglandin E(2) receptor subtype in the rat brain: relationship to sites of interleukin-1-induced cellular responsiveness. *J Comparat Neurol*, **428**, 5–20.

Ek, M., Kurosawa, M., Lundeberg, T., and Ericsson, A. (1998). Activation of vagal afferents after intravenous injection of interleukin-1beta: role of endogenous prostaglandins. *J Neurosci*, **18**, 9471–9.

Elmquist, J. K., Breder, C. D., Sherin, J. E., Scammell, T. E., Hickey, W. F., Dewitt, D., and Saper, C. B. (1997). Intravenous lipopolysaccharide induces cyclooxygenase 2-like immunoreactivity in rat brain perivascular microglia and meningeal macrophages. *J Comparat Neurol*, **381**, 119–29.

Elmquist, J. K. and Saper, C. B. (1996). Activation of neurons projecting to the paraventricular hypothalamic nucleus by intravenous lipopolysaccharide. *J Comparat Neurol*, **374**, 315–31.

Elmquist, J. K., Scammell, T. E., and Saper, C. B. (1997). Mechanisms of CNS response to systemic immune challenge: the febrile response. *Trends Neurosci*, **20**, 565–70.

Ericsson, A., Arias, C., and Sawchenko, P. E. (1997). Evidence for an intramedullary prostaglandin-dependent mechanism in the activation of stress-related neuroendocrine circuitry by intravenous interleukin-1. *J Neurosci*, **17**, 7166–79.

Ericsson, A., Kovács, K. J., and Sawchenko, P. E. (1994). A functional anatomical analysis of central pathways subserving the effects of interleukin-1 on stress-related neuroendocrine neurons. *J Neurosci*, **14**, 897–913.

Ericsson, A., Liu, C., Hart, R. P., and Sawchenko, P. E. (1995). Type 1 interleukin-1 receptor in the rat brain: distribution, regulation, and relationship to sites of IL-1-induced cellular activation. *J Comparat Neurol*, **361**, 681–98.

Evans, S. S., Wang, W. C., Bain, M. D., Burd, R., Ostberg, J. R., and Repasky, E. A. (2001). Fever-range hyperthermia dynamically regulates lymphocyte delivery to high endothelial venules. *Blood*, **97**, 2727–33.

Flower, R. J. and Vane, J. R. (1974). Inhibition of prostaglandin biosynthesis. *Biochem Pharmacol*, **23**, 1439–50.

Gaykema, R. P., Dijkstra, I., and Tilders, F. J. (1995). Subdiaphragmatic vagotomy suppresses endotoxin-induced activation of hypothalamic corticotropin-releasing hormone neurons and ACTH secretion. *Endocrinol*, **136**, 4717–20.

Givalois, L., Dornand, J., Mekaouche, M., Solier, M. D., Bristow, A. F., Ixart, G., *et al.* (1994). Temporal cascade of plasma level surges in ACTH, corticosterone, and cytokines in endotoxin-challenged rats. *Amer J Physiol*, **267**, R164–70.

Goehler, L. E., Gaykema, R. P., Nguyen, K. T., Lee, J. E., Tilders, F. J., Maier, S. F., and Watkins, L. R. (1999). Interleukin-1beta in immune cells of the abdominal vagus nerve: a link between the immune and nervous systems? *J Neurosci*, **19**, 2799–806.

Graham, J. C., Hoffman, G. E., and Sved, A. F. (1995). c-Fos expression in brain in response to hypotension and hypertension in conscious rats. *J Autonomic Nervous System*, **55**, 92–104.

Gross, P. M. (1992). Circumventricular organ capillaries. *Progress In Brain Research*, **91**, 219–33.

Hansen, M. K., Daniels, S., Goehler, L. E., Gaykema, R. P., Maier, S. F., and Watkins, L. R. (2000). Subdiaphragmatic vagotomy does not block intraperitoneal lipopolysaccharide-induced fever. **85**, 83–7.

Hansen, M. K., Nguyen, K. T., Fleshner, M., Goehler, L. E., Gaykema, R. P., Maier, S. F., and Watkins, L. R. (2000). Effects of vagotomy on serum endotoxin, cytokines, and corticosterone after intra-peritoneal lipopolysaccharide. *Amer J Physiol*, **278**, R331–6.

Hansen, M. K., O'Connor, K. A., Goehler, L. E., Watkins, L. R., and Maier, S. F. (2001). The contribution of the vagus nerve in interleukin-1beta-induced fever is dependent on dose. **280**, R929–34.

Hashimoto, M., Bando, T., Iriki, M., and Hashimoto, K. (1988). Effect of indomethacin on febrile response to recombinant human interleukin 1-alpha in rabbits. *Amer J Physiol*, **255**, R527–33.

Hau, T. (1990). Bacteria, toxins, and the peritoneum. *World Journal of Surgery*, **14**, 167–75.

Hinson, R. M., Williams J. A., and Shacter, E. (1996). Elevated interleukin 6 is induced by prostaglandin E2 in a murine model of inflammation: possible role of cyclooxygenase-2. *Proc Natl Acad Sci USA*, **93**, 4885–90.

Hiscott, J., Marois, J., Garoufalis, J., D'Addario, M., Roulston, A., Kwan, I., *et al.* (1993). Characterization of a functional NF-kappa B site in the human interleukin 1 beta promoter: evidence for a positive autoregulatory loop. *Mol Cell Biol*, **13**, 6231–40.

Horn, T., Wilkinson, M. F., Landgraf, R., and Pittman, Q. J. (1994). Reduced febrile responses to pyrogens after lesions of the hypothalamic paraventricular nucleus. *Amer J Physiol*, **267**, R323–8.

Huang, Q. H., Hruby, V. J., and Tatro, J. B. (1999). Role of central melanocortins in endotoxin-induced anorexia. *Amer J Physiol*, **276**, R864–71.

Husseini, R. H., Sweet, C., Collie, M. H., and Smith, H. (1982). Elevation of nasal viral levels by suppression of fever in ferrets infected with influenza viruses of differing virulence. *J Infect Dis*, **145**, 520–4.

Jepson, M. M., Millward, D. J., Rothwell, N. J., and Stock, M. J. (1988). Involvement of sympathetic nervous system and brown fat in endotoxin-induced fever in rats. *Amer J Physiol*, **255**, E617–20.

Kakucska, I., Qi, Y., Clark, B. D., and Lechan, R. M. (1993). Endotoxin-induced corticotropin-releasing hormone gene expression in the hypothalamic paraventricular nucleus is mediated centrally by interleukin-1. *Endocrinol*, **133**, 815–21.

Kapás, L., Hansen, M. K., Chang, H. Y., and Krueger, J. M. (1998). Vagotomy attenuates but does not prevent the somnogenic and febrile effects of lipopolysaccharide in rats. *Amer J Physiol*, **274**, R406–11.

Kapcala, L. P., He, J. R., Gao, Y., Pieper, J. O., and DeTolla, L. J. (1996). Subdiaphragmatic vagotomy inhibits intra-abdominal interleukin-1 beta stimulation of adrenocorticotropin secretion. *Brain Res*, **728**, 247–54.

Kent, S., Bluthe, R. M., Dantzer, R., Hardwick, A. J., Kelley, K.W., Rothwell, N. J., and Vannice, J. L. (1992). Different receptor mechanisms mediate the pyrogenic and behavioral effects of interleukin 1. *Proc Natl Acad Sci USA*, **89**, 9117–20.

Kent, S., Bluthé, R. M., Kelley, K. W., and Dantzer, R. (1992). Sickness behavior as a new target for drug development. *Trends Pharmacol Sci*, **13**, 24–28.

Kluger, M. J. (1991). Fever: role of pyrogens and cryogens. *Physiological Reviews*, **71**, 93–127.

Kluger, M. J. and Rothenburg, B. A. (1979). Fever and reduced iron: their interaction as a host defense response to bacterial infection. *Science*, **203**, 374–6.

Konsman, J. P., Kelley, K., and Dantzer, R. (1999). Temporal and spatial relationships between lipopolysaccharide-induced expression of Fos, interleukin-1beta and inducible nitric oxide synthase in rat brain. *Neuroscience*, **89**, 535–48.

Konsman, J. P., Luheshi, G. N., Bluthé, R. M., and Dantzer, R. (2000). The vagus nerve mediates behavioral depression, but not fever, in response to peripheral immune signals; a functional anatomical analysis. *Eur J Neurosci*, **12**, 4434–46.

Konsman, J. P., Rees, G., Ek, M., Dantzer, R., Ericsson-Dahlstrand, A., and Blomqvist, A. (2000). Distribution of interleukin-1 receptor type 1 mRNA and protein in rat brain. *Soc Neurosc Abstr*, **26**, 242.241.

Konsman, J. P., Tridon, V., and Dantzer, R. (2000). Diffusion and action of intracerebroventricularly injected interleukin-1 in the central nervous system. *Neuroscience*, **101**, 957–67.

Kovács, K. J. (1998). c-Fos as a transcription factor: a stressful (re)view from a functional map. *Neurochem Int*, **33**, 287–97.

Krukoff, T. L., MacTavish, D., Harris, K. H., and Jhamandas, J. H. (1995). Changes in blood volume and pressure induce c-fos expression in brainstem neurons that project to the paraventricular nucleus of the hypothalamus. *Brain Res. Mol Brain Res*, **34**, 99–108.

Lacroix, S., and Rivest, S. (1997). Functional circuitry in the brain of immune-challenged rats: partial involvement of prostaglandins. *J Comparat Neurol*, **387**, 307–24.

Lacroix, S. and Rivest, S. (1998). Effect of acute systemic inflammatory response and cytokines on the transcription of the genes encoding cyclooxygenase enzymes (COX-1 and COX-2) in the rat brain. *J Neurochem*, **70**, 452–66.

Laflamme, N. and Rivest, S. (2001). Toll-like receptor 4: the missing link of the cerebral innate immune response triggered by circulating gram-negative bacterial cell wall components. *FASEB J*, **15**, 155–63.

Layé, S., Gheusi, G., Cremona, S., Combe, C., Kelley, K., Dantzer, R., and Parnet, P. (2000). Endogenous brain IL-1 mediates LPS-induced anorexia and hypothalamic cytokine expression. *Amer J Physiol*, **179**, R93–8.

Lenczowski, M. J., Bluthé, R. M., Roth, J., Rees, G. S., Rushforth, D. A., van Dam, A. M., *et al.* (1999). Central administration of rat IL-6 induces HPA activation and fever but not sickness behavior in rats. *Amer J Physiol*, **276**, R652–8.

Lenczowski, M. J., Van Dam, A. M., Poole, S., Larrick, J. W., and Tilders, F. J. (1997). Role of circulating endotoxin and interleukin-6 in the ACTH and corticosterone response to intraperitoneal LPS. *Amer J Physiol*, **273**, R1870–7.

Li, Y. W. and Dampney, R. A. (1994). Expression of Fos-like protein in brain following sustained hypertension and hypotension in conscious rabbits. *Neuroscience*, **61**, 613–34.

Lipton, J. M., Ceriani, G., Macaluso, A., McCoy, D., Carnes, K., Biltz, J., and Catania, A. (1994). Antiinflammatory effects of the neuropeptide alpha-MSH in acute, chronic, and systemic inflammation. *Ann NY Acad Sci*, **741**, 137–48.

Long, N. C., Otterness, I., Kunkel, S. L., Vander, A. J., and Kluger, M. J. (1990). Roles of interleukin 1 beta and tumor necrosis factor in lipopolysaccharide fever in rats. *Amer J Physiol*, **259**, R724–8.

Lu, J., Zhang, Y. H., Chou, T. C., Gaus, S. E., Elmquist, J. K., Shiromani, P., and Saper, C. B. (2001). Contrasting effects of ibotenate lesions of the paraventricular nucleus and subparaventricular zone on sleep-wake cycle and temperature regulation. *J Neurosci*, **21**, 4864–74.

Luheshi, G., Miller, A. J., Brouwer, S., Dascombe, M. J., Rothwell, N. J., and Hopkins, S. J. (1996). Interleukin-1 receptor antagonist inhibits endotoxin fever and systemic interleukin-6 induction in the rat. *Amer J Physiol*, **270**, E91–5.

Luheshi, G. N., Bluthe, R. M., Rushforth, D., Mulcahy, N., Konsman, J. P., Goldbach, M., and Dantzer, R. (2000). Vagotomy attenuates the behavioural but not the pyrogenic effects of interleukin-1 in rats. *Autonomic Neurosci*, **85**, 127–32.

Luheshi, G. N., Stefferl, A., Turnbull, A. V., Dascombe, M. J., Brouwer, S., Hopkins, S. J., and Rothwell, N. J. (1997). Febrile response to tissue inflammation involves both peripheral and brain IL-1 and TNF-alpha in the rat. *Amer J Physiol*, **272**, R862–8.

Mackowiak, P. A., Bartlett, J. G., Borden, E. C., Goldblum, S. E., Hasday, J. D., Munford, R. S., *et al.* (1997). Concepts of fever: recent advances and lingering dogma. *Clin Infect Dis*, **25**, 119–38.

Martin, S. M., Malkinson, T. J., Veale, W. L., and Pittman, Q. J. (1990). Depletion of brain alpha-MSH alters prostaglandin and interleukin fever in rats. *Brain Res*, **526**, 351–4.

Miller, A. J., Hopkins, S. J., and Luheshi, G. N. (1997). Sites of action of IL-1 in the development of fever and cytokine responses to tissue inflammation in the rat. *Brit J Pharmacol*, **120**, 12 747–9.

Milton, A. S. and Wendlandt, S. (1970). A possible role for prostaglandin E1 as a modulator for temperature regulation in the central nervous system of the cat. *J Physiol*, **207**, 76P–77P.

Morimoto, A., Murakami, N., Nakamori, T., Sakata, Y., and Watanabe, T. (1989). Brain regions involved in the development of acute phase responses accompanying fever in rabbits. *J Physiol (Lond)*, **416**, 645–57.

Murakami, N. and Watanabe, T. (1989). Activation of ACTH release is mediated by the same molecule as the final mediator, PGE2, of febrile response in rats. *Brain Res*, **478**, 171–4.

Murray, M. J. and Murray, A. B. (1979). Anorexia of infection as a mechanism of host defense. *Amer J Clin Nutr*, **32**, 593–6.

Murray, M. J., Murray, A. B., Murray, M. B., and Murray, C. J. (1978). The adverse effect of iron repletion on the course of certain infections. *Brit Med J*, **2**, 1113–5.

Niijima, A. (1996). The afferent discharges from sensors for interleukin 1 beta in the hepatoportal system in the anesthetized rat. *J Autonomic Nerv Syst*, **61**, 287–91.

Oka, T., Oka, K., Scammell, T. E., Lee, C., Kelly, J. F., Nantel, F., Elmquist, J. K., and Saper, C. B. (2000). Relationship of EP(1-4) prostaglandin receptors with rat hypothalamic cell groups involved in lipopolysaccharide fever responses. *J Comparat Neurol*, **428**, 20–32.

O'Neill, C. (1994). The biochemistry of prostaglandins: a primer. *Aust N Z J Obstetr Gynaecol*, **34**, 332–7.

O'Neill, G. P., Kennedy, B. P., Mancini, J. A., Kargman, S., Ouellet, M., Yergey, J., *et al.* (1995). Selective inhibitors of COX-2. *Agents And Actions. Suppl*, **46**, 159–168.

O'Neill, L. A. and Greene, C. (1998). Signal transduction pathways activated by the IL-1 receptor family: ancient signaling machinery in mammals, insects, and plants. *J Leukocyte Biol*, **63**, 650–7.

Opp, M. R., Obal, F. Jr., Payne, L., and Krueger, J. M. (1990). Responsiveness of rats to interleukin-1: effects of monosodium glutamate treatment of neonates. *Physiol Behav*, **48**, 451–7.

Parsadaniantz, S. M., Lebeau, A., Duval, P., Grimaldi, B., Terlain, B., and Kerdelhue, B. (2000). Effects of the inhibition of cyclo-oxygenase 1 or 2 or 5-lipoxygenase on the activation of the hypothalamic-pituitary-adrenal axis induced by interleukin-1beta in the male Rat. *J Neuroendocrinol*, **12**, 766–73.

Philipp-Dormston, W. K. and Siegert, R. (1974). Identification of prostaglandin E by radioimmunoassay in cerebrospinal fluid during endotoxin fever. *Naturwissenschaften*, **61**, 134–5.

Quan, N., Sundar, S. K., and Weiss, J. M. (1994). Induction of interleukin-1 in various brain regions after peripheral and central injections of lipopolysaccharide. *J Neuroimmunol*, **49**, 125–34.

Reyes, T. M. and Sawchenko, P. E. (2000). Is the arcuate nucleus involved in cytokine-induced anorexia? *Soc Neurosci Abstr*, **26**, 441.443.

Ribardo, D. A., Crowe, S. E., Kuhl, K. R., Peterson, J. W., and Chopra, A. K. (2001). Prostaglandin levels in stimulated macrophages are controlled by phospholipase A2-activating protein and by activation of phospholipase C and D. *J Biol Chem*, **276**, 5467–75.

Rivest, S. (1999). What is the cellular source of prostaglandins in the brain in response to systemic inflammation? Facts and controversies. *Mol Psychiatr*, **4**, 500–7.

Rivest, S. and Laflamme, N. (1995). Neuronal activity and neuropeptide gene transcription in the brains of immune-challenged rats. *J Neuroendocrinol*, **7**, 501–25.

Rivier, C. and Vale, W. (1991). Stimulatory effect of interleukin-1 on adrenocorticotropin secretion in the rat: is it modulated by prostaglandins? *Endocrinology*, **129**, 384–388.

Roberts, N. J. (1991). Impact of temperature elevation on immunologic defenses. *Rev Infect Dis*, **13**, 462–72.

Romanovsky, A. A., Simons, C. T., Székely, M., and Kulchitsky, V. A. (1997). The vagus nerve in the thermoregulatory response to systemic inflammation. *Amer J Physiol*, **273**, R407–13.

Ross, G., Roth, J., Storr, B., Voigt, K., and Zeisberger, E. (2000). Afferent nerves are involved in the febrile response to injection of LPS into artificial subcutaneous chambers in guinea pigs. *Physiol Behav*, 71, 305–13.

Rothwell, N. J., Busbridge, N. J., Lefeuvre, R. A., Hardwick, A. J., Gauldie, J., and Hopkins, S. J. (1991). Interleukin-6 is a centrally acting endogenous pyrogen in the rat. *Can J Physiol Pharmacol*, 69, 1465–9.

Ruiter, D. J., van der Meulen, J., Brouwer, A., Hummel, M. J., Mauw, B. J., van der Ploeg, J. C., and Wisse, E. (1981). Uptake by liver cells of endotoxin following its intravenous injection. *Lab Invest*, 45, 38–45.

Sagar, S. M., Price, K. J., Kasting, N. W., and Sharp, F. R. (1995). Anatomic patterns of Fos immunostaining in rat brain following systemic endotoxin administration. *Brain Res Bull*, 36, 381–92.

Saper, C. B., Reis, D. J., and Joh, T. (1983). Medullary catecholamine inputs to the anteroventral third ventricular cardiovascular regulatory region in the rat. *Neurosci Lett*, 42, 285–91.

Schotanus, K., Tilders, F. J., and Berkenbosch, F. (1993). Human recombinant interleukin-1 receptor antagonist prevents adrenocorticotropin, but not interleukin-6 responses to bacterial endotoxin in rats. *Endocrinology*, 133, 2461–8.

Schwartz, M. W., Woods, S. C., Porte, D. Jr., Seeley, R. J., and Baskin, D. G. (2000). Central nervous system control of food intake. *Nature*, 404, 661–71.

Schöbitz, B., Reul, J. M., and Holsboer, F. (1994). The role of the hypothalamic–pituitary–adrenocortical system during inflammatory conditions. *Crit Rev Neurobiol*, 8, 263–91.

Sehic, E. and Blatteis, C. M. (1996). Blockade of lipopolysaccharide-induced fever by subdiaphragmatic vagotomy in guinea pigs. *Brain Res*, 726, 160–6.

Sehic, E., Li, S., Ungar, A. L., and Blatteis, C. M. (1998). Complement reduction impairs the febrile response of guinea pigs to endotoxin. *Amer J Physiol*, 274, R1594–603.

Sehic, E., Székely, M., Ungar, A. L., Oladehin, A., and Blatteis, C. M. (1996). Hypothalamic prostaglandin E2 during lipopolysaccharide-induced fever in guinea pigs. *Brain Res Bull*, 39, 391–9.

Sehic, E., Ungar, A. L., and Blatteis, C. M. (1996). Interaction between norepinephrine and prostaglandin E2 in the preoptic area of guinea pigs. *Amer J Physiol*, 271, R528–36.

Shih, S. T., Khorram, O., Lipton, J. M., and McCann, S. M. (1986). Central administration of alpha-MSH antiserum augments fever in the rabbit. *Amer J Physiol*, 250, R803–6.

Sirko, S., Bishai, I., and Coceani, F. (1989). Prostaglandin formation in the hypothalamus *in vivo*: effect of pyrogens. *Amer J Physiol*, 256, R616–24.

Swiergiel, A. H., Smagin, G. N., Johnson, L. J., and Dunn, A. J. (1997). The role of cytokines in the behavioral responses to endotoxin and influenza virus infection in mice: effects of acute and chronic administration of the interleukin-1-receptor antagonist (IL-1ra). *Brain Res*, 776, 96–104.

Takai, N., Kataoka, M., Higuchi, Y., Matsuura, K., and Yamamoto, S. (1997). Primary structure of rat CD14 and characteristics of rat CD14, cytokine, and NO synthase mRNA expression in mononuclear phagocyte system cells in response to LPS. *J Leukocyte Biol*, 61, 736–44.

Tewari, A., Buhles, W. C., and Starnes, H. F. (1990). Preliminary report: effects of interleukin-1 on platelet counts. *Lancet*, 336, 712–14.

Tkacs, N. C., Li, J., and Strack, A. M. (1997). Central amygdala Fos expression during hypotensive or febrile, nonhypotensive endotoxemia in conscious rats. *J Comparat Neurol*, 379, 592–602.

Uehara, A., Ishikawa, Y., Okumura, T., Okamura, K., Sekiya, C., Takasugi, Y., and Namiki, M. (1989). Indomethacin blocks the anorexic action of interleukin-1. *Eur J Pharmacol*, 170, 257–60.

Vallières, L. and Rivest, S. (1997). Regulation of the genes encoding interleukin-6, its receptor, and gp130 in the rat brain in response to the immune activator lipopolysaccharide and the proinflammatory cytokine interleukin-1beta. *J Neurochem*, 69, 1668–83.

Vaughn, L. K., Veale, W. L., and Cooper, K. E. (1980). Antipyresis: its effect on mortality rate of bacterially infected rabbits. *Brain Res Bull*, 5, 69–73.

Wan, W., Wetmore, L., Sorensen, C. M., Greenberg, A. H., and Nance, D. M. (1994). Neural and biochemical mediators of endotoxin and stress-induced c-fos expression in the rat brain. *Brain Res Bull*, **34**, 7–14.

Williams, J. A. and Shacter, E. (1997). Regulation of macrophage cytokine production by prostaglandin E2. Distinct roles of cyclooxygenase-1 and -2. *J Biol Chem*, **272**, 25 693–9.

Wing, E. J. and Young, J. B. (1980). Acute starvation protects mice against Listeria monocytogenes. *Infect Immunity*, **28**, 771–6.

Yin, M. J., Yamamoto, Y., and Gaynor, R. B. (1998). The anti-inflammatory agents aspirin and salicylate inhibit the activity of I(kappa)B kinase-beta. *Nature*, **396**, 77–80.

Zhang, J. and Rivest, S. (2000). A functional analysis of EP4 receptor-expressing neurons in mediating the action of prostaglandin E2 within specific nuclei of the brain in response to circulating interleukin-1beta. *J Neurochem*, **74**, 2134–45.

Zhang, Y., Lu, J., Elmquist, J. K., and Saper, C. B. (2000). Lipopolysaccharide activates specific populations of hypothalamic and brainstem neurons that project to the spinal cord. *J Neurosci*, **20**, 6578–86.

Chapter 6

Inflammatory events in focal cerebral ischaemia

Gregory J. del Zoppo and John M. Hallenbeck

Inflammation plays a central role in tissue and wound recovery/repair, as a part of the host immune defense system. Occlusion of a brain-supplying artery initiates responses in the downstream microvasculature and the surrounding ischaemic tissue which stimulate leucocyte invasion and accumulation, cellular activation, and neuronal and glial necrosis. These responses involve the rapid appearance of specific transcription factors (e.g. NF-kB), the release of cytokines and chemokines, activation of microvascular endothelial cells and leucocytes, the generation of reciprocal adhesion receptors, leucocyte transmigration, and changes in microvessel perfusion and integrity.

Tissue ischaemia generates biologically active substances, which promote leucocyte invasion following abrupt reduction in regional cerebral blood flow (rCBF). Many cellular responses have been noted at threshold CBF (6–22 mL/100 g/min). Individual neurones generally stop spontaneous electrical activity at CBF levels less than 18 mL/100 g/min. This corresponds to rCBF thresholds for electroencephalographic alterations of 18 mL/100 g/min in other models (Heiss *et al.* 1976a). The threshold reduction in rCBF responsible for leucocyte diapedesis is not known, however, mean blood transit times are longer (0.45–0.55 s) in the deep cortical microvessel beds than in the superficial beds (0.34 s) (Fenstermacher *et al.* 1991). However, the distribution of leucocyte invasion within the ischaemic zone suggests that with heterogeneity of flow reduction in the carotid artery territory of patients and experimental models there is a tendency to accumulate in areas of low flow (Heiss *et al.* 1976b; Heiss 1992; Baron 1999).

6.1 PMN leucocytes and cerebral injury

Leucocyte-containing infiltrates have been observed in the ischaemic areas of cerebral tissues from patients succumbing from ischaemic stroke (Adams and Sidman 1968; Graham 1992; Moossy 1985; Okazaki 1989; Zülch and Kleihves 1966). Imaging studies employing ^{111}In-labeled autologous leucocytes or ^{99}Tc-HMPAO-labelled granulocytes have suggested leucocyte accumulation within the jeoparized tissue in from 2 h to 5 weeks after the ischaemic insult (Pozilli *et al.* 1985; Wang *et al.* 1993; Stevens *et al.* 1998). Potentially important considerations to those observations are the uncertain application of the stroke diagnosis and the contribution of stroke subtypes (e.g. lacunes) to those intervention, difficulties with clinical diagnosis (Schmid-Schöbein 1990; Schmid-Schöbein *et al.* 1991; Abels *et al.* 1994), and the known variability in infarct volume. Postmortem studies suggest that after 24 h, leucocytes are abundant at the edge of an ischaemic lesion, but are rare in the central region (Graham 1992). Between 24 and 36 h, PMN leucocytes appear around small blood vessels and throughout the entire infarct (Adams and Sidman 1968). Zülch noted that leucocytes (not otherwise characterized) emigrate diffusely from veins about 16 h after the injury following experimental brain embolism in cats (Zülch and Kleihves 1966). Some groups have failed to find PMN leucocytes within the injured brain, indicating that the observation is not uniform.

Experimental studies on with focal central nervous system (CNS) ischaemia has suggested two related hypotheses: (1) PMN leucocytes participate in microvascular responses to ischaemia, and (2) PMN leucocytes contribute directly to brain tissue injury and neuronal death.

6.2 Infiltration of the brain parenchyma during cerebral ischaemia

PMN leucocytes can contribute to parenchymal injury by: (1) causing additional impairment of local blood flow by microvessel obstruction, (2) exacerbating endothelial cell and matrix injury by releasing hydrolytic enzymes and generating oxygen free radicals, (3) initiating intravascular thrombus formation, (4) emigrating into the ischaemic parenchyma to potentially injure neurones and glial cells.

PMN leucocytes have been implicated in the development of cerebral injury following experimental ischaemia and hypotension. Hallenbeck and colleagues demonstrated the accumulation within 1–4 h of ^{111}In-labeled autologous leucocytes in areas of low blood flow following intra-arterial air embolism (Hallenbeck et al. 1986). Anderson et al. (1990) found correlations among the reduction in brain ATP content, the extent of neuronal injury, and the number of PMN leucocytes in the brain vessels and parenchyma following hypotension, with reperfusion to normotensive levels.

6.3 Microvessel ultrastructure and leucocyte reactivity

Leucocyte-microvessel receptor interactions are critical to the inflammatory response, and require that the cerebral microvessel be intact initially (Haring et al. 1996a). The ultrastructural features of cerebral microvessels are unique in several respects (Peters et al. 1991). Cerebral capillaries consist of three elements: endothelial cells, basal lamina (a portion of the ECM), and the astrocyte end-feet. Anatomical and functional relationships support their consideration as a ternary complex (Haring et al. 1996b; Zülch 1985; Peters et al. 1991). In non-capillary microvessels, individual smooth muscle cells are encased in ECM, which is continuous with the basal lamina (Peters et al. 1991). The basal lamina is also one important barrier to the transmigration of circulating blood cells, including leucocytes (Hamman et al. 1996; Hamman et al. 1995). Penetrating arteries and arterioles of the cortex lack an adventitia, but are surrounded by a single cell layer, the tunica adventitia, which is of leptomeningeal origin (Peters et al. 1991). The glia limitans, formed by the astrocyte endfeet, microglial cells, and pericytes, is fused to the basal lamina in precapillary arterioles and capillaries (Jones 1970).

Endothelial cells of cerebral capillaries and postcapillary venules (Gimbrone 1986; Nagy et al. 1984; Shivers et al. 1984) are joined by interendothelial tight junctions that provide a high electrical resistance (Crone and Olesen 1982) and normally display little, if any, transcytotic activity (Brightman and Reese 1969). In addition to tight junctions, the basal lamina (as a portion of the ECM) and subjacent cells are also important to the maintenance of the blood–brain barrier (BBB) to leucocyte transmigration (Risau and Wolburg 1990).

The close proximity of astrocytes and other neuronal elements to the endothelium suggests a close functional relationship for communication and nutrient transfer. Integrin adhesion receptors on endothelial cells and on astrocyte end-feet are presumed to maintain close cell–cell apposition via matrix attachments (Haring *et al.* 1996; del Zoppo *et al.* 1996; Wagner *et al.* 1997). Communication or 'crosstalk' between the smooth muscle cells and endothelial cells in larger vessels (30–70 μm diameter) is suggested by the presence of myoendothelial bridges that traverse the elastic lamina (Aydin *et al.* 1991; Dahl 1973). The association of astrocytes with neurones suggests the presence of direct interactions between cerebral microvessels and the neurones they serve.

Because of their large size (10–11 μm diameter) and their viscoelastic properties, PMN leucocytes have restricted movement through the capillary portions of microvascular beds (Schmid-Schöbein 1990; Schmid-Schöbein *et al.* 1991; Schmid-Schönbein 1987). Recent studies of PMN leucocyte movement through the rat pial circulation indicate that, in the absence of ischaemia, few PMN leucocytes roll along venular segments after moving through the capillary bed (Abels *et al.* 1994). However, PMN leucocytes were observed to interact with cerebral microvessel endothelium in areas of injury (Härtl *et al.* 1996).

6.4 PMN leucocyte flux during focal cerebral ischaemia

Leucocyte invasion into the ischaemic CNS involves (i) leucocyte activation, (ii) altered microvascular reactivity and integrity, (iii) microvessel obstruction, (iv) leucocyte transmigration, and (v) the contributions of leucocyte-mediated phagocytosis to the evolving tissue injury. These events are modulated in part by the early recanalization of occluded cerebral arteries as demonstrated in experimental models and in atherothrombotic/embolic stroke in humans. Early recanalization can result in decreased infarct volume and improved neurological outcome (The National Institutes of Neurological Disorders and Strokert-PA Stroke Study Grouop 1995; del Zoppo *et al.* 1988; del Zoppo *et al.* 1992; Hacke *et al.* 1988; Mori *et al.* 1988; Mori *et al.* 1992). Garcia and co-workers explored vascular and parenchymal alterations following permanent MCA : O in primates, cats, and Wistar rats (Garcia *et al.* 1977; Garcia *et al.* 1983; Garcia *et al.* 1993; Zea-Longa *et al.* 1989). PMN leucocytes rapidly enter the brain tissue in the ischaemic territory (within 24 h in rodents), followed by the incursion of mononuclear cells (del Zoppo *et al.* 1991; Garcia 1994).

del Zoppo and colleagues examined the interplay of microvascular and parenchymal events induced by MCA : O/R in primates (del Zoppo *et al.* 1991; del Zoppo *et al.* 1992; Mori *et al.* 1992; Thomas *et al.* 1993), while other groups have explored a number of aspects of those observations (Zhang *et al.* 1995; Zhang *et al.* 1994; Zhang *et al.* 1996; Zhang *et al.* 1998; Chopp *et al.* 1994; Garcia *et al.* 1996). The initial steps in PMN leucocyte invasion of the ischaemic cerebral territory following MCA : O involve the lodgement of PMN leucocytes in select capillaries and their firm adhesion to postcapillary venules (del Zoppo *et al.* 1991; Garcia 1994).

Early studies of MCA : O in anesthetized primates did not identify microvessel occlusions in the ischaemic territory, but intravascular thrombi were occasionally noted (Little *et al.* 1975; Little *et al.* 1976). Carbon tracer techniques detected obstructions within microvessels of capillary diameter with periods of ischaemia exceeding 3 h, which were attributed to 'perivascular glial swelling and developing cerebral edema' (Little *et al.* 1975). But, in other experiments, microvessel occlusions were not observed in MCA : O time-course studies with anesthetized primates, although luminal encroachment by astrocyte swelling was identified

(Garcia *et al.* 1983). The failure to find such obstructions early after MCA:O, particularly in light of the apparent loss of microvascular patency, could reflect technical issues including the failure to uniformly reperfuse (or perfuse-fix) the MCA territory, initial obstruction involving capillaries not detectable by carbon black, use of perfusion fluids with low osmolality or temperature-related effects in open models, and the location of microvascular occlusions within the ischaemic territory.

6.5 **Focal no-reflow**

Ames *et al.* (1968) and Fischer *et al.* (1977) attributed patchy loss of carbon tracer (the 'no-reflow' phenomenon) in the cerebral hemispheres of rabbits subjected to transient pressure cuff-induced strangulation (global ischaemia) to microvascular events (Ginsberg and Myers 1972; Jander *et al.* 2000; Boutin *et al.* 2001; Shohami *et al.* 1999; Dawon *et al.* 1996). Focal 'no-reflow', under conditions of focal cerebral ischaemia/reperfusion (I/R), was described by del Zoppo and colleagues in unanesthetized primates (del Zoppo *et al.* 1991; Mori *et al.* 1992; Crowell and Olsson 1972; Crowell *et al.* 1970; Todd *et al.* 1986). Similar findings have been made in rodents (Tagaya *et al.* 2001). PMN leucocyte adhesion to the endothelium in post-capillary venules and their lodgement, by viscoelastic forces, in capillaries of the ischaemic territory in part contributes to microvascular obstruction (Haring *et al.* 1996; Garcia *et al.* 1993; Garcia 1994; Okada *et al.* 1994; Schmid-Schönbein 1987).

Loss of microvessel patency after focal cerebral ischaemia in an anesthetized primate MCA:O/R model was first suggested by Crowell *et al.* (Crowell and Olsson 1972; Crowell *et al.* 1970). The consistency of its appearance in nonhuman primate focal I/R preparations implies certain necessary conditions (del Zoppo *et al.* 1991; Barone *et al.* 1997). The reproducibility of this phenomenon in some hands has been variable, and at least one source has considered it a postmortem artefact (de la Torre *et al.* 1992). In addition to intravascular cell-mediated microvascular flow obstruction, the 'no-reflow' phenomenon has been attributed to extravascular compression (Garcia *et al.* 1983; Yoshida *et al.* 1992), intraluminal endothelial projections (Betz *et al.* 1994), endothelial cell swelling (del Zoppo *et al.* 1986), aggregated platelets (del Zoppo *et al.* 1991; Okada *et al.* 1994), and fibrin formation (del Zoppo *et al.* 1991; Thomas *et al.* 1993). In view of the appearance of astrocyte end-foot swelling, platelet accumulation, and fibrin deposition, intravascular PMN leucocyte adherence is one contributor to focal 'no-reflow.'

The known interactions of activated PMN leucocytes and platelets with their endothelial cell adhesion receptors suggest that interventions which block leucocyte adhesion, platelet–fibrin interactions, and could limit or inhibit post-I/R microvessel occlusion, and subsequent events. del Zoppo *et al.* (1991) documented that PMN leucocytes can obstruct cerebral microvessels early during reperfusion (del Zoppo *et al.* 1991; Mori *et al.* 1992). Mori *et al.* (1992) demonstrated that focal 'no-reflow' could be significantly abrogated by blockade of PMN leucocyte adhesion to activated endothelium using (Mori *et al.* 1992) pharmacological grade murine antihuman monoclonal antibody (MoAb) IB4 (60.3) to the granulocyte β_2-integrin CD18, infused before reperfusion. Degranulated platelets and fibrin were also found in close juxtaposition to PMN leucocytes within obstructed capillaries and larger non-capillary microvessels within the ischaemic zone (del Zoppo *et al.* 1991). Fibrin deposition has also been documented within the vascular wall and lumina of capillaries within the ischaemic zones, independent of leucocyte adhesion (Okada *et al.* 1994). Hence, post-ischaemic microvascular obstruction is a complex product of leucocyte dynamics and local activation of haemostasis.

Another interpretation of those observations is that leucocytes may have been trapped in the experimental preparation (Härtl *et al.* 1996; Garcia 1994). Observations in cerebral and other systems identify vascular columns of cell-free plasma, probably caused by transient obstruction of the vessel by transitting leucocytes(s). The low density of microvessels (<15 per cent) displaying leucocyte adhesion receptors or adherent cells following MCA : O at any one time suggests the alternative concept that within the subcortex obstructed microvessels are bounded by those with cellular/plasma flow. The local 'no-reflow' may incorporate normal vessels with flow into an enlarging injury zone by secondary mechanisms (including inflammatory cell invasion (Tagaya *et al.* 2001)).

6.6 **Endothelial cell leucocyte adhesion receptor upregulation**

The initial movement of inflammatory cells into the ischaemic CNS coincides with the appearance of the leucocyte adhesion receptors P-selectin, ICAM-1, and E-selectin on microvessel endothelium, together with their counter-receptors (e.g. PSGL-1, the β_2-integrin CD18 group) on leucocytes (Haring *et al.* 1996; Mori *et al.* 1992; Okada *et al.* 1994). In the non-human primate basal ganglia, endothelial cell leucocyte adhesion receptors respond to focal ischaemia in a rapid and orderly way. P-selectin appears on the endothelium by 2 h MCA : O, followed by ICAM-1 by 4 h, and E-selectin between 7 and 24 h following MCA : O (during reperfusion) in the ischaemic regions of the awake non-human primate (Haring *et al.* 1996; Okada *et al.* 1994).

P-selectin appears on an increasing number of microvessels up to 24 h post-MCA : O, and derives from both vascular and platelet sources. In isolated systems, P-selectin expression occurs in response to hypoxia or thrombin stimulation (McEver 1991; McEver *et al.* 1995). Platelet accumulation within the ischaemic territory was confirmed by an increase in the platelet integrin $\alpha_{IIb}\beta_3$ antigen in a subpopulation of microvessels beginning within 2 h MCA : O (Okada *et al.* 1994). Non-platelet P-selectin appeared on 5.5–9.5 per cent of microvessels throughout 24 h post-MCA : O (Garcia *et al.* 1993). The persistence of P-selectin on the luminal vascular surface could be explained by continued local thrombin generation (Roberts 1992). In contrast, ICAM-1 appeared maximally on 10.0 ± 6.8 per cent of (non-capillary) microvessels at 4 h after MCA : O (Kawamura *et al.* 1990). E-selectin upregulation in the same territory was delayed, and marked by the appearance of the receptor on microvessels in the contralateral non-ischaemic hemisphere by 24 h following MCA : O (Haring *et al.* 1996). Both P- and E-selectin expression following MCA : O occurred only on microvessels with an intact basal lamina (Haring *et al.* 1996; Okada *et al.* 1994).

Observations in kind have been made in rodent models of focal cerebral ischaemia that indicate that these receptors appear simultaneously (Zhang *et al.* 1995; Zhang *et al.* 1994; Zhang *et al.* 1998).

6.7 **Inflammatory cytokine generation and release during focal cerebral ischaemia**

Cytokines with their redundant, overlapping, and pleiotropic effects play an integral role in the signalling that regulates cellular responses to various forms of stress including ischaemia.

Proinflammatory cytokines, tumour neurosis factor (TNF-α), and interleukin-1 (IL-1) are expressed in ischaemic brain and influence the early progression of injury (Barone and Feuerstein 1999). Both TNF and IL-1 convert the luminal surface of endothelium from an antithrombotic, anticoagulant, anti-inflammatory interface to an interface that is pro-thrombotic and pro-inflammatory (Pober and Cotran 1999; Hallenbeck 1996; Ruetzler et al. 2001).

In addition to endothelium (Gourin and Shackford 1997), the pro-inflammatory cytokines can be produced by perivascular macrophages (Woodroofe and Cuzner 1993; Buttini et al. 1994), microglia (Buttini et al. 1996), astrocytes (Rieberman et al. 1989), and neurones (Gourin and Shackford 1997; Saito et al. 1996; Davies et al. 1999). Following brain ischaemia, IL-1 increases within 3–6 h and peaks between 3–5 days (Saito et al. 1996; Legos et al. 2000). Corresponding times for TNF-α are appearance within 30 min to 1 h after ischaemia and a peak at 8–24 h with a substantial decline by 4 days (Buttini et al. 1996; Liu et al. 1994). IL-1 and TNF-α can affect microglia, astrocytes and neurones through signalling mediated by their receptors, the 80 kDa IL-1 receptor I (Touzani et al. 1999), the 55 kDa TNF-α receptor 1, and the 75 kDa TNF-α receptor 2 (Botchkina et al. 1997). In microglia, these cytokines stimulate further production of cytokines, expression of adhesion molecules, activation of the arachidonic acid cascade, production of nitric oxide (NO) by inducible nitric oxide syntheses (iNOS), production of quinolinic acid (neurotoxic), activation of NF-kB, and production of free radicals. Astrocytes can be similarly stimulated and in addition can be induced to proliferate and release growth factors. These cytokines can also potentiate NMDA receptor-mediated neurotoxicity and conversely NMDA receptor-mediated signalling can activate inflammatory gene expression with production of cytokines such as IL-1β (Jander et al. 2000).

IL-1 has been clearly implicated in the progression of ischaemic brain injury (Boutin et al. 2001). Central administration of IL-1β exacerbates brain damage in animal stroke models. Injection or over-expression of interleukin-1 receptor antagonist IL-1 ra the natural IL-1 inhibitor, or blockade of IL-1β converting enzyme activity, which inhibits IL-1 synthesis, dramatically reduce infarction volumes in preclinical stroke models. Although somewhat more controversial, there is abundant evidence that TNF also contributes to ischaemic brain damage (Shohami et al. 1999). TNF-α inhibition with a recombinant type I soluble TNF receptor, TNF binding protein (TNFbp), significantly attenuated impairment of micro-vascular perfusion in the ischaemic injury zone and reduced infarct volume in a model of focal brain ischaemia (Dawon et al. 1996). Also, several groups have demonstrated clear-cut cytoprotection by TNFbp or neutralizing anti-TNF antibodies in preclinical stroke models (Barone et al. 1997; Meistrell et al. 1997; Nawashiro et al. 1997; Yang et al. 1998).

The observed effects of IL-1 and TNF-α in injured brain have not been uniformly cytotoxic. Both of these inflammatory cytokines can serve as a preconditioning stress and induce tolerance to brain ischaemia. IL-1 has been shown to be necessary and sufficient to produce ischaemic tolerance in a model of global brain ischaemia in the gerbil (Ohtsuki et al. 1996). Similarly, TNF-α has been shown to be necessary and sufficient to produce ischaemic tolerance in focal brain ischaemia models in the rat and mouse (Tasaki et al. 1997; Nawashiro et al. 1997). Introduction of TNF-α into cortical neuronal cultures 24 h before they are subjected to a potentially lethal exposure to hypoxia or combined hypoxia and glucose deprivation 'in vitro ischaemia' also preconditions those cells such that they become tolerant and display reduced cytotoxicity (Liu et al. 2000). Similarly, primary cortical neurone cultures pretreated with IL-1 24 h prior to exposure to excitatory amino acid (EAA)-induced neurodegeneration exhibited increased resistance consistent with the development of tolerance (Strijbos and Rothwell 1995). In these paradigms, the inflammatory cytokines may be functioning as mediators of sublethal stress that induce pleiotropic adaptations to a subsequent potentially lethal stress rather than acting as direct neuroprotectants.

Mice lacking both IL-1α and IL-1β show a dramatic, 70 per cent reduction in infarct volume compared to wild-type mice after standardized brain ischaemia (Boutin *et al.* 2001). In contrast, mice genetically deficient in the p55 and p75 TNF receptors (TNFR-KO) develop larger infarcts than their wild-type counterparts in response to standardized brain ischaemia (Bruce *et al.* 1996). This was interpreted to show that TNF-α is neuroprotective in acute ischaemic stroke. In genetically deficient mouse models, the effects of chronic deprivation or molecular adaptation can be variables that introduce uncertainty, however. Available data provide strong support for a cytotoxic effect of the inflammatory cytokines as well as evidence to support a neuroprotective role for these intercellular signalling molecules. Resolution and clarification of these apparent discrepancies will require further study.

6.8 Platelet-activating factor (PAF)

Platelet-activating factor has been detected by biochemical assay in experimental hemispheric cerebral ischaemia, and in rodent species under the conditions of focal cerebral ischaemia (Lindsberg *et al.* 1991; Uchiyama *et al.* 1991; Lindsberg *et al.* 1990). Bazan and colleagues have described both the generation and the metabolism of PAF from ischaemic tissue (Spinnewyn *et al.* 1987; Birkle *et al.* 1998; Marcheselli *et al.* 1990; Bazan and Allan 1996; Serou *et al.* 1999). A potent phospholipid platelet activator, PAF is released from stimulated leucocytes and also activates granulocytes, monocytes, endothelial cells, smooth muscle cells, neurones, and mesangial cells (Valone 1988).

6.9 Transmigration of polymorphonuclear leucocytes

Leucocyte transmigration in the CNS occurs both at interendothelial tight junctions and through endothelial cells, without apparent disruption of the interface. Activated leucocytes expressing VEGF antigen have been detected as early as 1 h after MCA:O on the abluminal side of select microvessels (Abumiya *et al.* 1999). But, the specific endothelial cell adhesion requirements for transmigration in the cerebral microvasculature have not been identified. Dereski *et al.* noted the appearance of PMN leucocytes into both the intravascular and parenchymal compartments from several minutes to 8 h after MCA:O, reaching a maximum at 72 h during focal ischaemic in anesthetized Wistar rats (Dereski *et al.* 1992). Very few PMN leucocytes were seen within the ischaemic territory after 7 days. Transmigration across postcapillary venules began 4–6 h after MCA occlusion, with maximum invasion into the ischaemic parenchyma by 24 h after MCA occlusion (Garcia *et al.* 1993). Coagulation necrosis was apparent in the ischaemic area 24–48 h after MCA:O (Garcia *et al.* 1993). Separate studies using the closed cranial model of Zea Longa, confirmed the appearance of granulocytes into the ischaemic zone within 30 min of proximal MCA:O (Garcia *et al.* 1993; Zea-Longa *et al.* 1989; Garcia *et al.* 1994). Those data suggest a temporal sequence of PMN leucocyte invasion followed by neuronal necrosis; however, it is yet unclear whether the two biological phenomena are causally related.

In contrast to striatal and cortical beds, evidence for leucocyte adhesion in the pial microvasculature during focal ischaemia (which affects the cortical tissue) is conflicting

(Härtl et al. 1996; Ritter et al. 2000; Heinel et al. 1994). Abels and co-workers did not observe an increase in the number of PMN leucocytes that rolled in the pial vasculature after 20 min of carotid occlusion and reperfusion in a rat model of MCA territory ischaemia (Abels et al. 1994). Environmental risks, particularly exposure to products of cigarette incineration, can stimulate PMN leucocyte activation and rolling (Ono et al. 1991).

Differences in leucocyte infiltration into the ischaemic zone may reflect species differences, and the contributions of anaesthesia (Tagaya et al. 1997; Bowers et al. 1977; Moudgil et al. 1981) in anaesthetized rodent MCA:O models, the zone of ischaemic injury, defined histologically or by cellular injury, extends as a wavefront along the occluded vessel but is fixed at early times in the non-human primate (Tagaya et al. 2001; Tagaya et al. 1997).

6.10 Microvascular thrombosis

Fibrin is generated and deposited within and surrounding microvessels in the ischaemic core following MCA:O (del Zoppo et al. 1991). This implies the generation of thrombin which derives in part from activation of the extrinsic coagulation pathway, initiated by the tissue factor (TF) : Factor VIIa complex. TF is found particularly in the grey matter, where it provides a static procoagulant reservoir (del Zoppo et al. 1992), suggesting the exposure of plasma to TF because of enhanced vascular permeability. Also, circulating monocytes express functional TF antigen on their surface within 2 h of stimulation (Gregory et al. 1989), after exposure to endotoxin (Drake et al. 1989; Niemetz and Morrison 1977; Niemetz 1972), C5a (Muhlfelder et al. 1979), and plasma lipoproteins (Levy et al. 1981). The contribution of TF-mediated coagulation to 'focal no-reflow' was tested by the infusion of the murine anti-human MoAb TF9-6B4 directed against TF prior to MCA occlusion in the non-human primate (Thomas et al. 1993). A modest increase in the patency of microvessels of all size classes, but particularly in those of 7.5–30.0 μm and 30.0–50.0 μm diameters resulted, consistent with the known cerebrovascular distribution of TF antigen (del Zoppo et al. 1992).

6.11 Matrix degradation and microvessel activation

During focal cerebral ischaemia, ECM components of the basal lamina (laminin-1, laminin-5, collagen IV, and fibronectin) disappear together during MCA : O/R (Hamman et al. 1996; Hamman et al. 1995). Their fate may be due to proteolysis, blockade of transcription, inhibition of translation, or a combination of these. Remodelling of the ECM involves secreted proteases such as the MMPs and plasminogen activators (Krome 1994; Levin del Zoppo 1994), as well as activated serine proteases. Among serine proteases, thrombin stimulates MMP-2 and MMP-9 secretion by vascular smooth muscle cells (Fabunmi et al. 1996; Galis et al. 1997). Both pro-MMP-2 and MMP-9 are generated rapidly by the parenchyma following MCA : O, as are u-PA, and its inhibitor, PAI-1 (Rosenberg et al. 1996; Clark et al. 1997; Fujimura et al. 1999; Heo et al. 1999; Hosomi et al. 2001). Also, PMN leucocyte granule enzymes, including collagenase (MMP-8), gelatinase (MMP-9), elastase, and cathepsin G are released during the inflammatory phase following ischaemia and can degrade laminins and collagens (Krome 1994; Murphy et al. 1987; Watanabe et al. 1990; Heck et al. 1990; Pike et al. 1989). A clear dichotomy between the expression of pro-MMP-2 and pro-MMP-9 in primates and rodents has been seen following MCA:O (G. J. del Zoppo and E. L. Lo, unpublished data). The compartmentalization of these activities is still under study (Heo et al. 1999).

The changes in protease expression and vascular matrix integrity are consistent with leucocyte infiltration and/or vascular remodelling (Abumiya *et al.* 1999). VEGF and integrin $\alpha_V\beta_3$ occur on microvessels displaying antigens of cellular activation (e.g. PCNA) (Abumiya *et al.* 1999). VEGF transcripts also appear in cells with the morphology of PMN leucocytes which penetrate the vascular wall or on histiocyte-appearing cells localized within the vascular wall of select microvessels within 1–2 h following MCA : O (Abumiya *et al.* 1999). Although coupled to HIF expression (Fang *et al.* 2001; Laughner *et al.* 2001; Kimura *et al.* 2001), it is known that VEGF can be expressed by activated leucocytes (Salven *et al.* 1999; Scalia *et al.* 1999; Webb *et al.* 1998).

6.12 Genetic manipulation of leucocyte adhesion/activation

Support for a tissue-damaging role for leucocytes is provided by observations in murine transgenic models in which the genes for P-selectin, ICAM-1, and NADPH oxidase are deleted (Connolly *et al.* 1997; Soriano *et al.* 1996; Walder *et al.* 1997). In the NADPH oxidase$^{(-/-)}$ murine models, the phagocyte oxidase is absent, so that the respiratory burst does not occur, specifically impairing PMN leucocyte-mediated tissue injury. Other studies with P-selectin$^{(-/-)}$ and ICAM-1$^{(-/-)}$ transgenics displaying reduced expression of the respective leucocyte adhesion receptors indicated cytotoxic effects of leucocyte–endothelial cell interactions in ischaemia-induced inflammation (Connolly *et al.* 1997; Soriano *et al.* 1996).

6.13 Alteration of secondary injury

Various forms of sublethal stress (e.g. ischaemia (Kitigawa *et al.* 1990), oxidative stress (Ohtsuki *et al.* 1992), hyperthermia, or hypoxia (Wada *et al.* 1999)) can precondition brain cells and induce a state of resistance to a subsequent challenge that would otherwise be lethal. Ischaemic tolerance of this type appears to involve stress responses for which certain cytokines may mediate sublethal preconditioning. IL-1 and TNF-α have been implicated in the signalling that regulates tolerance to brain ischaemia in stroke models (Ohtsuki *et al.* 1996; Tasaki *et al.* 1997; Nawashiro *et al.* 1997). There is limited evidence that sublethal stress (e.g. hypothermia) affects leucocyte-mediated inflammation in experimental ischaemia (Kawai *et al.* 2000).

6.14 Leucocytes and cerebrovascular vasomotor reactivity

The effects of activated PMN leucocytes on cerebral vascular motor responses have not been well studied. It has been proposed that leucocytes contribute to the regulation of cerebral vascular tone (Akopov *et al.* 1994; Morita *et al.* 1993; Hamann and del Zoppo 1994). Endothelial cells contribute to arterial vasomotor reactivity through the prostacyclin (PGI$_2$), NO, and perhaps other pathways (Akopov *et al.* 1994; Hamann and del Zoppo 1994; Vanhoutte and Shimokawa 1989; Rosenblum 1986; Brenner *et al.* 1986). Endothelin-1 (ET-1), which stimulates vasoconstriction, can be induced by PMN leucocytes (Morita *et al.* 1993), while leucocytes together with platelets can alter vascular tone (Hamann and del Zoppo 1994). Akopov *et al.* (1994) reported that vasoconstriction of isolated rabbit MCA segments was increased by exposure to activated platelets after leucocyte activation, but not in leucocyte-depleted animals. Activation of platelets by release of PAF in the vicinity of activated leucocytes may lead to platelet release of the vasoconstrictors thromboxane A$_2$ and 5-HT. Platelet release products can also injure neurones (Joseph *et al.* 1992; Joseph *et al.* 1991; Joseph *et al.* 1992).

6.15 Outcome measures and antileucocyte strategies

A legion of experiments have indirectly suggested that altered PMN leucocyte function or induced leucopenia can improve defined responses to cerebrovascular obstruction (reperfusion), including oedema formation, neuronal injury, infarction volume, and neurological outcome. Strategies that block granulocyte adhesion can affect transmigration of PMN leucocytes and decrease oedema formation. Bednar *et al.* found a substantial decrease in oedema formation after using an anti-CD18 MoAb in a rabbit multivessel occlusion/hypotension model of focal cerebral ischaemia (Bednar *et al.* 1992). Their finding can be explained by the abrogation of granulocyte adhesion to the postcapillary venule endothelium, reduced endothelial permeability, and decreased PMN leucocyte egress. This is in keeping with the known interaction between activated granulocytes and venule endothelium, and the appearance of blood–brain permeability after MCA:O/R (Kuroiwa *et al.* 1985). However, recent studies suggest other contributors to oedema formation (e.g. bradykinin) (Sarkar *et al.* 2000). In separate experiments, cerebral infarct volume was reduced by a polyclonal antineutrophil serum given before the onset of focal/hemispherical ischaemia in a complex rabbit model of thromboembolism/induced hypotension (Bednar *et al.* 1991). Vasthare *et al.* demonstrated that leucopenia induced in a rodent carotid artery ligation model of reversible forebrain ischaemia was accompanied by preserved electroencephalographic activity and evoked potential peak amplitude, in contrast to control animals (Heinel *et al.* 1994; Vasthare *et al.* 1990).

Blockade of the leucocyte β_2-integrin CD18 following MCA:O and prior to reperfusion significantly increased microvascular patency in post-capillary venules relative to control (Mori *et al.* 1992). Similarly, specific inhibitors of the platelet integrin $\alpha_{IIb}\beta_3$-fibrin receptor reduced microvascular 'no-reflow' in the non-human primate (Abumiya *et al.* 2000) and injury volume in the mouse (Coudhri *et al.* 1998). Those studies support the contribution of leucocytes and platelets to postcapillary venular occlusion. Antileucocyte strategies which can decrease injury have included the antineutrophil antibody RP-3 and antibodies against leucocyte CD11b and CD18, or endothelial cell ICAM-1 (Zhang *et al.* 1995; Chopp *et al.* 1994; Matsuo *et al.* 1994). Kogure and colleagues described a beneficial effect of leucopenia on oedema formation and infarct volume after I/R in a well-characterized experimental model (Matsuo *et al.* 1994). Many of the leucocyte inhibition studies have shown reductions in injury volume ranging from about 30 to 60 per cent. However, there are also negative studies. Härtl *et al.* (1996) have examined some of these studies critically (Härtl *et al.* 1996).

A recent study in established rat stroke models employing a much used murine antibody directed against rat ICAM-1 (1A29) when infused twice prior to MCA:O induced rat antimouse antibodies, and activated complement, PMN leucocytes, and vascular endothelium. The approach, which mimicked a previous clinical trial (see Section 6.16) overwhelmed any potential benefit from inhibition of leucocyte accumulation, and increased infarct volume (Furuya *et al.* 2000). That study suggested that single or multiple exposures to intravenously administered heterologous proteins might activate local inflammatory mechanisms which increase ischaemic brain injury.

6.16 Inflammation in clinical stroke

Two phase III clinical trials of anti-inflammatory approaches in acute ischaemic stroke have been undertaken. Enlimomab, a murine anti-human ICAM-1 MoAb antibody, increased mortality in a prospective placebo-controlled multicentre acute stroke trial (Sherman 1997).

The reasons for the increased intervention-related mortality have not been published, but appear to *not* be due to fever as has been stated in one report but may have been due to continuous exposure of the injured brain to non-autologous proteins. Another recent trial utilizing a humanized MoAb to CD18 (Hu23F2G, Leukarrest) was stopped when it was claimed to be safe, but showed no benefit in an interim futility analysis (ICOS Stroke Trial 2000). Those apparent failures of anti-adhesion therapy in stroke do not negate the hypothesis that inflammation plays a role in ischaemic brain injury, as supported by the battery of animal model studies. They do, however, highlight the complexities of the immune system and significant problems in clinical trial design in this arena. Based on the experimental work, and identified difficulties with the two clinical trials, in future carefully designed clinical studies that incorporate lessons from past failures are in order.

6.17 Summary

Inflammation accompanies ischaemic brain injury and contributes to the injury process. The sequence and nature of PMN leucocyte-mediated events in the CNS following MCA : O appear to depend on (1) the location of the initial arterial obstruction and occlusion duration, (2) post-occlusion reperfusion, (3) the presence and efficiency of leptomeningeal collaterals, and (4) the presence of concurrent cellular inflammation. Differences in the rCBF and the three-dimensional microvascular architecture of microvessels in the cortex, subjacent white matter, striatum, and pia may contribute to differential involvement of activated granulocytes in tissue injury in those areas. Many questions about the effects of PMN leucocytes and their functional alterations on cerebral tissues during ischaemia are still unanswered.

The general hypothesis that leucocyte-dependent and humoural inflammatory processes set in motion by the initial ischaemic insult can produce harm (or benefit) in the CNS, and that abrogation of those processes may reduce the ultimate injury remains clinically untested. Because of the redundancy and overlap of inflammatory mediator effects, it is uncertain whether a specific inhibitor of a single step or interaction will have a clinically detectable beneficial effect (Hallenbeck and Frerichs 1993). Among the unanswered questions are which anti-inflammatory agents (singly or in combination) might be efficacious in patients, realizing that ill-timed delivery, prolonged administration, or inappropriate formulation of anti-inflammatory agents could potentially worsen outcome. However, there is strong evidence that a search for the upstream activators/mediators of inflammation or the intracellular signalling steps that confer broad suppression of inflammatory mechanisms may offer new targets for intervention. Furthermore, the roles that coagulation system activation play in leucocyte–vascular interactions suggest additional targets. Well-designed preclinical and clinical trials of anti-inflammatory approaches for ischaemic stroke together are necessary to bring potential benefit to patients.

Acknowledgment

Supported in part by grants RO1 NS26945 and RO1 38710 (GJdZ) of the National Institutes of Health (NINDS).

References

Abels, C., Röhrich, F., Uhl, E., Corvin, S., Villringer, A., Dirnagl, U., *et al.* (1994). Current evidence on a pathophysiological of leukocyte/endothelial interactions in cerebral ischemia. In *Brain*

Ischemia and Basic Mechanisms, (ed. A. Hartmann, F. Yatsu, and W. Kuschinsky), Springer-Verlag, Heidelberg, pp. 366–72.

Abumiya, T., Lucero, J., Heo, J. H., Tagaya, M., Koziol, J. A., Copeland, B. R., and del Zoppo, G. J. (1999). Activated microvessels express vascular endothelial growth factor and integrin $\alpha_v\beta_3$ during focal cerebral ischemia. *J Cereb Blood Flow Metab*, 19, 1038–50.

Abumiya, T., Fitridge, R., Mazur, C., Copeland, B. R., Koziol, J. A., Tschopp, J. F., *et al.* (2000). Integrin $\alpha_{IIb}\beta_3$ inhibitor preserves microvascular patency in experimental acute focal cerebral ischemia. *Stroke*, 31, 1402–10.

Adams, R. D. and Sidman, R. L. (1968). Cerebrovascular disease. In *Introduction to Neuropathology*, (ed. R. D. Adams and R. L. Sidman), McGraw-Hill, New York, pp. 171–83.

Akopov, S. E., Sercombe, R., and Seylaz, J. (1994). Leukocyte-induced acute endothelial dysfunction in middle cerebral artery in rabbits: Response to aggregating platelets. *Stroke*, 25, 2246–52.

Ames, A. III, Wright, R. C., Kowada, M., Thurston, J. M., and Majno, G. (1968). Cerebral ischemia. The non-reflow phenomenon. *Am J Pathol*, 52, 437–53.

Anderson, M. L., Smith, D. S., Nioka, S., Subramanian, H., Garcia, J. H., Halsey, J. H., and Chance, B. (1990). Experimental brain ischemia: Assessment of injury by magnetic resonance spectroscopy and histology. *Neurol Res*, 12, 195–204.

Aydin, F., Rosenblum, W. I., and Povlishock, J. T. (1991). Myoendothelial junctions in human brain arterioles. *Stroke*, 22, 1592–7.

Barone, F. C., Arvin, B., White, R. F., Miller, A., Webb, C. L., Willette, R. N., *et al.* (1997). Tumor necrosis factor-A mediator of focal ischemic brain injury. *Stroke*, 28, 1233–44.

Baron, J. (1999). Mapping the ischaemic penumbra with PET: implications for acute stroke treatment. *Cerebrovasc Dis*, 9(4), 193–201.

Barone, F. C. and Feuerstein, G. Z. (1999). Inflammatory mediators and stroke: New opportunities for novel therapeutics. *J Cereb Blood Flow Metab*, 19, 819–34.

Bazan, N. G. and Allan, G. (1996). Platelet-activating factor in the modulation of excitatory amino acid neurotransmitter release and of gene expression. *J. Lipid Mediators & Cell Signalling*, 14(1–3), 321–30.

Bednar, M. M., Raymond, S., McAuliffe, T., Lodge, P. A., and Gross, C. E. (1991). The role of neutrophils and platelets in a rabbit model of thromboembolic stroke. *Stroke*, 22, 44–50.

Bednar, M. M., Gross, C. E., Raymond, S., Wright, S. D. and Kohut, J. J. (1992). IB4, a monoclonal antibody against the CD18 adhesion complex of leukocytes, attenuates intracranial hypertension in a rabbit stroke model. *Stroke*, 23, 152 (Abstract).

Betz, A. L., Keep, R. F., Beer, M. E., and Ren, X. D. (1994). Blood-brain permeability and brain concentration of sodium, potassium, and chloride during focal ischemia. *J Cereb Blood Flow Metab*, 14, 29–37.

Birkle, D. L., Kurian, P., Braquet, P., and Bazan, N. G. (1998). Platelet-activating factor antagonist BN529021 decreased accumulation of free polyunsaturated fatty acid in mouse brain during ischemia and electroconvulsive shock. *J. Neurochems*, 51, 1900–5.

Botchkina, G. I., Meistrell, M. E., Botchkina, I. L., and Tracey, K. J. (1997). Expression of TNF and TNF receptors (p55 and p75) in therat brain after focal cerebral ischemia. *Mol Med*, 3, 765–81.

Boutin, H., LeFeuvre, R. A., Horai, R., Asano, M., Iwakura, Y., and Rothwell, N. J. (2001). Role of IL-1 alpha and IL-1 beta in ischemic brain damage. *J Neurosci*, 21, 5528–34.

Bowers, T. K., O'Flaherty, J., Simmons, R. L., and Jacob, H. S. (1997). Postsurgical granulocyte dysfunction: Studies in healthy kidney donors. *J Lab Clin Med*, 90, 720–7.

Brenner, B. M., Troy, J. L., and Balterman, B. J. (1986). Endothelium-dependent vascular responses: Mediators and mechanisms. *J Clin Invest*, 84, 1373–7.

Brightman, M. W. and Reese, T. S. (1969). Junctions between intimately apposed cell membranes in the vertebrate. *J Cell Biol*, 40, 648–77.

Bruce, A. J., Boling, W., Kindy, M. S., Peschon, J., Kraemer, P. J., Carpenter, M. K., *et al.* (1996). Altered neuronal and microglial responses to excitotoxic and ischemic brain injury in mice lacking TNF receptors. *Nat Med*, 2, 788–94.

Buttini, M., Sauter, A., and Boddeke, H. W. (1994). Induction of interleukin-1 beta mRN after focal cerebral ischaemia in the rat. *Mol Brain Res*, 23, 126–34.

Buttini, M., Appel, K., Sauter, A., Gebicke-Haerter, P. J., and Boddeke, H. W. G. M. (1996). Expression of tumor necrosis factor alpha after focal cerebral ischaemia in the rat. *Neuroscience*, 71, 1–16.

Chopp, M., Zhang, R. L., Chen, H., Li, Y., Jiang, N., and Rusche, J. R. (1994). Postischemic administration of an anti-Mac-1 antibody reduces ischemic cell damage after transient middle cerebral artery occlusion in rats. *Stroke*, 25, 869–75.

Clark, A. W., Krekoski, C. A., Bou Shao-Sun, Chapman, K. R., and Edwards, D. R. (1997). Increased gelatinase A (MMP-2) and gelatinase B (MMP-9) activities in human brain after focal ischemia. *Neurosci Lett*, 238, 53–6.

Connolly, E. S. Jr., Winfree, C. J., Prestigiacomo, C. J., Kim, S. C., Choudri, T. F., Hoh, B. L., *et al.* (1997). Exacerbation of cerebral injury in mice that express the P-selectin gene: Identification of P-selectin blockade as a new target for the treatment of stroke. *Circ Res*, 81, 304–10.

Coudhri, T. F., Hoh, B. L., Zerwes, H. G., Prestigiacomo, C. J., Kim, S. C., and Connolly, E., (1998). Reduced microvascular thrombosis and improved outcome in acute murine stroke by inhibiting GP IIb/IIIa receptor-mediated platelet aggregation. *J Clin Invest*, 102, 1301–10.

Crowell, R. M., Olsson, Y., Klatzo, I., and Ommaya, A. (1970). Temporary occlusion of the middle cerebral artery in monkeys. Clinical and pathological observations. *Stroke*, 1, 439–48.

Crowell, R. M. and Olsson, Y. (1972). Impaired microvascular filling after focal cerebral ischemia in the monkey. *Neurology*, 22, 500–04.

Crone, C. and Olesen, S-P. (1982). Electrical resistance of brain microvascular endothelium. *Brain Res*, 241, 49–55.

Dahl, E. (1973). The fine structure of intracerebral vessels. *L Zellforsch Mikrosk Anat*, 145, 577–86.

Davies, C. A., Loddick, S. A., Toulmond, S., Stroemer, R. P., Hunt, J., and Rothwell, N. J. (1999). The progression and topographic distribution of interleukin-1 β expression after permanent middle cerebral artery occlusion in the rat. *J Cereb Blood Flow Metab*, 19, 87–98.

Dawon, D. A., Martin, D., and Hallenbeck, J. M. (1996). Inhibition of tumor necrosis factor-alpha reduces focal cerebral ischemic injury in the spontaneously hypertensive rat. *Neuroscience Lett*, 218, 41–4.

de la Torre, J. C., Fortin, T., Saunders, J. K., Butler, K., and Richard, M. T. (1992). The no-reflow phenomenon is a post-mortem artifact. *Acta Neurochir*, 115, 37–42.

del Zoppo, G. J., Copeland, B. R., Harker, L. A., Waltz, T. A., Zyroff, J., Hanson, S. R., and Battenberg, E. (1986). Experimental acute thrombotic stroke in baboons. *Stroke*, 17, 1254–65.

del Zoppo, G. J., Ferbert, A., Otis, S., Brückmann, H., Hacke, W., Zyroff, J., *et al.* (1988). Local intra-arterial fibrinolytic therapy in acute carotid territory stroke: A pilot study. *Stroke*, 19, 307–13.

del Zoppo, G. J., Schmid-Schönbein, G. W., Mori, E., Copeland, B. R., and Chang, C-M. (1991). Polymorphonuclear leukocytes occlude capillaries following middle cerebral artery occlusion and reperfusion in baboons. *Stroke*, 22, 1276–84.

del Zoppo, G. J., Poeck, K., Pessin, M. S., Wolpert, S. M., Furlan, A. J., Ferbert, A., *et al.* (1992). Recombinant tissue plasminogen activator in acute thrombotic and embolic stroke. *Ann Neurol*, 32, 78–86.

del Zoppo, G., Yu, J-Q., Copeland, B. R., Thomas, W. S., Schneiderman, J., and Morrissey. J. (1992). Tissue factor location in non-human primate cerebral tissue. *Thromb Haemost*, 68, 642–7.

del Zoppo, G. J., Haring, H-P., Tagaya, M., Wagner, S., Akamine, P., and Hamann, G. F. (1996). Loss of $\alpha_1\beta_1$ integrin immunoreactivity on cerebral microvessels and astrocytes following focal cerebral ischemia/reperfusion. *Cerebrovasc Dis*, 6, 9. (Abstract)

Dereski, M. O., Chopp, M., Knight, R. A., Chen, H., and Garcia, J. H. (1992). Focal cerebral ischemia in the rat: Temporal profile of neutrophil responses. *Neurosci Res Commun*, 11, 179–86.

Drake, T. A., Morrissey, J. H., and Edgington, T. S. (1989). Selective cellular expression of tissue factor in human tissues: Implications for disorders of hemostasis and thrombosis. *Am J Pathol*, 134, 1087–97.

Fabunmi, R. P., Baker, A. H., Murray, E. J., Booth, R. F. G., and Newby, A. C. (1996). Divergent regulation by growth factors and cytokines of 95 kDa and 72 kDa gelatinases and tissue inhibitors of metalloproteinases-1, -2, and -3 in rabbit aortic smooth muscle cells. *Biochem J*, 315, 335–42.

Fang, J., Yan, L., Shing, Y., and Moses, M. A. (2001). HIF-1alpha-medicated up-regulation of vascular endothelial growth factor, independent of basic fibroblast growth factor, is important in the switch to the angiogenic phenotype during early tumorigenesis. *Cancer Res*, 61(15), 5731–5.

Fenstermacher, J., Nakata, H., Tajima, A., Lin, S-Z., Otsuka, T., Acuff, V., *et al.* (1991). Functional variations in parenchymal microvascular systems within the brain. *Magn Reson Med*, 19, 217–20.

Fischer, E. G., Ames, A., Hedley-White, E. T., and O'Gorman, S. (1977). Reassessment of cerebral capillary changes in acute global ischemia and their relationship to the 'no-reflow phenomenon'. *Stroke*, 8, 36–9.

Fujimura, M., Gasche, Y., Morita-Fujimura, Y., Massengale, J., Kawase, M., and Chan, P. H. (1999). Early appearance of activated matrix metalloproteinase-9 and blood-brain barrier disruption in mice after focal cerebral ischemia and reperfusion. *Brain Res*, 842, 92–100.

Furuya, K., Takeda, H., Azhar, S., DeGraba, T. J., Rothlein, R., Hugli, T. E., *et al.* (2000). Some potentially harmful side effects of anti-ICAM-1 antibody administration in preclinical animal studies of stroke. *Stroke* 31, 277. (Abstract)

Galis, Z. S., Kranzhöfer, R., Fenton, J. W. I. I., and Libby, P. (1997). Thrombin promotes activation of matrix metalloproteinase-2 produced by cultured vascular smooth muscle cells. *Arterioscler Thromb Vasc Biol*, 17, 483–9.

Garcia, J. H., Kalimo, H., and Kamijyo, Y. (1977). Cellular events during partial cerebral ischemia. 1. Electron microscopy of feline cerebral cortex after middle cerebral artery occlusion. *Virchows Arch [B]*, 25, 191–206.

Garcia, J. H., Mitchem, H. L., Briggs, L., Morawetz, R., Hudetz, A. G., Hazelrig, J. B., *et al.* (1983). Transient focal ischemia in subhuman primates: Neuronal injury as a function of local cerebral blood flow. *J Neuropathol Exp Neurol*, 42, 44–60.

Garcia, J. H., Yoshida, Y., Chen, H., Li, Y., Zhang, Z. G., Liam, J., *et al.* (1993). Progression from ischemic injury to infarct following middle cerebral artery occlusion in the rat. *Am J Pathol*, 142, 623–35.

Garcia, J. H., Yoshida, Y., Lian, J., Chen, S., Chen, H., Li, Y., and Chopp, M. (1993). Experimental occlusion of a middle cerebral artery (MCA) is accompanied by early polymorphonuclear leukocyte infiltration. *Stroke*, 24, 166. (Abstract)

Garcia, J. H., Liu, K. F., Yoshida, Y., Lian, J., Chen, S., and del Zoppo, G. J. (1994). Influx of leukocytes and platelets in an evolving brain infarct (Wistar rat). *Am J Pathol*, 144, 188–99.

Garcia, J. H., Liu, K-F., and Bree, M. P. (1996). Effects of CD11b/18 monoclonal antibody on rats with permanent middle cerebral artery occlusion. *Am J Pathol*, 148, 241–48.

Gimbrone, M. A., Jr. (1986). Nature's blood container. In *Vascular Endothelium in Hemostasis and Thrombosis*, (ed. M. A. Gimbrone Jr.). Churchill-Livingstone, Edinburgh, pp. 1–13.

Ginsberg, M. D. and Myers, R. E. (1972). The topography of impaired microvascular perfusion in the primate brain following total circulatory arrest. *Neurology* 22, 998–1011.

Gourin, C. G. and Shackford, S. R. (1997). Production of tumor necrosis factor A and interleukin-1β by human cerebral microvascular endothelium after percussive trauma. *J Trauma*, 42, 1101–7.

Graham, D. I. (1992). Hypoxia and vascular disorders. In *Greenfield's Neuropathology*, (ed. J. H. Adams and L. W. Duchen) 5th edn, Oxford University Press, New York, pp. 198–200.

Gregory, S. A., Morrissey, J. H., and Edgington, T. S. (1989). Regulation of tissue factor expression in the monocyte procoagulant response to endotoxin. *Mol Cell Biol*, 9, 2752–5.

Hacke, W., Zeumer, H., Ferbert, A., Brückmann, H., and del Zoppo, G. J. (1988). Intra-arterial thrombolytic therapy improves outcome in patients with acute vertebrobasilar occlusive disease. *Stroke*, 19, 1216–22.

Hallenbeck, J. M., Dutka, A. J., Tanishima, T., Kochanek, P. M., Kumaroo, K. K., and Thompson, C. B., *et al.* (1986). Polymorphonuclear leukocyte accumulation in brain regions with low blood flow during the early postischemic period. *Stroke*, 17, 246–53.

Hallenbeck, J. M., and Frerichs, K. U. (1993). Stroke therapy: It may be time for an integrated approach. *Arch Neurol*, 50, 768–70.

Hallenbeck, J. M. (1996). Cellular and Molecular Mechanisms of Ischemic Brain Damage. In *Inflammatory reactions at the blood-endothelial interface in acute stroke.*, (ed. B. K. Siesjo and T. Wieloch) 71 edn, Lippincott-Raven, Philadelphia, pp. 281–300.

Hamann, G. F., Okada, Y., Fitridge, R., and del Zoppo, G. J. (1995). Microvascular basal lamina antigens disappear during cerebral ischemia and reperfusion. *Stroke*, 26, 2120–6.

Hamann, G. F. and del Zoppo, G. J. (1994). Leukocyte involvement in vasomotor reactivity of the cerebral vasculature. *Stroke*, 25, 2117–19.

Hamann, G. F., Okada, Y., and del Zoppo, G. J. (1996). Hemorrhagic transformation and microvascular integrity during focal cerebral ischemia/reperfusion. *J Cereb Blood Flow Metab*, 16, 1373–8.

Haring, H-P., Berg, E. L., Tsurushita, N., Tagaya, M., and del Zoppo, G. J. (1996a). E-selectin appears in non-ischemic tissue during experimental focal cerebral ischemia. *Stroke* 27, 1386–92.

Haring, H-P., Akamine, P., Habermann, R., Koziol, J. A., and del Zoppo, G. J. (1996b). Distribution of the integrin-like immunoreactivity on primate brain microvasculature. *J Neuropathol Exp Neurol*, 55, 236–45.

Härtl, R., Schürer, L., Schmid-Schonbein, G. W., and del Zoppo, G. J. (1996). Experimental antileukocyte interventions in cerebral ischemia. *J Cereb Blood Flow Metab*, 16, 1108–19.

Heiss, W-D., Hayakawa, T., and Waltz, A. G. (1976a). Cortical neuronal function during ischaemia. *Arch Neurol*, 33, 813–20.

Heiss, W. D., Hayakawa, T., and Waltz, A. G. (1976b). Patterns of changes of blood flow and relationships to infarction in experimental cerebral ischemia. *Stroke*, 7, 454–459.

Heiss, W. D. (1992). Experimental evidence of ischemic thresholds and functional recovery. *Stroke*, 23, 1668–72.

Heinel, L., Rubin, S., Rosenwasser, R., Vasthare, U., and Tuma, R. (1994). Leukocyte involvement in cerebral infarct generation after ischemia and reperfusion. *Brain Res Bull*, 34, 137–41.

Heck, L. W., Blackburn, W. D., Irwin, M. H., and Abrahamson, D. R. (1990). Degradation of basement membrane laminin by human neutrophil elastase and cathepsin G. *Am J Pathol*, 136, 1267–74.

Heo, J. H., Lucero, J., Abumiya, T., Koziol, J. A., Copeland, B. R., and del Zoppo, G. J. (1999). Matrix metalloproteinases increase very early during experimental focal cerebral ischemia. *J Cereb Blood Flow Metab*, 19, 624–33.

Hosomi, N., Lucero, J., Heo, J. H., Koziol, J., Copeland, B. R., and del Zoppo, G. J. (2001). Rapid differential endogenous plasminogen activator expression after acute middle cerebral artery occlusion. *Stroke*, 32, 1341–8.

ICOS Stroke Trial. (2000). ICOS Halts Trial of Stroke Drug, Reports Q1 Net Loss. http://biz.yahoo.com/rf/ooo420/mf.html 2000.

Jander, S., Schroeter, M., and Stoll, G. (2000). Role of NMDA receptor signaling in the regulation of inflammatory gene expression after focal brain ischemia. *J Neuroimmunology*, 109, 181–7.

Jones, E. G. (1970). On the mode of entry of blood vessels into the cerebral cortex. *J Anat*, 106, 507–20.

Joseph, R., Tsering, C., Grunfeld, S., and Welch, K. M. (1992). Further studies on platelet-mediated neurotoxicity. *Brain Res* 577, 268–75.

Joseph, R., Tsering, C., Grunfeld, S., and Welch, K. M. (1991). Platelet secretory products may contribute to neuronal injury. *Stroke*, 22, 1448–51.

Joseph, R., Tsering, C., and Welch, K. M. (1992). Study of platelet-mediated neurotoxicity in rat brain. *Stroke*, 23, 394–8.

Kawamura, S., Schürer, L., Goetz, A., Kempirski, O., Schmucker, B., and Baethmann, A. (1990). An improved closed cranial window technique for investigations of blood-brain barrier function and cerebral vasomotor control in the rat. *Int J Microcirc Clin Exp*, 9, 369–83.

Kawai, N., Okauchi, M., Morisaki, K., and Nagao, S. (2000). Effects of delayed intraischemic and postischemic hypothermia on a focal model of transient cerebral ischemia in rats. *Stroke*, 31(8), 1982–9.

Kimura, H., Weisz, A., Ogura, T., Hitomi, Y., Kurashima, Y., Hashimoto, K., *et al.* (2001). Identification of hypoxia-inducible factor 1 ancillary sequence and its function in vascular endothelial growth actor gene inducction by hypoxia an nitric oxide. *J Biol Chem* 276(3), 2292–8.

Kitigawa, K., Matsumoto, M., Tagaya, M., Hata, R., Ueda, H., Niinobe, M., *et al.* (1990). 'Ischemic tolerance' phenomenon found in the brain. *Brain Res*, 528, 21–4.

Krane, S. M. (1994). Clinical importance of metalloproteinases and their inhibitors. In *Inhibition of matrix metalloproteinases: therapeutic potential* (ed. R. A. Greenwald and L. M. Golub). *Ann N Y Acad Sci*, 732, 1–10.

Kuroiwa, T., Ting, P., Martinez, H., and Klatzo, I. (1985). The aphasic opening of the blood-brain barrier to proteins following temporary middle cerebral artery occlusions. *Acta Neuropathol (Berl)*, 68, 122–9.

Laughner, E., Taghavi, P., Chiles, K., Mahon, P. C., and Semenza, G. L. (2001). HER2 (neu) signaling increases the rate of hypoxia-inducible factor 1alpha (HIF-1alpha) synthesis:novel mechanism for HIF-1-medicated vascular endothelial growth factor expression. *Mol Cell Biol*, 21(12), 3995–4004.

Legos, J. J., Whitmore, R. G., Erhardt, J. A., Parsons, A. A., Tuma, R. F., and Barone, F. C. (2000). Quantitative changes in interleukin proteins following focal stroke in the rat. *Neuroscience Lett*, 282, 189–92.

Levy, G. A., Schwartz, B. S., Curtiss, L. K., and Edgington, T. S. (1981). Plasma lipoprotein induction and suppression of the generation of cellular procoagulant activity *in vitro*. *J Clin Invest*, 67, 1614–22.

Levin, E. G. and del Zoppo, G. J. (1994). Localization of tissue plasminogen activator in the endothelium of a limited number of vessels. *Am J Pathol*, 144, 855–61.

Lieberman, A. P., Pitha, P. M., Shin, H. S., and Shin, M. L. (1989). Production of tumor necrosis factor and other cytokines by astrocytes stimulated with lipopolysaccharide or a neurotopic virus. *Proc Natl Acad Sci USA*, 86, 6348–52.

Lindsberg, P. J., Yue, T-L., Frerichs, K. U., Hallenbeck, J. M., and Feuerstein, G. (1990). Evidence for platelet-activating factor as a novel mediator in experimental stroke in rabbits. *Stroke*, 21, 1452–7.

Lindsberg, P. J., Hallenbeck, J. M., and Feuerstein, G. (1991). Platelet activating factor in stroke and brain injury. *Ann Neurol*, 30, 117–29.

Little, J. R., Kerr, F. W. L., and Sundt, T. M., Jr. (1975). Microcirculatory obstruction in focal cerebral ischemia. Relationship to neuronal alterations. *Mayo Clin Proc*, 50, 264–70.

Little, J. R., Kerr, F. W. L., and Sundt, T. M., Jr. (1976). Microcirculatory obstruction in focal cerebral ischemia: An electron microscopic investigation in monkeys. *Stroke*, 7, 25–30.

Liu, T., Clark, R. K., McDonnell, P. C., Young, P. R., White, R. F., Barone, F. C., and Feuerstein, G. Z. (1994). Tumor necrosis factor-α expression in ischemic neurons. *Stroke*, 25, 1481–8.

Liu, J., Ginis, I., Spatz, M., and Hallenbeck, J. M. (2000). Hypoxic preconditioning protects culturedneurons against hypoxic stress via TNF-(and ceramide. *Am J Physiol Cell Physiol*, 278, C144–C153.

Marcheselli, V. L., Rossowska, M. J., Domingo, M. T., Braquet, P., and Bazan, N. G. (1990). Distinct platelet-activiating factor binding sites in synaptic endings and in intracellular memebrans of rat cerebral cortex. *J Biol Chem*, **265**(16), 9140–5.

Matsuo, Y., Onodera, H., Shiga, Y., Nakamura, M., Ninomiya, M., Kihare, T., and Kogure, K. (1994). Correlation between myeloperoxidase-quantified neutrophil accumulation and ischemic brain injury in the rat. Effects of neutrophil depletion. *Stroke*, **25**, 1469–75.

McEver, R. P. (1991). Selectins: Novel receptors that mediate leukocyte adhesion during inflammation. *Thromb Haemost*, **65**, 223–8.

McEver, R. P., Moore, K. L., and Cummings, R. D. (1995). Leukocyte trafficking mediated by selectin-carbohydrate interactions. *J Biol Chem*, **270**, 11 025–8.

Meistrell, M. E., Botchkina, G. I., Wang, H., Di Santo, E., Cockroft, K. M., Bloom, O., *et al.* (1997). Tumor necrosis factor is a brain damaging cytokine in cerebral ischemia. *Shock*, **8**, 341–8.

Moossy, J. (1985). Pathology of ischemic cerebrovascular disease. In *Neurosurgery/Volume II*, (ed. R. H. Wilkins and S. S. Rengachary), McGraw-Hill, New York, pp. 1193–8.

Mori, E., Tabuchi, M., Yoshida, T., and Yamadori, A. (1988). Intracarotid urokinase with thromboembolic occlusion of the middle cerebral artery. *Stroke*, **19**, 802–12.

Mori, E., Yoneda, Y., Tabuchi, M., Yoshida, T., Ohkawa, S., Ohsumi, Y., *et al.* (1992). Intravenous recombinant tissue plasminogen activator in acute carotid artery territory stroke. *Neurology*, **42**, 976–82.

Mori, E., Chambers, J. D., Copeland, B. R., Arfors, K-E., and del Zoppo, G. J. (1992). Inhibition of polymorphonuclear leukocyte adherence suppresses no-reflow after focal cerebral ischemia. *Stroke*, **23**, 712–18.

Morita, T., Kurihara, H., Yoshizumi, M., Maemura, K., Sugiyama, T., Nagai, R., and Yazaki, Y. (1993). Human polymorphonuclear leukocytres have dual efects on endothelium-1: The induciton of endothelin-1 mRNA expression in vascular endothelial cells and modification of the endothelin-1 molecule. *Heart Vessels*, **8**, 1–6.

Moudgil, G. C., Pandya, A. R., and Ludlow, D. J. (1981). Influence of anaesthesia and surgery on neutrophil chemotaxis. *Can Anaesth Soc J*, **28**, 232–8.

Muhlfelder, T. W., Niemetz, J., Kreutzer, D., Beebe, D., Ward, P. A., and Rosenfeld, S. I. (1979). C5 chemotactic fragment induces monocyte production of tissue factor activity. *J Clin Invest*, **63**, 147–50.

Murphy, G., Reynolds, J. J., Bretz, U., and Baggiolini, M. (1987). Collagenase is a component of the specific granules of human neutrophil leukocytes. *Biochem J*, **162**, 195–7.

Nagy, Z., Peters, H., and Huther, I. (1984). Fracture faces of cell junctions in cerebral endothelium during normal and hyperosmotic conditions. *Lab Invest*, **50**, 313–22.

Nawashiro, H., Martin, D., and Hallenbeck, J. M. (1997). Neuroprotective effects of TNF-binding protein in focal cerebral ischemia. *Brain Res*, **778**, 265–71.

Nawashiro, H., Tasaki, K., Ruetzler, C. A., and Hallenbeck, J. M. (1997). TNF-alpha pretreatment induces protective effects against focal cerebral ischemia in mice. *J Cereb Blood Flow Metab*, **17**, 483–90.

Niemitz, J. (1972). Coagulant activity of leukocytes. Tissue factor activity. *J Clin Invest*, **51**, 307–13.

Niemetz, J. and Morrison, D. C. (1977). Lipid A as the biologically active moiety in bacterial endotoxin (LPS)-initiated generation of procoagulant activity by peripheral blood leukocytes. *Blood*, **49**, 947–55.

Ohtsuki, T., Matsumoto, M., Kuwabara, K., Kitagawa, K., Suzuki, K., Taniguchi, N., and Kamada, T. (1992). Influence of oxidative stress on induced tolerance to ischemia in gerbil hippocampal neurons. *Brain Res*, **599**, 246–52.

Ohtsuki, T., Ruetzier, C. A., Tasaki, M., and Hallenbeck, J. M. (1996). Interleukin-1 mediators induction of tolerance to global ischemia in gerbil hippocampal CA 1 neurones. *J Cereb Blood Flow Metab*, **16**, 1137–42.

Okazaki, H. (1989). Cerebrovascular disease. In *Fundamentals of Neuropathology*, 1st edn, Igaku-Shoin, New York, pp. 25–45.

Okada, Y., Copeland, B. R., Mori, E., Tung, M-M., Thomas, W. S., and del Zoppo, G. J. (1994). P-selectin and intercellular adhesion molecule-1 expression after focal brain ischemia and reperfusion. *Stroke*, 25, 202–11.

Okada, Y., Copeland, B. R., Fitridge, R., Koziol, J. A., and del Zoppo, G. J. (1994). Fibrin contributes to microvascular obstructions and parenchymal changes during early focal cerebral ischemia and reperfusion. *Stroke*, 25, 1847–54.

Ono, N., Koyama, T., Suehiro, A., Oku, K-I., Fujikake, K., and Kakishita, E. (1991). Clinical significance of new coagulation and fibrinolytic markers in ischemic stroke patients. *Stroke* 22, 1369–73.

Peters, H., Palay, S. L., and Webster, H. D. (1991). *The Fine Structure of the Nervous System. Neurons and Their Supporting Cells*, 3rd edn, Oxford University Press, New York.

Pike, M. C., Wicha, M. S., Yoon, P., Mayo, L., and Boxer, L. A. (1989). Laminin promotes the oxidative burst in human neutrophils via increased chemoattractant receptor expression. *J Immunol*, 142, 2004–11.

Pober, J. S. and Cotran, R. S. (1999). Cytokines and Endothelial Cell Biology. *Physiol Rev*, 70, 427–51.

Pozilli, C., Lenzi, G. L., Argentino, C., Carolei, A. S., Rasura, M., Signore, A., *et al*. (1985). Imaging of leukocytic infiltration in human cerebral infarcts. *Stroke*, 16, 251–5.

Risau, W. and Wolburg, H. (1990). Development of the blood-brain barrier. *TINS*, 13, 174–8.

Ritter, L., Orozco, J., Coull, B., McDonagh, P., and Rosenblum, W. (2000). Leukocyte accumulation and hemodynamic changes in the cerebral microcirculation during early reperfusion after stroke. *Stroke*, 31(5), 1153–61.

Roberts, H. R. (1992). New perspectives on the coagulation cascade. *Hosp Pract*, 15, 97.

Rosenblum, W. I. (1986). Endothelial dependent relaxation demonstrated *in vivo* in cerebral arterioles. *Stroke*, 17, 494–7.

Rosenberg, G. A., Navratil, M., Barone, F., and Feuerstein, G. (1996). Proteolytic cascade enzymes increase in focal cerebral ischemia in rat. *J Cereb Blood Flow Metab*, 16, 360–6.

Ruetzler, C. A., Furuya, K., Takeda, H., and Hallenbeck, J. M. (2001). Brain vessels normally undergo cyclic activation and inactivation: evidence from tumor necrosis factor-alpha, heme oxygenase-1, and manganese superoxide dismutase immunostaining of vessels and perivascular brain cells. *J Cereb Blood Flow Metab*, 21, 244–52.

Saito, K., Suyama, K., Nishida, K., Sei, Y., and Basile, A. S. (1996). Early increases in TNF-(IL-6 and IL-1) levels following transient cerebral ischemia in gerbil brain. *Neuroscience Lett*, 206, 149–52.

Salven, P., Orpana, A., and Joensuu, H. (1999). Leukocytes and platelets of patients with cancer contain high levels of vascular endothelial growth factor. *Clin Cancer Res*, 5, 487–91.

Sarker, M. H., Hu, D. E., and Fraser, P. A. (2000). Acute effects of bradykinin on cerebral microvascular permeability in the anaesthetized rat. *J Physiol*, 528, (Pt 1) 177–87.

Scalia, R., Booth, G., and Lefer, D. (1999). Vascular endothelial growth factor attenuates leukocyte-endothelium interaction during acute endothelial dysfunction: Essential role of endothelium-derived nitric oxide. *FASEB J*, 13, 1039–46.

Schmid-Schönbein, G. W. (1987). Leukocyte kinetics in the microcirculation. *Biorheology*, 24, 139–51.

Schmid-Schönbein, G. W. (1987). Capillary plugging by granulocytes and the no-reflow phenomenon in the microcirculation. *Fed Proc* 46, 2397–401.

Schmid-Schönbein, G. W. (1990). Leukocyte biophysics. *Cell Biophys*, 17, 107–135.

Schmid-Schönbein, G. W., Skalak, R., Simon, S. I., and Engler, R. L. (1991). The interaction between leukocytes and endothelium *in vivo*. *Ann N Y Acad Sci*, 516, 348–361.

Serou, M. J., DeCoster, M. A., and Bazan, N. G. (1999). Interleukin-1 beta activates expression of cyclooxygenase-2 and inducible nitric oxide synthase in primary hippocampal neuronal culture:

platelet-activating factor as a preferential mediator of cyclooxygenase-2 expression. *J Neurosci Res,* 58(4), 593–8.

Sherman, D. G. (1997). The enlimomab acute stroke trial. *Neurology,* 48, A270. (Abstract)

Shivers, R. R., Betz, A. L., and Goldstein, G. W. (1984). Isolated rat brain capillaries possess intact, structurally complex, interendothelial tight junctions; freeze-fracture verification of tight junction integrity. *Brain Res,* 324, 313–22.

Shohami, E., Ginis, I., and Hallenbeck, J. M. (1999). Dual role of tumor necrosis factor alpha in brain injury. *Cytokine and Growth Factor Reviews,* 10, 119–30.

Soriano, S. G., Lipton, S. A., Wang, Y. F., Xiao, M., Springer, T. A., Gutierrez-Ramos, J-C., and Hickey, P.R. (1996). Intercellular adhesion molecule-1-deficient mice are less susceptible to cerebral ischemia-reperfusion injury. *Ann Neurol,* 39, 618–24.

Spinnewyn, B., Blavet, N., Clostre, F., Bazan, N., and Braquet, P. (1987). Involvement of platelet-activating factor (PAF) in cerebral post-ischemic phase in Mongolian gerbils. *Prosstaglandins,* 34, 337–49.

Stevens, H., Van de Wiele, C., Santens, P., Jansen, H. M., De Reuck, J., Dierckx, R., and Korf, J. (1998). Cobalt-57 and technetium-99m-HMPAO-labeled leukocytes for visualization of ischemic infarcts. *J Nucl Med,* 39, 495–8.

Strijbos, P. J. and Rothwell, N. J. (1995). Interleukin-1 beta attenuates excitatory amino acid-induced neurodegeneration in vitro: involvment of nerve growth factor. *J Neuroscience* 15, 3468–74.

Tagaya, M., Liu, K-F., Copeland, B., Seiffert, D., Engler, R., Garcia, J. H., and del Zoppo, G. J. (1997). DNA scission after focal brain ischemia: Temporal differences in two species. *Stroke,* 28, 1245–54.

Tagaya, M., Haring, H-P., Stuiver, I., Wagner, S., Abumiya, T., Lucero, J., *et al.* (2001). Rapid loss of microvascular integrin expression during focal brain ischemia refects neuron injury. *J Cereb Blood Flow Metabol,* 21, 835–46.

Tasaki, K., Ruetzler, C., Ohtsuki, T., Martin, D., Nawashiro, J., and Hallenbeck, J. (1997). Lipopolysaccharide pretreatment induces resistance against subsequent focal cerebrael ischemic damage in spontaneously hypertensive rats. *Brain Res,* 748, 267–70.

The National Institutes of Neurological Disorders and Stroke rt-PA Stroke Study Group. (1995). Tissue plasminogen activator for acute ischemic stroke. *N Engl J Med,* 333, 1581–7.

Thomas, W. S., Mori, E., Copeland, B. R., Yu, J-Q., Morrissey, J. H., and del Zoppo, G. J. (1993). Tissue factor contributes to microvascular defects following cerebral ischemia. *Stroke,* 24, 847–53.

Todd, N. V., Picozzi, P., Crockard, H. A., and Russell, R. W. R. (1986). Duration of ischemia influences the development and resolution of ischemic brain edema. *Stroke,* 17, 466–71.

Touzani, O., Boutin, H., Chuquet, J., and Rothwell, N. (1999) Potential mechanisms of interleukin-1 involvement in cerebral ischaemia. *J Neuroimmunol,* 100, 203–15.

Uchiyama, S., Yamazaki, M., and Maruyama, S. (1991). Role of platelet-activating factor in aggregation of leukocytes and platelets in cerebral ischemia. *Lipids,* 26, 1247–9.

Valone, F. H. (1988). Interrelationships among platelet-activating factor binding and metabolism and induction of platelet activation. In *Platelet Membrane Receptors: Molecular Biology, Immunology, Biochemistry, and Pathology,* (ed. G. A. Jameson) Alan R. Liss, Inc., New York, pp. 319–40.

Vanhoutte, P. M, and Shimokawa, H. (1989). Endothelium-derived relaxing factor and coronary spasm. *Circulation,* 80, 1–9.

Vasthare, U. S., Heinel, L. A., Rosenwasser, R. H., and Tuma, R. F. (1990). Leukocyte involvement in cerebral ischemia and reperfusion injury. *Surg Neurol,* 33, 261–5.

Wada, T., Kondoh, T., and Tamaki, N. (1999). Ischemic 'cross' tolerance in hypoxic ischemia of immature rat brain. *Brain Res,* 847, 299–307.

Wagner, S., Tagaya, M., Koziol, J. A., Quaranta, V., and del Zoppo, G. J. (1997). Rapid disruption of an astrocyte interaction with the extracellular matrix mediated by integrin $\alpha_6\beta_4$ during focal cerebral ischemia/reperfusion. *Stroke,* 28, 858–65.

Walder, C. E., Green, S. P., Darbonne, W. C., Mathias, J., Rae, J., Dinauer, M. C., and Curnutte, J. T. (1997). Ischemic stroke injury is reduced in mice lacking a functional NADPH oxidate. *Stroke*, 28, 2252–8.

Wang, P. Y., Kao, C. H., Mui, M. Y., and Wang, S. J. (1993). Leukocytic infiltration in acute hemispheric ischemic stroke. *Stroke*, 24, 236–40.

Watanabe, H., Hattori, S., Katsuda, S., Nakanishi, I., and Nagai Y. (1990). Human neutrophil elastase: Degradation of basement membrane components and immunolocalization in the tissue. *J Biochem*, 108, 753–9.

Webb, N., Myers, C., Watson, C., Bottomley, M., and Brenchley P. (1998). Activated human neutrophils express vascular endothelial growth factor (VEGF). *Cytokine*, 10, 254–7.

Woodroofe, M. N. and Cuzner, M. L. (1993). Cytokine mRNA expression in inflammatory multiple sclerosis lesions: Detection by non-radioactive *in situ* hybridization. *Cytokine*, 5, 583–8.

Yang, G-Y., Gong, C., Quin, Z., Ye, W., Mao, Y., and Bertz, A. L. (1998). Inhibition of TNF (attenuates infarct volume and ICAM-1 expression in ischemic mouse brain. *Neuroreport*, 9, 2131–4.

Yoshida, Y., Dereski, M. O., Garcia, J. H., Hetzel, F. W., and Chopp, M. (1992). Photoactivated photofrin II: Astrocytic swelling precedes endothelial injury in rat brain. *J Neuropathol Exp Neurol*, 51, 91–100.

Zea-Longa, E., Weinstein, P. R., Carlson, S., and Cummins, R. (1989). Reversible middle cerebral artery occlusion without craniectomy in rats. *Stroke*, 20, 84–91.

Zhang, R. L., Chopp, M., Li, Y., Zaloga, C., Jiang, N., Jones, M. L., *et al.* (1994). Anti-ICAM-1 antibody reduces ischemic cell damage after transient middle cerebral artery occlusion in the rat. *Neurology*, 44, 1747–51.

Zhang, R. L., Chopp, M., Tang, W. X., Prostak, I., Manning, A. M., and Anderson, D. C. (1995). Anti-ICAM-1 antibody (1A29) reduces ischemic tissue damage after transient but not permanent middle cerebral artery (MCA) occlusion in rat. *Stroke*, 26, 1438–42.

Zhang, R. L., Chopp, M., Zhang, Z. G., Phillips, M. C., Rosenbloom, C. L., Cruz, R., and Manning, A. (1996). E-selectin focal cerebral ischemia and reperfusion in the rat. *J Cereb Blood Flow Metab*, 16, 1126–36.

Zhang, R., Chopp, M., Zhang, Z., Jiang, N., and Powere, C. (1998). The expression of P- and E-selectins in three models of middle cerebral artery occlusion. *Brain Res*, 785, 207–14.

Zülch, K-J. and Kleihues, P. (1966). Neuropathology of cerebral infarction. In *Stroke. Thule International Symposia 1966*, Nordiska Bokhandelns, Stockholm, pp. 57–75.

Zülch, K-J. (1985). *The Cerebral Infarct: Pathology, Pathogenesis, and Computed Tomography*, Springer-Verlag, Heidelberg.

Chapter 7

Cytokines and neurodegeneration

Sarah Loddick and Nancy Rothwell

7.1 Introduction

The term cytokine describes a large and rapidly expanding group of polypeptides which can be expressed by most cell types and have diverse actions on numerous biological processes. Cytokines include the families of interleukins (IL), chemokines, tumour necrosis factors (TNF), interferons, and growth factors. There is some debate about whether neurotrophins might be included within the cytokine family but they will not be discussed here.

Most cytokines are expressed constitutively at low levels, but are produced rapidly in response to infection, injury, or inflammation. They tend to act locally in an autocrine or paracrine manner to influence cell growth and differentiation, inflammation, immune activation, and responses to disease and injury. These actions are often interdependent; many cytokines act in synergy and induce each other, and may exert similar effects suggesting significant redundancy. In contrast, some cytokines have opposing actions. For example, cytokines such as IL-1, IL-6 and TNF-α have been defined as pro-inflammatory, while others exert largely 'anti-inflammatory' actions, for example, IL-1ra, IL-4, IL-10. Such definitions do, however, need to be treated with some caution, particularly in the central nervous system (CNS).

Cytokines are established mediators of local and systemic responses to injury and infection in peripheral tissues, where their roles are quite well defined. In contrast, the CNS has been considered as 'immune privileged', and thus the involvement of cytokines in CNS disease was not recognized until some time after their peripheral actions had been established. Nevertheless, many cytokines are expressed within, and act on, cells of the CNS. It is not possible to review in depth all aspects of the contribution of cytokines to immune and inflammatory responses within the CNS which may influence neurodegeneration. Thus, we will focus on those cytokines for which there is substantial evidence supporting their role in neurodegeneration rather than recovery, and cytokines implicated in acute neurodegeneration. We will consider the methodological approaches and evidence for their contribution, likely mechanisms of expression and action, and clinical relevance.

7.2 Experimental approaches

Early studies focused on the presence of cytokine(s) in brain tissue and cerebrospinal fluid (CSF) after experimental and clinical brain injury, and studied the effect of exogenous administration of recombinant cytokines. More recently, studies have attempted to determine the effect of endogenous cytokines using specific inhibitors (e.g. receptor antagonist, specific antibodies) and genetically modified mice.

For most cytokines there are no specific receptor antagonists; thus a number of strategies have been employed to block the action of the endogenous protein in the brain. Passive immunoneutralization has been successful in some studies, but the lack of high affinity, species-specific neutralizing antibodies to cytokines has limited the success of this approach. Other approaches include the use of recombinant forms of soluble receptors and binding proteins (Barone *et al.* 1997; Ruocco *et al.* 1999). IL-1 is unusual among cytokines in that a naturally occurring, selective receptor antagonist (IL-1ra) exists, and recombinant IL-1ra has been used in numerous experimental studies to acutely block the actions of IL-1α and β in the brain (see Section 7.6 and Touzani *et al.* 1999). More recent studies have employed genetically modified mice that enable the functions of individual cytokines and receptors to be investigated (e.g. Boutin *et al.* 2001; Bruce *et al.* 1996; Gary *et al.* 1998). However, data from these mice must be interpreted with caution because in most cases the genetic modification is present throughout life and compensatory changes may have occurred during development (Taverne, 1993).

7.3 Neurodegeneration

7.3.1 Causes of neurodegeneration

Neuronal death in the brain occurs naturally during development, and in response to insults to the brain which may be exogenous (e.g. traumatic injury or exposure to toxins) or endogenous (e.g. hypoxia, ischaemia or neurodegenerative disease). The major clinical causes of neurodegeneration are traumatic brain injury, cerebral ischaemia (stroke, hypoxia, or cardiac arrest), and chronic neurodegenerative disorders such as Alzheimer's disease (AD), Parkinson's and related movement disorders, amyotrophic lateral sclerosis (ALS) and multiple sclerosis (MS). While the aetiologies of these conditions vary considerably, the pathways and mechanisms that result in neuronal death may be similar.

Until fairly recently, neuronal death in the adult CNS was thought to be necrotic in nature with cells undergoing swelling, organelle dissolution and membrane rupture with release of cell debris. However, there is now increasing evidence that neuronal apoptosis occurs in the adult brain during neurodegeneration (Mattson *et al.* 2001).

7.3.2 Mechanisms of neurodegeneration

Current understanding of the mechanisms leading to neuronal death have been reviewed extensively (e.g. Dirnagl *et al.* 1999; Rogers and Shen 2000; Zipfel *et al.* 2000), but a brief and simplistic overview may usefully set the scene for discussion of the actions of cytokines on neuronal survival and degeneration.

The initial disruptive event in the brain depends largely on the nature of the stimulus (e.g. mechanical damage, hypoxia, ischaemia, exposure to a toxin), but these insults all cause disruption of ionic gradients, increased neuronal activity, reduced energy (ATP) availability, and excessive release of neurotransmitters. In particular, release of excitatory amino acids (EAA) such as glutamate has been identified as a key event in the cascade of neural death. Consequently, inhibitors of glutamate release or antagonists of *N*-methyl-D-aspartate (NMDA) and non-NMDA receptors have been shown to attenuate various forms of experimentally induced neurodegeneration and several are being developed for clinical application, though none have yet proved effective in patients (De Keyser *et al.* 1999).

Potential interventions to block the mechanisms leading to neuronal injury include inhibitors of glutamate release or action (see previous paragraph) or calcium entry, which is essential for many forms of neuronal death and leads to severe disruption of intracellular function, activation of proteolytic enzymes and damage to intracellular organelles (Hunter 1997). Modulation of cell death may also be achieved by inhibition of arachidonic acid release, since this forms the precursor of potentially damaging eicosanoids, which can directly modify glutamate release and actions, and modulate synthesis of platelet-activating factor (PAF) and nitric oxide (Farooqui et al. 1997).

There is now increasing awareness of the role of non-neuronal cells in neurodegeneration. Glia are an important source and site of action of neurotoxic (e.g. cytokines, nitric oxide, EAAs) and neuroprotective molecules (e.g. growth factors); they can modulate local ion and transmitter concentrations and exert direct effects on neurones via electrical contacts. Similarly, endothelial cells express cytokines, adhesion molecules, growth factors, and nitric oxide, all of which could influence neuronal survival.

7.4 Synthesis of cytokines in neurodegenerative conditions

The expression of most cytokines in normal brain, like that in other tissues, is very low, leading to problems of detection by standard techniques, and questions over their physiological relevance under basal conditions. The expression of numerous cytokines (e.g. specific neurotrophins and growth factors, IL-1, IL-1ra, IL-6, TNF-α, IL-10, TGF-β) is increased rapidly in response to diverse insults such as ischaemia, traumatic injury and neurotoxins in rodent brain (e.g. Allan and Rothwell 2001; Barone and Feuerstein 1999; del Zoppo et al. 2000; Flanders et al. 1998; Iadecola and Alexander 2001). Marked and very rapid increases in cytokines have also been reported in brain tissue or CSF of patients with conditions associated with damage to neurones (e.g. Asensio and Campbell 1999; Perrella et al. 2001; Rostasy et al. 2000).

Interleukin-1 and TNF-α mRNA expression has been detected as early as 15–30 min after induction of cerebral ischaemia, while other cytokines' mRNAs increase within 24 h and cytokine expression can be sustained for many days (see Allan and Rothwell 2001; Barone and Feuerstein 1999; Iadecola and Alexander 2001). It seems that virtually all resident CNS cells as well as invading immune cells can express cytokines. Glia, especially microglia and astrocytes, produce many cytokines (e.g. IL-1, IL-6, TNF-α, granulocyte-macrophage colony-stimulating factor (GMCSF), macrophage colony-stimulating factor (MCSF), transforming growth factor (TGF)-β in vitro, suggesting that they are an important source of cytokines in response to brain damage (e.g. Giulian et al. 1994; Raivich et al. 1999b). However, neurones, endothelial, and ependymal cells as well as invading cells, may also synthesize cytokines. Macrophages, lymphocytes, and neutrophils can invade the CNS after damage, inflammation or breakdown of the blood–brain barrier (BBB) (Merrill and Murphy 1997; Perry et al. 1998), but since significant immune cell invasion is usually delayed by several hours after damage to the brain, they are unlikely to be involved in the very early production of cytokines after CNS injury.

The regulation of cytokine expression is complex. Many cytokines can induce or inhibit the expression of other cytokines and in some cases (e.g. the IL-1 family) it is necessary to consider several molecules (e.g. IL-1 ligands, IL-1ra, IL-1 binding proteins) in assessing overall bioactivity. In addition to cellular injury and invading pathogenesis, cytokine expression can be influenced by peripheral injury and infection, possibly via afferent vagal signals (see Rothwell and Luheshi 2000). Hypoxia *per se*, excessive neuronal activation (e.g. spreading depression or seizures), and chronic disruption may also influence early cytokine expression (see Allan and Rothwell 2001).

Cytokines such as IL-1, TNF-α and TGF-β are expressed as biologically inactive precursors which must be cleaved enzymatically to generate the active protein. TNF-α convertase (which releases TNF-α) and caspase-1 (which cleaves pro IL-1β) are present in the CNS where expression is regulated after brain injury (Hurtado *et al.* 2001; Zhu *et al.* 1999). Little is known about the latency associated proteins and latent TGF-β binding proteins (which regulate activity of released TGF-β) in the CNS. Cleavage and release of IL-1β (which lacks a classical leader sequence) is believed to be regulated through actions of a purinergic, P2$\times$7 receptor on primed microglia, which results in potassium efflux and activation of caspase-1 (Ferrari *et al.* 1997) though the precise means by which cellular release occurs is uncertain.

7.5 Neurotrophic and neuroprotective effects of cytokines

In vitro studies suggest that many cytokines can exert potent neuroprotective effects (Araujo and Cotman 1993; Bruce-Keller *et al.* 1999; Prehn *et al.* 1993; Strijbos and Rothwell 1995). However, in many cases, data from *in vivo* studies conflict with *in vitro* data, and relatively few cytokines have been proven as endogenous neuroprotectants.

Interleukin-1 protects cultured neurones from ischaemic and excitotoxic injury (Carlson *et al.* 1999; Pringle *et al.* 2001; Strijbos and Rothwell 1995), and treating animals with IL-1β *prior* to an ischaemic insult reduces neuronal death through a mechanism similar to ischaemic 'pre-conditioning' (Ohtsuki *et al.* 1996). However, the overwhelming evidence from *in vivo* studies suggests that IL-1β is neurotoxic and contributes directly to neuronal injury (see Section 7.6). Most of these data derive from studies using a recombinant form of the IL-1 receptor antagonist (IL-1ra) which is one of the few cytokines that has been shown to act as an endogenous neuroprotective agent. Expression of IL-1ra is increased in the brain after experimentally induced injury and injection of anti-IL-1ra antiserum increases ischaemic brain injury (Loddick *et al.* 1997).

The role of TNF-α in neurodegeneration appears to be complex. *In vitro*, TNF-α has neuroprotective actions (Barger *et al.* 1995; Bruce-Keller *et al.* 1999), and as with IL-1, pretreatment with TNF-α *in vivo* can protect the brain from subsequent ischaemic injury (Nawashiro *et al.* 1997). TNF-α acts by binding to two different receptors, the p55 and the p75 receptor, both of which are present in brain (Cheng *et al.* 1994; Kinouchi *et al.* 1991). A variety of approaches have been employed to elucidate the role of endogenous TNF-α in neurodegeneration, including the use of TNF-α antibodies, soluble receptors, and genetically modified animals which lack one or both of these receptors. These *in vivo* studies suggest that TNF-α may protect the brain via activation of the p55 receptor (Bruce *et al.* 1996; Gary *et al.* 1998). However, several lines of evidence suggest that TNF-α is neurotoxic (see Section 7.6).

Similar controversies exist over the role of IL-6 in neurodegeneration, and both neuroprotective and neurodegenerative effects of this cytokine have been described. Neurotrophic effects of exogenous IL-6 have been described *in vitro* (Hama *et al.* 1989; Hama *et al.* 1991; Kushima *et al.* 1992). In addition, IL-6 protects the brain from excitotoxic and ischaemic injury *in vitro* and *in vivo* (Ali *et al.* 2000; Loddick *et al.* 1998; Matsuda *et al.* 1996; Yamada and Hatanaka 1994). Efforts to determine the role of endogenous IL-6 in neurodegeneration have been hampered by the lack of specific inhibitors for use *in vivo*. In addition, two studies using IL-6 knock out mice have yielded conflicting data, describing an increased (Penkowa *et al.* 1999) or unaltered susceptibility (Clark *et al.* 2000) to brain injury *in vivo*. Thus, further studies are needed to clarify the role of IL-6 in neurodegeneration.

Interleukin-4 (IL-4) is an anti-inflammatory cytokine which appears to have protective effects in experimental allergic encephalomyelitis (EAE), a model for MS (Falcone *et al.* 1998). *In vitro*, IL-4 enhances neuronal survival, but it is not clear whether this effect is due to neuroprotective or neurotrophic effects of IL-4 (Araujo and Cotman 1993). Our recent data suggest that endogenous IL-4 inhibits brain damage since mice lacking IL-4 have enhanced damage after stroke (Boutin and Rothwell, unpublished observations). IL-10 expression is increased in the brain in response to several experimental and clinical neuro-degenerative conditions (Bell *et al.* 1997; Csuka *et al.* 1999; Tarkowski *et al.* 1997). This expression may be of benefit to the injured brain since IL-10 prevents EAE relapse in rats (Crisi *et al.* 1995) and improves outcome after ischaemic and traumatic brain injury (Knoblach and Faden 1998; Spera *et al.* 1998). Furthermore, IL-10 knockout in mice increases injury after experimental stroke (Gahtan and Overmier 1999). These neuropro-tective effects of IL-4 and IL-10 may be mediated via modulation of IL-1ra expression (Vannier *et al.* 1992).

Transforming growth factor-β protects cultured neurones from hypoxic, excitotoxic, and β-amyloid induced neuronal death (Buisson *et al.* 1998; Prehn *et al.* 1993; Ren and Flanders 1996). Although neurotoxic effects of TGF-β have also been described (Prehn and Krieglstein 1994; Prehn and Miller 1996), the majority of evidence points to protective effects of TGF-β. Injection of TGF-β1 reduces neuronal death caused by experimentally induced ischaemic and excitotoxic brain damage in rodents *in vivo* (Pratt and McPherson 1997; Ruocco *et al.* 1999). Furthermore, injection of a soluble TGF-β receptor inhibits the effects of the endogenous cytokine and worsens ischaemic and excitotoxic injury, indicating that TGF-β is an *endogenous* neuroprotective agent (Ruocco *et al.* 1999).

7.6 Neurotoxic actions of cytokines

In vitro, several cytokines (e.g. TNF-α, IL-1, IFNγ) can induce cell death, usually at quite high doses and often in a synergistic manner (Chao *et al.* 1995; Jeohn *et al.* 1998). In addition to direct effects on neuronal survival, cytokines can act on glia to release neurotoxic sub-stances (Allan and Rothwell 2001; Giulian *et al.* 1994; Raivich *et al.* 1999*a*), and IL-1 may cause the release of neurotoxic substances from glial cells since conditioned medium from IL-1β treated glial cultures is toxic to cultured neurones (Martin *et al.* 1998).

Infusion of cytokines in to the brain parenchyma can elicit responses characteristic of those seen after brain damage, for example marked gliosis (Giulian *et al.* 1988), oedema (Holmin and Mathiesen 2000), damage to the BBB (Holmin and Mathiesen 2000), and expression of molecules (e.g. major histocompatibility complex (MHC) class II antigens), characteristic of inflammation and immune activation in the CNS (Fabry *et al.* 1994; O'Keefe *et al.* 1999). However, there is little direct evidence to indicate that acute administration of cytokines into the brain in normal animals induces overt neurodegeneration. Nevertheless, sustained administration of some cytokines, or co-application with another insult, may induce or enhance neurodegeneration. Transgenic mice over-expressing IL-6 in the brain exhibit profound neuropathology, including oedema, encephalopathy, demyelination, and neuronal damage (Campbell *et al.* 1993; Heyser *et al.* 1997). These data indicate that, in contrast to the acute neuroprotective effects of IL-6, chronic over-expression in the brain may be highly detrimental, but this may reflect actions of the cytokine on neuronal development.

Several pieces of evidence indicate that cytokines can *exacerbate* neurodegenerative conditions. Clinical trials of IFN-γ in MS showed a marked increase in clinical symptoms (see Clanet *et al.* 1989). Indeed, IFN-γ has now been implicated in the development and/or progression of MS, and the beneficial effects of IFN-β in patients with MS have been ascribed, at least in part, to inhibition of the synthesis or actions of IFN-γ (Khademi *et al.* 2000).

Intracerebral injection of IL-1 markedly enhances neurodegeneration caused by experimentally induced excitotoxic or ischaemic injury in rodents (Lawrence *et al.* 1998; Loddick and Rothwell 1996; Yamasaki *et al.* 1995). Such exacerbation may reflect non-specific, pro-inflammatory or pyrogenic actions of IL-1, since increased body temperature markedly increases ischaemic damage, particularly in global ischaemia (Ginsberg *et al.* 1993). However, although IL-1 can cause significant fever (Loddick and Rothwell 1996), icv injection of IL-6, which has similar pyrogenic potency, inhibits, rather than enhances, damage caused by focal ischaemia (Loddick *et al.* 1998).

The most direct evidence for the role of endogenous cytokines in neurodegeneration derives from studies in which expression or action of the endogenous protein is inhibited, and here the most extensive data exist for IL-1.

Interleukin-1ra has been used extensively to investigate the role of IL-1 in neurodegeneration, and markedly inhibits neuronal injury caused by ischaemic, excitotoxic or traumatic insults in the rat. Icv injection of IL-1ra inhibits damage resulting from focal ischaemia (induced by middle cerebral artery occlusion, MCAO) in the rat by approximately 50 per cent, an effect that is comparable with or greater than that of NMDA receptor antagonists such as MK801 (Loddick and Rothwell 1996). Systemic administration of high doses of IL-1ra is also effective at reducing infarct size and oedema induced by MCAO (Relton *et al.* 1996). These effects of IL-1ra are not due to changes in physiological parameters such as blood pressure, heart rate, or body temperature, suggesting a fundamental role of IL-1 in the development of ischaemic damage (Loddick and Rothwell 1996). IL-1ra also inhibits excitotoxic and traumatic brain damage, and improves neurological outcome as well as reducing infarct volume (Garcia *et al.* 1995; Lawrence *et al.* 1998; Toulmond and Rothwell 1995). Injection (icv) of an anti-IL-1β antibody similarly inhibits oedema, neuronal damage, and neutrophil invasion caused by transient forebrain ischaemia in the rat (Yamasaki *et al.* 1995), suggesting that IL-1β may be the major form of IL-1 which contributes to neurodegeneration. However, mice lacking IL-1α or IL-1β or the IL-1R1 receptor exhibit normal ischaemic brain damage (Boutin *et al.* 2001; Touzani *et al.* 2002), but in mice lacking both forms of IL-1 infarct volume is reduced by about 80 per cent (see Fig. 7.1, Boutin *et al.* 2001).

Lateral fluid percussion injury in the rat is followed by increased local expression of IL-1, TNF-α, and IL-6 (Taupin *et al.* 1993). Central injection of IL-1ra inhibits the extent of traumatic brain damage in the rat (Toulmond and Rothwell 1995) and the neuroprotective effects are apparent even when IL-1ra is administered 4 h after injury, and are sustained for at least 7 days (Toulmond and Rothwell 1995). In view of the key role of EAAs in many forms of acute and chronic neurodegeneration, it is likely that cytokines such as IL-1 interact in some way with EAAs or their receptors. Brain damage caused by pharmacological activation of either NMDA or AMPA receptors in the rat striatum is markedly attenuated by co-infusion of IL-1ra (Lawrence *et al.* 1998). However, although IL-1 may modulate release

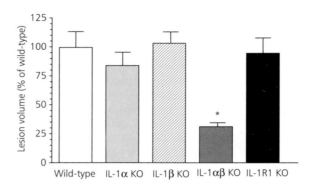

Fig. 7.1 Brain injury (lesion volume expressed as a percentage of wild-type) measured 24 h after induction of transient (30 min) cerebral ischaemia in wild-type, IL-1α knockout, IL-1β knockout, IL-1αβ double knockout, and IL-1 receptor (IL-1R1) knockout mice. Data are expressed as mean ± SEM of 8–9 animals. *Significantly different compared to wild-type, $p < 0.05$, ANOVA followed by Scheffes *post hoc* test. (Data adapted from Boutin *et al.* 2001; Touzani *et al.* 2002).

or re-uptake of glutamate or other EAAs, it appears to act mainly at a step in the cascade of cell death beyond the point of EAA receptor activation (Allan and Rothwell 2001).

For TNF-α and IL-6 the data are somewhat complex. Acute inhibition of TNF-α, for example, using a neutralizing antibody or a soluble receptor which limits the biological activity of TNF-α, reduces ischaemic and traumatic brain injury in rodents (see Shohami *et al.* 1999), indicating that endogenous TNF-α contributes to neuronal injury. Recent studies of TNF-deficient embryos have revealed that fewer sympathetic and sensory neurones die during development implicating TNF in developmental neuronal death (Barker *et al.* 2001). However, mice lacking TNF-α or its signalling receptors have worse neuronal damage suggesting a neuroprotective action (Scherbel *et al.* 1999). This discrepancy may relate to the time course of TNF-α expression and/or the presence of other mediators which may act in concert with TNF-α (Shohami *et al.* 1999).

7.6.1 Mechanisms of cytokine involvement in neurotoxicity

The mechanisms involved in the actions of cytokines described above remain to be fully elucidated, but appear to depend on complex interactions with multiple cell types. The observation that IL-1ra does not protect primary cultured neurones (Strijbos and Rothwell 1995) may indicate that IL-1 acts on non-neuronal cells in the CNS to influence neuronal survival indirectly, a hypothesis that is supported by the fact that conditioned media from IL-1β treated glial cells is toxic to neurones (Martin *et al.* 1998). Glial cells respond to a variety of cytokines, and can in turn mediate potentially detrimental or protective effects via the release of growth factors, cytokines, arachidonic acid, and NO (see above and Giulian *et al.* 1993).

Cytokines have several actions on the cerebro-vascular system that could contribute to neuronal injury (see Fig. 7.2). IL-1 and TNF-α can release neurotoxins such as NO from endothelial cells (Bonmann *et al.* 1997), and increase expression of adhesion molecules which may facilitate leucocyte infiltration and subsequent progression of neuronal death

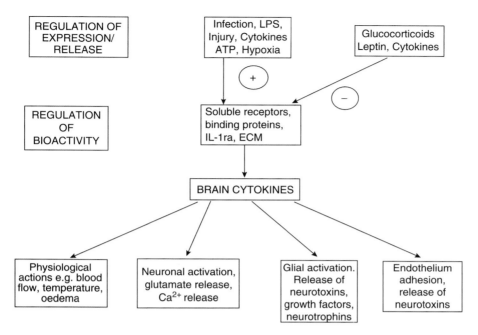

Fig. 7.2 Cytokine involvement in acute neurodegeneration.

(Wong and Dorovini-Zis 1996). Venters *et al.* recently reported that TNF-α can mediate neuronal death indirectly via inhibition of survival signals (Venters *et al.* 1999), a mechanism that could apply to other cytokines and explain their minimal effects on normal brain (see Loddick and Rothwell 1999). The effects of IL-1 on neuronal death appear to be mediated by specific brain regions and involve complex pathways which could explain the lack of IL-1β toxicity in cell culture systems (Allan *et al.* 2000; Allan and Rothwell 2001). Thus, the precise mechanism of action of cytokines in neurodegeneration remains to be determined, but appears to depend on complex interactions between different cytokines, and multiple cell types.

7.7 **Role of cytokines in chronic neurodegeneration**

The data implicating cytokines in chronic neurological disorders such as AD, Down syndrome, Parkinson's disease, Huntington's chorea, MS, AIDS dementia, and epileptic damage is largely indirect and/or circumstantial, but intriguing. Some aspects of this topic are dealt with in Chapters 8 and 9. Increased expression of cytokines has been reported in each of these conditions and, in some cases, in relevant animal models of the disease (see Allan and Rothwell 2001; Rothwell and Luheshi 2000). However, it is difficult to distinguish cause and effect in these disorders. Neuronal damage can increase cytokine expression rapidly, but this does not necessarily imply causal involvement in neurodegeneration, and does not indicate whether any effect is beneficial or detrimental.

7.7.1 **Alzheimer's disease**

There is now considerable, and growing evidence that AD is associated with an inflammatory response in the brain (Halliday *et al.* 2000; McGeer *et al.* 2000). Several studies
suggest that acute head trauma is a risk factor of AD (e.g. Lye and Shores 2000; O'Meara *et al.*
1997), and there is a potentially strong, but unproven link between these events since IL-1β
expression is increased in brain injury, inflammation, and AD (see Section 7.4). Furthermore, cytokines can elicit many of the responses observed in the brains of patients with
AD or Down syndrome, such as glial activation, complement and MHC class II antigen
expression, and perhaps most importantly synthesis of β-APP (Panegyres and Hughes 1998;
Yang *et al* 1998). However, it is still unclear whether such inflammatory responses result
from or contribute to the pathogenesis of AD. Polymorphisms in IL-1 genes have been
associated with early onset AD and several other pieces of indirect evidence suggest but do
not prove a causal link between IL-1 and AD (see Allan and Rothwell 2001).

7.7.2 **Multiple sclerosis**

Multiple sclerosis is associated with a progressive inflammatory response in the brain,
probably of immune origin, although the aetiology and mechanisms of progression, relapse,
and remission of the disease are largely unknown. However, there is now compelling evidence that cytokines can mediate or modulate the clinical symptoms and progression of MS.
This evidence has been derived largely from studies of EAE in animals, which is accepted as a
relevant model of MS, and from clinical trials with interferons. IFN-β is now established as a
treatment for MS, and its effects are likely to depend on modification of other cytokines
such as TGF-β, IL-1, IL-1ra, IL-6, and IL-10 (Karp *et al.* 2001; Ozenci *et al.* 2000). The
severity of EAE is attenuated by inhibition of the actions of IL-1 (Jacobs *et al.* 1991) or
TNF-α (Taupin *et al.* 1997) or by administration of 'anti-inflammatory' cytokines such as
TGF-β (Jin *et al.* 2000).

7.7.3 **HIV dementia**

Central nervous system dysfunction is a common feature of AIDS, and up to 80 per cent of
patients show neurological abnormalities at post-mortem examination (Sotrel and Dal
Canto 2000). HIV, or its envelope coat protein gp120, can induce expression of cytokines
such as IL-1, TNF-α, IL-6, IL-8, TGF-β, and GMCSF in human monocytes (Merrill and
Chen 1991). It has been postulated that gp120 may be involved directly in neurodegeneration, since it causes neuronal damage when injected into the brain of rodents, possibly via
release of endogenous cytokines (Lipton 1994). Since several cytokines potentiate HIV-1
replication, a positive feedback loop may exist in which cytokines play a key role (Kinter *et al.*
2000; Poli and Fauci 1993).

7.7.4 **Parkinson's disease**

Parkinson's disease has not traditionally been linked to inflammatory responses, but
given the importance of excitotoxic mechanisms to this disease (Bezard *et al.* 2001),
cytokines may contribute either to the onset, or progression of Parkinson's, and other
movement disorders.

Polymorphisms in IL-1α and IL-1β have been recently linked with Parkinson's (Dodel *et al.* 2001; Nishimura *et al.* 2000) and many cytokines (IL-1, 2, 4, 6, TNF-α, EGF, BDNF, TGF-β) are increased in CSF or brains of Parkinson's patients (Mogi and Nagatsu 1999; Nagatsu *et al.* 2000), but it remains unclear whether these changes play a causal role in the disease or reflect a secondary response to ongoing brain damage.

7.8 Summary and conclusions

Cytokines and neurodegeneration have become an intense area of research with major clinical implications and there seems little doubt that most insults to the CNS elicit expression of a variety of cytokines. What is less certain is the specific role(s) these molecules play in the subsequent damage and repair, or in chronic neurological disorders. For some cytokines such as TNF-α and IL-6, data are equivocal, whereas for others (e.g. inhibition of IL-1 or activation of TGF-β) clear neuroprotection has been reported. The mechanisms of these actions are still largely unknown, and may reflect multiple and often conflicting actions. In view of the discrepancy between some *in vivo* and *in vitro* studies (particularly in primary neuronal cultures), caution needs to be exercised in extrapolation of data derived from *in vitro* studies, and attention focused on the causes of these discrepancies and the development of relevant *in vitro* systems.

Excitement over the clinical potential for modulating cytokines in neurological disorders is tempered by the relatively poor brain penetration and short half-life of these molecules, and the fact that most cytokines have apparently both beneficial and detrimental effects. Nevertheless, many cytokines or their inhibitors can and do gain access to the CNS and therefore provide therapeutic targets. Of the cytokines, IL-1 is probably the most advanced as a therapeutic target with several possible interventions (e.g. P2×7 or caspase-1 inhibitors, IL-1 antibodies, IL-1ra). IL-1ra has proven to be safe in a number of non-CNS disorders and is now in early clinical trials in stroke; other cytokine inhibitors are likely to follow shortly.

References

Ali, C., Nicole, O., Docagne, F., Lesne, S., MacKenzie, E. T., Nouvelot, A., *et al.* (2000). Ischemia-induced interleukin-6 as a potential endogenous neuroprotective cytokine against NMDA receptor-mediated excitotoxicity in the brain. *J Cereb Blood Flow Metab*, 20, 956–66.

Allan, S. M., Parker, L. C., Collins, B., Davies, R., Luheshi, G. N., and Rothwell, N. J. (2000). Cortical cell death induced by IL-1 is mediated via actions in the hypothalamus of the rat. *Proc Natl Acad Sci USA*, 97, 5580–5.

Allan, S. M. and Rothwell, N. J. (2001). Cytokines and acute neurodegeneration. *Nat Rev Neurosci*, 2, 734–44.

Araujo, D. M. and Cotman, C. W. (1993). Trophic effects of interleukin-4, -7 and -8 on hippocampal neuronal cultures: potential involvement of glial-derived factors. *Brain Res*, 600, 49–55.

Asensio, V. C. and Campbell, I. L. (1999). Chemokines in the CNS: plurifunctional mediators in diverse states. *Trends Neurosci*, 22, 504–12.

Barger, S. W., Horster, D., Furukawa, K., Goodman, Y., Krieglstein, J., and Mattson M. P. (1995). Tumor necrosis factors alpha and beta protect neurones against amyloid beta-peptide toxicity: evidence for involvement of a kappa B-binding factor and attenuation of peroxide and Ca^{2+} accumulation. *Proc Natl Acad Sci USA*, 92, 9328–32.

Barker, V., Middleton, G., Davey, F., and Davies, A. M. (2001). TNFalpha contributes to the death of NGF-dependent neurones during development. *Nat Neurosci*, 4, 1194–8.

Barone, F. C., Arvin, B., White, R. F., Miller, A., Webb, C. L., Willette, R. N., et al. (1997). Tumor necrosis factor-alpha. A mediator of focal ischemic brain injury. Stroke, 28, 1233–44.

Barone, F. C. and Feuerstein, G. Z. (1999). Inflammatory mediators and stroke: new opportunities for novel therapeutics. J Cereb Blood Flow Metab, 19, 819–34.

Bell, M. J., Kochanek, P. M., Doughty, L. A., Carcillo, J. A., Adelson, P. D., Clark, R. S. B., et al. (1997). Interleukin-6 and interleukin-10 in cerebrospinal fluid after severe traumatic brain injury in children. Journal of Neurotrauma, 14, 451–7.

Bezard, E., Brotchie, J. M., and Gross, C. E. (2001). Pathophysiology of levodopa-induced dyskinesia: potential for new therapies. Nat Rev Neurosci, 2, 577–88.

Bonmann, E., Suschek, C., Spranger, M., and Kolb-Bachofen, V. (1997). The dominant role of exogenous or endogenous interleukin-1 beta on expression and activity of inducible nitric oxide synthase in rat microvascular brain endothelial cells. Neurosci Lett, 230, 109–12.

Boutin, H., LeFeuvre, R. A., Horai, R., Asano, M., Iwakura, Y., and Rothwell, N. J. (2001). Role of IL-1alpha and IL-1beta in ischemic brain damage. J Neurosci, 21, 5528–34.

Bruce-Keller, A. J., Geddes, J. W., Knapp, P. E., McFall, R. W., Keller, J. N., Holtsberg, F. W., et al. (1999). Anti-death properties of TNF against metabolic poisoning: mitochondrial stabilization by MnSOD. J Neuroimmunol, 93, 53–71.

Bruce, A. J., Boling, W., Kindy, M. S., Peschon, J., Kraemer, P. J., Carpenter, M. K., et al. (1996). Altered neuronal and microglial responses to excitotoxic and ischemic brain injury in mice lacking TNF receptors. Nat Med, 2, 788–94.

Buisson, A., Nicole, O., Docagne, F., Sartelet, H., MacKenzie, E. T., and Vivien, D. (1998). Up-regulation of a serine protease inhibitor in astrocytes mediates the neuroprotective activity of transforming growth factor beta1. FASEB J, 12, 1683–91.

Campbell, I. L., Abraham, C. R., Masliah, E., Kemper, P., Inglis, J. D., Oldstone, M. B., and Mucke, L. (1993). Neurologic disease induced in transgenic mice by cerebral overexpression of interleukin 6. Proc Natl Acad Sci USA 90, 10061–5.

Carlson, N. G., Wieggel, W. A., Chen, J., Bacchi, A., Rogers, S. W., and Gahring, L. C. (1999). Inflammatory cytokines IL-1 alpha, IL-1 beta, IL-6, and TNF-alpha impart neuroprotection to an excitotoxin through distinct pathways. J Immunol, 163, 3963–8.

Chao, C. C., Hu, S., Ehrlich, L., and Peterson, P. K. (1995). Interleukin-1 and tumor necrosis factor-alpha synergistically mediate neurotoxicity: involvement of nitric oxide and of N-methyl-D-aspartate receptors. Brain Behav Immun, 9, 355–65.

Cheng, B., Christakos, S., and Mattson, M. P. (1994). Tumor necrosis factors protect neurons against metabolic- excitotoxic insults and promote maintenance of calcium homeostasis. Neuron, 12, 139–53.

Clanet, M., Blancher, A., Calvas, P., and Rascol, O. (1989). Interferons and multiple sclerosis. Biomed Pharmacother, 43, 355–60.

Clark, W. M., Rinker, L. G., Lessov, N. S., Hazel, K., Hill, J. K., Stenzel-Poore, M., and Eckenstein, F. (2000). Lack of Interleukin-6 expression is not protective against focal central nervous system ischemia. Stroke, 31, 1715–20.

Crisi, G. M., Santambrogio, L., Hochwald, G. M., Smith, S. R., Carlino, J. A., and Thorbecke G. J. (1995). Staphylococcal enterotoxin B and tumor-necrosis factor-alpha-induced relapses of experimental allergic encephalomyelitis: protection by transforming growth factor-beta and interleukin-10. Eur J Immunol, 25, 3035–40.

Csuka, E., Morganti-Kossmann, M. C., Lenzlinger, P. M., Joller, H., Trentz, O., and Kossmann, T. (1999). IL-10 levels in cerebrospinal fluid and serum of patients with severe traumatic brain injury: relationship to IL-6, TNF-alpha, TGF-beta1 and blood–brain barrier function. J Neuroimmunol, 101, 211–21.

De Keyser, J., Sulter, G., and Luiten, P. G. (1999). Clinical trials with neuroprotective drugs in acute ischaemic stroke: are we doing the right thing? Trends Neurosci, 22, 535–40.

del Zoppo, G., Ginis, I., Hallenbeck, J. M., Iadecola, C., Wang, X., and Feuerstein, G. Z. (2000). Inflammation and stroke: putative role for cytokines, adhesion molecules and iNOS in brain response to ischemia. *Brain Pathol,* 10, 95–112.

Dirnagl, U., Iadecola, C., and Moskowitz, M. A. (1999). Pathobiology of ischaemic stroke: an integrated view. *Trends Neurosci,* 22, 391–7.

Dodel, R. C., Lohmuller, F., Du, Y., Eastwood, B., Gocke, P., Oertel, W. H., and Gasser, T. (2001). A polymorphism in the intronic region of the IL-1alpha gene and the risk for Parkinson's disease. *Neurology,* 56, 982–3.

Fabry, Z., Raine, C. S., and Hart, M. N. (1994). Nervous tissue as an immune compartment: the dialect of the immune response in the CNS. *Immunol Today,* 15, 218–24.

Falcone, M., Rajan, A. J., Bloom, B. R., and Brosnan, C. F. (1998). A critical role for IL-4 in regulating disease severity in experimental allergic encephalomyelitis as demonstrated in IL-4-deficient C57BL/6 mice and BALB/c mice. *J Immunol,* 160, 4822–30.

Farooqui, A. A., Yang, H. C. and Horrocks, L. (1997). Involvement of phospholipase A2 in neurodegeneration. *Neurochem Int,* 30, 517–22.

Ferrari, D., Chiozzi, P., Falzoni, S., Dal Susino, M., Melchiorri, L., Baricordi, O. R., and Di Virgilio, F. (1997). Extracellular ATP triggers IL-1 beta release by activating the purinergic P2Z receptor of human macrophages. *J Immunol,* 159, 1451–8.

Flanders, K. C., Ren, R. F., and Lippa, C. F. (1998). Transforming growth factor-betas in neurodegenerative disease. *Prog Neurobiol,* 54, 71–85.

Gahtan, E. and Overmier, J. B. (1999). Inflammatory pathogenesis in Alzheimer's disease: biological mechanisms and cognitive sequeli. *Neurosci Biobehav Rev,* 23, 615–33.

Garcia, J. H., Liu, K. F., and Relton, J. K. (1995). Interleukin-1 receptor antagonist decreases the number of necrotic neurons in rats with middle cerebral artery occlusion. *Am J Pathol,* 147, 1477–86.

Gary, D. S., Bruce-Keller, A. J., Kindy, M. S., and Mattson, M. P. (1998). Ischemic and excitotoxic brain injury is enhanced in mice lacking the p55 tumor necrosis factor receptor. *J Cereb Blood Flow Metab,* 18, 1283–7.

Ginsberg, M. D., Globus, M. Y. T., Dietrich, W. D., and Busto, R. (1993). Temperature modulation of ischemic brain injury - a synthesis of recent advances. *Progress in Brain Research,* 96, 13–22.

Giulian, D., Beth Leara, J. L., and Keenen, C. (1994). Phagocytic microglia release cytokines and cytotoxins that regulate the survival of astrocytes and neurones in culture. *Neurochemistry International,* 25, 227–33.

Giulian, D., Vaca, K., and Corpuz, M. (1993). Brain glia release factors with opposing actions on neuronal survival. *J Neurosci,* 13, 29–37.

Giulian, D., Woodward, J., Young, D. G., Krebs, J. F., and Lachman, L. B. (1988). Interleukin-1 injected into mammalian brain stimulates astrogliosis and neovascularisation. *J Neurosci,* 8, 2485–90.

Halliday, G., Robinson, S. R, Shepherd, C., and Kril, J. (2000). Alzheimer's disease and inflammation: a review of cellular and therapeutic mechanisms. *Clin Exp Pharmacol Physiol,* 27, 1–8.

Hama, T., Kushima, Y., Miyamoto, M., Kubota, M., Takei, N., and Hatanaka, H. (1991). Interleukin-6 improves the survival of mesencephalic catecholaminergic and septal cholinergic neurons from postnatal, two-week-old rats in cultures. *Neuroscience,* 40, 445–52.

Hama, T., Miyamoto, M., Tsukui, H., Nishio, C., and Hatanaka, H. (1989). Interleukin-6 as a neurotrophic factor for promoting the survival of cultured basal forebrain cholinergic neurons from postnatal rats. *Neurosci Lett,* 104, 340–4.

Heyser, C. J., Masliah, E., Samimi, A., Campbell, I. L., and Gold L. H. (1997). Progressive decline in avoidance learning paralleled by inflammatory neurodegeneration in transgenic mice expressing interleukin 6 in the brain. *Proc Natl Acad Sci USA,* 94, 1500–5.

Holmin, S. and Mathiesen, T. (2000). Intracerebral administration of interleukin-1beta and induction of inflammation, apoptosis, and vasogenic edema. *J Neurosurg,* 92, 108–20.

Hunter, A. J. (1997). Calcium antagonists: their role in neuroprotection. *Int Rev Neurobiol*, **40**, 95–108.

Hurtado, O., Cardenas, A., Lizasoain, I., Bosca, L., Leza, J. C., Lorenzo, P., and Moro, M. A. (2001). Up-regulation of TNF-alpha convertase (TACE/ADAM17) after oxygen-glucose deprivation in rat forebrain slices. *Neuropharmacology*, **40**, 1094–102.

Iadecola, C. and Alexander, M. (2001). Cerebral ischemia and inflammation. *Curr Opin Neurol*, **14**, 89–94.

Jacobs, C. A., Baker, P. E., Roux E. R., Picha, K. S., Toivola, B., Waugh, S., and Kennedy, M. K. (1991). Experimental autoimmune encephalomyelitis is exacerbated by IL- 1α and suppressed by soluble IL-1 receptor. *J Immunol*, **146**, 2983–9.

Jeohn, G. H., Kong, L. Y., Wilson, B., Hudson, P., and Hong, J. S. (1998). Synergistic neurotoxic effects of combined treatments with cytokines in murine primary mixed neuron/glia cultures. *J Neuroimmunol*, **85**, 1–10.

Jin, Y. X., Xu, L. Y., Guo, H., Ishikawa, M., Link, H., and Xiao, B. G. (2000). TGF-beta1 inhibits protracted-relapsing experimental autoimmune encephalomyelitis by activating dendritic cells. *J Autoimmun*, **14**, 213–20.

Karp, C. L., Boxel-Dezaire, A. H., Byrnes, A. A., and Nagelkerken, L. (2001). Interferon-beta in multiple sclerosis: altering the balance of interleukin-12 and interleukin-10? *Curr Opin Neurol*, **14**, 361–8.

Khademi, M., Wallstrom, E., Andersson, M., Piehl, F., Di Marco, R., and Olsson, T. (2000). Reduction of both pro- and anti-inflammatory cytokines after 6 months of interferon beta-1a treatment of multiple sclerosis. *J Neuroimmunol*, **103**, 202–10.

Kinouchi, K., Brown, G., Pasternak, G., and Donner, D. B. (1991). Identification and characterization of receptors for tumor necrosis factor-α in the brain. *Biochem Biophys Res Commun*, **181**, 1532–8.

Kinter, A., Arthos, J., Cicala, C., and Fauci, A. S. (2000). Chemokines, cytokines and HIV: a complex network of interactions that influence HIV pathogenesis. *Immunol Rev*, **177**, 88–98.

Knoblach, S. M. and Faden, A. I. (1998). Interleukin-10 improves outcome and alters proinflammatory cytokine expression after experimental traumatic brain injury. *Exp Neurol*, **153**, 143–51.

Kushima, Y., Hama, T., and Hatanaka, H. (1992). Interleukin-6 as a neurotrophic factor for promoting the survival of cultured catecholaminergic neurons in a chemically defined medium. *Neuroscience Research*, **13**, 267–80.

Lawrence, C. B., Allan, S. M., and Rothwell N. J. (1998). Interleukin-1beta and the interleukin-1 receptor antagonist act in the striatum to modify excitotoxic brain damage in the rat. *Eur J Neurosci*, **10**, 1188–95.

Lipton, S. A. (1994). Ca^{2+}, N-methyl-D-aspartate receptors, and AIDS-related neuronal injury. *Int Rev Neurobiol*, **36**, 1–27.

Loddick, S. A. and Rothwell, N. J. (1996). Neuroprotective effects of human recombinant interleukin-1 receptor antagonist in focal cerebral ischaemia in the rat. *J Cereb Blood Flow Metab*, **16**, 932–40.

Loddick, S. A. and Rothwell, N. J. (1999). Mechanisms of tumor necrosis factor alpha action on neurodegeneration: interaction with insulin-like growth factor-1. *Proc Natl Acad Sci USA*, **96**, 9449–51.

Loddick, S. A., Turnbull, A. V., and Rothwell, N. J. (1998). Cerebral interleukin-6 is neuroprotective during permanent focal cerebral ischemia in the rat. *J Cereb Blood Flow Metab*, **18**, 176–9.

Loddick, S. A., Wong, M. L., Bongiorno, P. B., Gold, P. W., Licinio, J., and Rothwell, N. J. (1997). Endogenous interleukin-1 receptor antagonist is neuroprotective. *Biochem Biophys Res Commun*, **234**, 211–15.

Lye, T. C. and Shores, E. A. (2000). Traumatic brain injury as a risk factor for Alzheimer's disease: a review. *Neuropsychol Rev*, **10**, 115–29.

Martin, D., Miller, G., Neuberger, T., Relton, J., and Fischer, N. (1998). Role of IL-1 in neurodegeneration. Pre-clinical findings with IL-1ra and ICE inhibitors. In *Neuroinflammation: mechanisms and management* (ed. P. L. Wood) Humana Press Inc., Totowa, pp. 197–219.

Matsuda, S., Wen, T. C., Morita, F., Otsuka, H., Igase, K., Yoshimura, H., and Sakanaka, M. (1996). Interleukin-6 prevents ischemia-induced learning disability and neuronal and synaptic loss in gerbils. *Neurosci Lett*, **204**, 109–12.

Mattson, M. P., Duan, W., Pedersen, W. A., and Culmsee, C. (2001). Neurodegenerative disorders and ischemic brain diseases. *Apoptosis*, **6**, 69–81.

McGeer, P. L., McGeer, E. G., and Yasojima, K. (2000). Alzheimer disease and neuroinflammation. *J Neural Transm Suppl*, **59**, 53–7.

Merrill, J. E. and Chen, I. S. (1991). HIV-1, macrophages, glial cells and cytokines in AIDS nervous system disease. *FASEB J*, **5**, 2391–7.

Merrill, J. E. and Murphy, S. P. (1997). Inflammatory events at the blood brain barrier: regulation of adhesion molecules, cytokines, and chemokines by reactive nitrogen and oxygen species. *Brain Behav Immun*, **11**, 245–63.

Mogi, M. and Nagatsu, T. (1999). Neurotrophins and cytokines in Parkinson's disease. *Adv Neurol*, **80**, 135–9.

Nagatsu, T., Mogi, M., Ichinose, H., and Togari, A. (2000). Cytokines in Parkinson's disease. *J Neural Transm Suppl*, **58**, 143–51.

Nawashiro, H., Tasaki, K., Ruetzler, C. A., and Hallenbeck, J. M. (1997). TNF-alpha pretreatment induces protective effects against focal cerebral ischemia in mice. *J Cereb Blood Flow Metab*, **17**, 483–90.

Nishimura, M., Mizuta, I., Mizuta, E., Yamasaki, S., Ohta, M., and Kuno, S. (2000). Influence of interleukin-1beta gene polymorphisms on age-at-onset of sporadic Parkinson's disease. *Neurosci Lett*, **284**, 73–6.

O'Keefe, G. M, Nguyen, V. T., and Benveniste, E. N. (1999). Class II transactivator and class II MHC gene expression in microglia: modulation by the cytokines TGF-beta, IL-4, IL-13 and IL-10. *Eur J Immunol*, **29**, 1275–85.

O'Meara E. S., Kukull, W. A., Sheppard, L., Bowen, J. D., McCormick, W. C., Teri, L., et al. (1997). Head injury and risk of Alzheimer's disease by apolipoprotein E genotype. *Am J Epidemiol*, **146**, 373–84.

Ohtsuki, T., Ruetzler, C. A., Tasaki, K., and Hallenbeck, J. M. (1996). Interleukin-1 mediates induction of tolerance to global ischemia in gerbil hippocampal CA1 neurons. *J Cereb Blood Flow Metab*, **16**, 1137–42.

Ozenci, V., Kouwenhoven, M., Teleshova, N., Pashenkov, M., Fredrikson, S., and Link, H. (2000). Multiple sclerosis: pro- and anti-inflammatory cytokines and metalloproteinases are affected differentially by treatment with IFN-beta. *J Neuroimmunol*, **108**, 236–43.

Panegyres, P. K. and Hughes, J. (1998). The neuroprotective effects of the recombinant interleukin-1 receptor antagonist rhIL-1ra after excitotoxic stimulation with kainic acid and its relationship to the amyloid precursor protein gene. *J Neurol Sci*, **154**, 123–32.

Penkowa, M., Moos, T., Carrasco, J., Hadberg, H., Molinero, A., Bluethmann, H., and Hidalgo, J. (1999). Strongly compromised inflammatory response to brain injury in interleukin-6-deficient mice. *Glia*, **25**, 343–57.

Perrella, O., Carreiri, P. B., Perrella, A., Sbreglia, C., Gorga, F., Guarnaccia, D., and Tarantino, G. (2001). Transforming growth factor beta-1 and interferon-alpha in the AIDS dementia complex (ADC): possible relationship with cerebral viral load? *Eur Cytokine Netw*, **12**, 51–5.

Perry, V. H., Bolton, S. J., Anthony, D. C., and Betmouni, S. (1998). The contribution of inflammation to acute and chronic neurodegeneration. *Res Immunol*, **149**, 721–5.

Poli, G. and Fauci, A. S. (1993). Cytokine modulation of HIV expression. *Semin Immunol*, **5**, 165–73.

Pratt, B. M. and McPherson, J. M. (1997). TGF-beta in the central nervous system: potential roles in ischemic injury and neurodegenerative diseases. *Cytokine Growth Factor Rev*, **8**, 267–92.

Prehn, J. H., Backhauss, C., and Krieglstein, J. (1993). Transforming growth factor-beta 1 prevents glutamate neurotoxicity in rat neocortical cultures and protects mouse neocortex from ischemic injury in vivo. *J Cereb Blood Flow Metab*, **13**, 521–5.

Prehn, J. H. and Krieglstein, J. (1994). Opposing effects of transforming growth factor-beta 1 on glutamate neurotoxicity. *Neuroscience*, **60**, 7–10.

Prehn, J. H. and Miller, R. J. (1996). Opposite effects of TGF-beta 1 on rapidly- and slowly-triggered excitotoxic injury. *Neuropharmacology*, **35**, 249–56.

Pringle, A. K., Niyadurupola, N., Johns, P., Anthony, D. C., and Iannotti, F. (2001). Interleukin-1beta exacerbates hypoxia-induced neuronal damage, but attenuates toxicity produced by simulated ischaemia and excitotoxicity in rat organotypic hippocampal slice cultures. *Neurosci Lett*, **305**, 29–32.

Raivich, G., Bohatschek, M., Kloss, C. U., Werner, A., Jones, L. L., and Kreutzberg, G. W. (1999*a*). Neuroglial activation repertoire in the injured brain: graded response, molecular mechanisms and cues to physiological function. *Brain Res Brain Res Rev*, **30**, 77–105.

Raivich, G., Jones, L. L., Werner, A., Bluthmann, H., Doetschmann, T., and Kreutzberg, G. W. (1999*b*). Molecular signals for glial activation: pro- and anti-inflammatory cytokines in the injured brain. *Acta Neurochir Suppl (Wien)*, **73**, 21–30.

Relton, J. K., Martin, D., Thompson, R. C., and Russell, D. A. (1996). Peripheral administration of Interleukin-1 Receptor antagonist inhibits brain damage after focal cerebral ischemia in the rat. *Exp Neurol*, **138**, 206–13.

Ren, R. F. and Flanders, K. C. (1996). Transforming growth factors-beta protect primary rat hippocampal neuronal cultures from degeneration induced by beta-amyloid peptide. *Brain Res*, **732**, 16–24.

Rogers, J. and Shen, Y. (2000). A perspective on inflammation in Alzheimer's disease. *Ann N Y Acad Sci*, **924**, 132–5.

Rostasy, K., Monti, L., Yiannoutsos, C., Wu, J., Bell, J., Hedreen, J., and Navia, B. A. (2000). NFkappaB activation, TNF-alpha expression, and apoptosis in the AIDS-Dementia-Complex. *J Neurovirol*, **6**, 537–43.

Rothwell, N. J. and Luheshi, G. N. (2000). Interleukin 1 in the brain: biology, pathology and therapeutic target. *Trends Neurosci*, **23**, 618–25.

Ruocco, A., Nicole, O., Docagne, F., Ali, C., Chazalviel, L., Komesli, S., *et al.* (1999). A transforming growth factor-beta antagonist unmasks the neuroprotective role of this endogenous cytokine in excitotoxic and ischemic brain injury. *J Cereb Blood Flow Metab*, **19**, 1345–53.

Scherbel, U., Raghupathi, R., Nakamura, M., Saatman, K. E., Trojanowski, J. Q., Neugebauer, E., *et al.* (1999). Differential acute and chronic responses of tumor necrosis factor-deficient mice to experimental brain injury. *Proc Natl Acad Sci USA*, **96**, 8721–6.

Shohami, E., Ginis, I., and Hallenbeck, J. M. (1999). Dual role of tumor necrosis factor alpha in brain injury. *Cytokine Growth Factor Rev*, **10**, 119–30.

Sotrel, A. and Dal Canto, M. C. (2000). HIV-1 and its causal relationship to immunosuppression and nervous system disease in AIDS: a review. *Hum Pathol*, **31**, 1274–98.

Spera, P. A., Ellison, J. A., Feuerstein, G. Z., and Barone, F. C. (1998). IL-10 reduces rat brain injury following focal stroke. *Neurosci Lett*, **251**, 189–92.

Strijbos, P. J. and Rothwell, N. J. (1995). Interleukin-1 beta attenuates excitatory amino acid-induced neurodegeneration in vitro: involvement of nerve growth factor. *J Neurosci*, **15**, 3468–74.

Tarkowski, E., Rosengren, L., Blomstrand, C., Wikkelso, C., Jensen, C., Ekholm, S., and Tarkowski, A. (1997). Intrathecal release of pro- and anti-inflammatory cytokines during stroke. *Clin Exp Immunol*, **110**, 492–9.

Taupin, V., Renno, T., Bourbonniere, L., Peterson, A. C., Rodriguez, M., and Owens, T. (1997). Increased severity of experimental autoimmune encephalomyelitis, chronic macrophage/microglial reactivity, and demyelination in transgenic mice producing tumor necrosis factor-alpha in the central nervous system. *Eur J Immunol*, **27**, 905–13.

Taupin, V., Toulmond, S., Serrano, A., Benavides, J., and Zavala, F. (1993). Increase in IL-6, IL-1 and TNF levels in rat brain following traumatic lesion. Influence of pre-and-post-traumatic treatment with Ro54864, a peripheral-type (p site) benzodiazepine ligand. *J Neuroimmunol*, **42**, 177–85.

Taverne, J. (1993). Transgenic mice in the study of cytokine function. *International Journal of Experimental Pathology*, **74**, 525–46.

Toulmond, S. and Rothwell, N. (1995). Interleukin-1 receptor antagonist inhibits neuronal damage caused by fluid percussion injury in the rat. *Brain Res*, **671**, 261–6.

Touzani, O., Boutin, H., LeFeuvre, R., Parker, L., Miller, A., Luheshi, G. and Rothwell, N. (2002). Interleukin-1 influences ischaemic brain damage in the mouse independently of the interleukin-1 type 1 receptor. *J Neurosci*, **22**, 38–43.

Touzani, O., Boutin, H., Chuquet, J., and Rothwell, N. (1999). Potential mechanisms of interleukin-1 involvement in cerebral ischaemia. *J Neuroimmunol*, **100**, 203–15.

Vannier, E., Miller, L. C., and Dinarello, C. A. (1992). Coordinated antiinflammatory effects of interleukin 4: Interleukin 4 suppresses interleukin 1 production but up-regulates gene expression and synthesis of interleukin 1 receptor antagonist. *Proc Natl Acad Sci USA*, **89**, 4076–80.

Venters, H. D., Tang, Q., Liu, Q., VanHoy, R. W, Dantzer, R., and Kelley, K. W. (1999). A new mechanism of neurodegeneration: a proinflammatory cytokine inhibits receptor signaling by a survival peptide. *Proc Natl Acad Sci USA*, **96**, 9879–84.

Wong, D. and Dorovini-Zis, K. (1996). Regulation by cytokines and lipopolysaccharide of E-selectin expression by human brain microvessel endothelial cells in primary culture. *J Neuropathol Exp Neurol*, **55**, 225–35.

Yamada, M. and Hatanaka, H. (1994). Interleukin-6 protects cultured rat hippocampal neurons against glutamate-induced cell death. *Brain Res*, **643**, 173–80.

Yamasaki, Y., Matsuura, N., Shozuhara, H., Onodera, H., Itoyama, Y., and Kogure, K. (1995). Interleukin-1 as a pathogenetic mediator of ischemic brain damage in rats. *Stroke*, **26**, 676–80.

Yang, Y., Quitschke, W. W., and Brewer, G. J. (1998). Upregulation of amyloid precursor protein gene promoter in rat primary hippocampal neurons by phorbol ester, IL-1 and retinoic acid, but not by reactive oxygen species. *Brain Res Mol Brain Res*, **60**, 40–9.

Zhu, S. G., Sheng, J. G., Jones, R. A., Brewer, M. M., Zhou, X. Q., Mrak, R. E., and Griffin, W. S. (1999). Increased interleukin-1beta converting enzyme expression and activity in Alzheimer disease. *J Neuropathol Exp Neurol*, **58**, 582–7.

Zipfel, G. J., Babcock, D. J., Lee, J. M., and Choi, D. W. (2000). Neuronal apoptosis after CNS injury: the roles of glutamate and calcium. *J Neurotrauma*, **17**, 857–69.

Chapter 8

Inflammatory responses to traumatic brain injury: an overview for the new millennium

Maria-Cristina Morganti-Kossmann, Mario Rancan, Philip F. Stahel, and Thomas Kossmann

8.1 Introduction

In recent decades, science has made huge strides, increasing human possibilities and extending man's reach with undreamed-of inventions. From the medical point of view—although diseases of other aetiologies receive more media attention, biomedical research and supporting foundations—traumatic brain injury (TBI) will remain the leading cause of death in individuals up to the age of 45 (Kraus *et al.* 1996). Even if patients survive a severe cerebral injury, the disabilities affect the familiar and economical aspects of social life.

Primary brain injury has been classified into two main categories, focal and diffuse damage. Focal brain injury is easily identified through the available diagnostic methodologies, while diffuse brain damage is more difficult to recognize, especially in the absence of focal lesions. Clinically, both focal and diffuse injuries are often present simultaneously in TBI patients (Graham *et al.* 2000; Maxwell *et al.* 1997). Secondary brain injury begins at the time of trauma, but can appear with a delay of hours or days from the primary insult, and is the result of a complex network of vascular, cellular and biochemical cascades leading to inflammation, swelling, raised intracranial pressure, and ischaemia (Baethmann *et al.* 1988; Graham *et al.* 2000; McIntosh *et al.* 1996). Extensive research revealed that focal and diffuse brain damage possess individual pathophysiologies. While much effort has been dedicated to focal brain injury, the pathophysiology of diffuse brain injury and the mechanisms leading to axonal disruption and dysfunction, still remain poorly understood. In this regard, the diversity and combination of the injury patterns found in TBI patients makes the search for an appropriate therapy a difficult task.

The major obstacle facing researchers and clinicians is the complex pathophysiology of secondary TBI which is characterized by activation of distinct cascades causing the release of excitatory aminoacids, proteases, reactive oxygen intermediates, ions, complement proteins, and other immune mediators (Baethmann *et al.* 1988; McIntosh *et al.* 1996). In addition, breakdown of the blood–brain barrier (BBB) contributes to the disturbance of normal physiology by allowing the passage of serum proteins and blood cells into the intrathecal compartment. The perturbation of cerebral homeostasis is at the basis of defective cerebral perfusion, brain edema formation, increased intracranial pressure, and ultimately neurological deficit, which are all clinical features of severe TBI. The management of TBI patients has been improved considerably in recent decades in particular due to advanced concepts of critical care (Neugebauer *et al.* 2000; Stocker *et al.* 1995). However, this progress is not sufficient to control the onset and degree of secondary insults which exacerbate the primary damage of the brain tissue and affect neurological outcome. The failure of several clinical trials based on the previous success in animal models of TBI, has brought profound scepticism in the development of effective therapy (Reinert and Bullock 1999).

The impact of neuroinflammation on the onset of secondary brain damage is a controversial issue due to the accepted dual role of cytokines in neuropathology (Allan and Rothwell 2001; Morganti-Kossmann *et al.* 1997; Morganti-Kossmann *et al.* 2000; Shohami *et al.* 1999). There is experimental evidence for a beneficial as well as a detrimental role of immunoactivation in the injured brain, which can contribute to tissue destruction and promote tissue repair. This chapter will review the controversial role of inflammatory responses after TBI resulting from clinical and experimental studies. Emphasis will be given to the interaction of immune-competent cells of the central nervous system (CNS) with the systemic immune system, the characterization of mediators and factors participating in the immunological processes as well as the controversy of the protective versus the deleterious consequences of immunoactivation will be discussed.

8.2 The inflammatory cascade

8.2.1 Cell activation and cell death

The previous definition of the nervous system as a 'immunologically priviledged site' is essentially based on its separation from the blood circulation mediated by a unique type of endothelium forming the BBB (Rubin and Staddon 1999). Tight junctions established between endothelial cells of cerebral microvessels, supported by astrocytes, play a fundamental role in mediating the exchange between the systemic circulation and the nervous tissue. Under normal circumstances, the function of the BBB is to provide a relative impermeability to most proteins, peptides, amino acids, and haematopoietic cells. Rupture of the BBB occurs rapidly following TBI allowing leakage of serum components and blood cells into the cerebral parenchyma, thereby initiating a cascade of molecular events contributing to immunoactivation (Clark *et al.* 1994; Soares *et al.* 1995). Extravasation of blood-derived leucocytes requires secretion of chemotactic factors (or chemokines) (Asensio and Campbell 1999) which attract these cells to the inflammatory foci, and upregulation of adhesion molecules necessary for promoting cellular adherence to the endothelium (Sobel *et al.* 1990). Neutrophils are the first cells entering the brain after trauma, followed by monocytes/macrophages and later, resident microglia, astrocytes and neurones become activated. Once recruited into the brain, leucocytes secrete many pro-inflammatory cytokines, oxygen radicals, nitric oxide, proteinases as well as neurotrophic factors and display an enhanced expression of major histocompatibility complex (MHC) antigen. Activated cells go through a process of cytoskeletal reorganization which allows motility (neutrophils, monocytes/macrophages), whereas others phagocytose the debris of damaged tissue (macrophages/microglia), proliferate to form a scar (fibroblasts/astrocytes), or undergo necrotic/apoptotic cell death (neurones). Altogether, these changes promote a complex intercellular communication between peripheral leucocytes accumulated in the brain and resident cells of the CNS mediated by the interaction of multiple ligand-receptor systems.

In the last decade, the mechanisms of cell death after TBI have received increased attention. Processes leading to brain atrophy and neuronal loss persist for a long time after trauma in humans and in rodents subjected to experimental head injury (Conti *et al.* 1998; Fox *et al.* 1998; Smith *et al.* 1997). The processes which remain chronically activated in the post-traumatic period need to be identified. Evidence for apoptotic as well as necrotic cell death involving neurones, astrocytes and endothelial cells, has been reported in the brain of rats subjected to fluid percussion injury and controlled cortical impact injury (Fox *et al.* 1998; Kaya *et al.* 1999; Newcomb *et al.* 1999; Rink *et al.* 1995). Neuronal cell death is a very complex phenomenon possibly resulting from events occurring simultaneously in response to trauma. Among these, the release of excitatory amino acids and reactive oxygen species, mitochondrial dysfunction and consequent energy failure as well as sequestration of neuro-trophins have been recognized following TBI. Within the cascade of apoptotic cell death, the involvement of Fas/Fas-ligand(L), the tumor suppressor gene p53 and caspases, (in particular of caspase-3) as also of anti-apoptotic factors like Bcl-2 have been found in various experimental models of TBI and in patients (Beer *et al.* 2000; Clark *et al.* 1997; Clark *et al.* 2000*a*; Clark *et al.* 1999; Clark *et al.* 2000*b*; Ertel *et al.* 1997; Kaya *et al.* 1999; Napieralski *et al.* 1999; Yakovlev *et al.* 1997). Although apoptosis has been defined as a process of cell death independent from immunoactivation, in experimental TBI, apoptotic cell death has been observed at time points corresponding to the elevation of cerebral cytokine produc-tion. Whether or not inflammatory mediators can be considered as potential factors mediating neuronal cell death after TBI is still awaiting further experimental evidence (Morganti-Kossmann and Kossmann 1995; Morganti-Kossmann *et al.* 1997; Morganti-Kossmann *et al.* 2000). However, inflammation seems at least to modulate apoptosis indirectly, as the cytokines IL-1, IL-6, tumour necrosis factor (TNF), and IFN-γ have been shown to enhance the constitutive expression of Fas and FasL by cultured human astrocytes. FasL-bearing astrocytes also undergo apoptosis *in vitro*, and induce apoptosis of co-cultured lymphocytes, suggesting that this mechanism of cell death may also occur after brain injury possibly involving neuronal cells (Choi *et al.* 1999). After controlled cortical impact injury, Fas expression has been identified on cortical astrocytes and neurones, while FasL increased also in microglial cells, and both stainings overlapped with the regions displaying the highest distribution of TUNEL positive cells. Further downstream in the apoptotic cascade, the activation of poly-ADP-ribose-synthase by DNA strands, an enzyme mediating DNA repair, has been demonstrated early (30 min) in the injured cortex and is cleaved later on (1 week) when it may impair delayed repair of damaged DNA (LaPlaca *et al.* 1999). Particularly after experimental axonal injury, the alterations caused by tear-shearing injury of axonal membrane lead to Ca^{++} influx, cytoskeleton changes and mitochondrial swelling which is determined by the opening of the membrane permeability transition pores. Expression of cytochrome-c and caspase-3 has been associated with brain regions with greater mitochondrial damage, thus converging the cascade of apoptotic cell death and energy failure. Administration of the immunosuppressive agent cyclosporin A, by inhibiting mitochondrial membrane permeability, protects the mitochondria, decreases significantly axonal cytoskeletal changes and augments axonal survival (Buki *et al.* 1999; Buki *et al.* 2000).

Studies on neuronal cell death induced by TBI may offer the opportunity to develop novel therapeutical strategies based on the administration of factors which inhibit cell death at different levels of the pathway. For instance, cerebral protection may be obtained by applying anti-apoptotic factors like Bcl-2 since transgenic mice overexpressing this molecule exhibit a significant decrease in the lesion size after controlled cortical impact injury (Raghupathi *et al.* 1998).

8.2.2 The cytokine cascade

The role cytokines play in the CNS has been investigated in various CNS pathologies (Allan and Rothwell 2001; Benveniste 1995; Morganti-Kossmann *et al.* 2000). They are secreted rapidly and are the main regulators of the initiation, propagation and termination of the inflammatory response. Cytokines are usually defined as pro- or anti-inflammatory based on their ability to promote or suppress immunoactivation. Their binding counterparts are high affinity receptors which transduce signals resulting in the induction of distinct and often opposite biological activities (Otero and Merrill 1994). The expression of cytokines and cytokine-receptors during the development of the nervous system as well as in normal adult brain has indicated that, besides their classical role as immune mediators, these molecules are also involved in embryogenesis and maintainance of normal functions of the CNS. Several reports from clinical as well as experimental studies have demonstrated that numerous immune mediators are upregulated in response to TBI, as seen from immuno-histochemical analysis and/or ELISA, and mRNA expression by either northern blot analysis or *in situ* hybridization. IL-6, TNF, ICAM-1, IL-8, transforming growth factor (TGF)-β and IL-10 represent the most investigated factors acting as pro-, anti-inflammatory or chemo-tactic agents and as adhesion molecules. The association of elevated immune parameters with the extent of cerebral damage, BBB dysfunction, leucocyte infiltration and neurological impairment suggested a detrimental role of neuroinflammation. However, recent data based mainly on the blockade of cytokines in TBI models through the administration of specific antagonists or on the use of transgenic mice, have demonstrated that cytokines possess a dual action and that their presence is fundamental for the process of tissue repair, regen-eration, and neurological recovery (Morganti-Kossmann *et al.* 1997).

8.2.3 Interleukin-6: how the brain influences the periphery

Interleukin-6 (IL-6) is a pleiotropic cytokine which is produced by a variety of immune and non-immune cells (Taga and Kishimoto 1997). This potent inducer of B-cell differentiation and immunoglobulin synthesis as well as of the acute phase response (Akira and Kishimoto 1992) is produced within the CNS by glial cells and also by cultured neuronal cells upon the exposure to different stimuli (Marz *et al.* 1998; Schobitz *et al.* 1995). Upregulation of IL-6 synthesis has been reported in various disorders of the CNS such as stroke, viral and bacterial meningitis, brain tumours, AIDS-related dementia complex, multiple sclerosis (MS) and Alzheimer's disease (Gruol and Nelson 1997; Morganti-Kossmann *et al.* 2000).

Several reports have demonstrated that IL-6 production is elevated after TBI in patients and in rodents subjected to various types of focal and diffuse brain injury (Hans *et al.* 1999*a*; Kossmann *et al.* 1995; McClain *et al.* 1991; Shohami *et al.* 1994; Taupin *et al.* 1993; Woodroofe *et al.* 1991). Our group reported previously that IL-6 is significantly elevated in the cerebrospinal fluid (CSF) compared to serum of patients with severe isolated head trauma. Interestingly, maximal concentrations of IL-6 in serum correlated with the peak levels of the acute phase proteins C-reactive protein, α1-antitrypsin and fibrinogen (Kossmann *et al.* 1995). This suggests that IL-6 produced in higher amounts intrathecally may cross the disrupted BBB, enter the peripheral circulation and induce the acute phase response.

This novel concept that cytokines produced in the injured brain may influence peripheral tissue is further corroborated by the correlation between CSF- and serum-IL-6 only with simultaneous BBB dysfunction in these patients. Furthermore, cerebral immunoactivation induced in rats can modulate IL-6 production in the periphery as well as the acute phase response (De Simoni *et al.* 1993). Thus, it is conceivable that IL-6 produced intrathecally may induce BBB dysfunction, enter the peripheral circulation and then activate other organs. The work by our group reported here was one of the first suggesting that some clinical manifestations observed in patients with severe head trauma may be initiated by cerebral immunoactivation.

8.2.4 IL-6 is a potential neurotrophic factor after traumatic brain injury

Interleukin-6 is the first cytokine to which a neurotrophic activity has been attributed through direct actions on neuronal cultures or indirectly through the induction of the nerve growth factor (NGF) by astrocytes (Frei *et al.* 1989). However, IL-6 also seems to be neurotoxic under certain circumstances depending on the type of neuronal cells (Gruol and Nelson 1997). An association of IL-6 with NGF was demonstrated in patients with severe TBI, since NGF was only present in the CSF of those individuals with higher IL-6 concentrations (Kossmann *et al.* 1996). To test this molecular dependency, primary mouse astrocytes were stimulated *in vitro* with human CSF containing IL-6 with and without pretreatment with anti-IL-6 antibodies. These experiments showed that human CSF induced NGF by astrocytes and that pre-incubation of CSF with neutralizing IL-6 antibodies attenuated the production of NGF by these cells (Kossmann *et al.* 1996). Taken together, these experiments suggest that the elevation of NGF in the CSF of patients with severe TBI may derive by astrocyte production stimulated by IL-6 which, in turn, could be released by reactive glial cells as well as leucocytes infiltrated into the brain parenchyma.

Several studies have addressed the physiological or pathological role of IL-6 in CNS disease. Two different kinds of transgenic mice with overexpression of IL-6 in the brain have been generated, one specifically expressed by neurones via the neurone specific enolase promotor (NSE-IL-6) and the other by astrocytes via the glial fibrillary acidic protein (GFAP) promotor (GFAP-IL-6) (Campbell *et al.* 1993; Fattori *et al.* 1995). Although both types of transgenic animals showed increased astrogliosis and activated microglia, the NSE-IL-6 mice did not exhibit neurological abnormalities. In contrast, GFAP-IL-6 animals exhibited severe neurological dysfunction in conjunction with neuronal loss, BBB breakdown and vascular pathology. These data show that chronic and dysregulated expression of IL-6 by astrocytes may contribute to neuropathology and that different biological responses may occur depending on the cell type producing this cytokine.

The elevation of cytokines in the CSF of TBI patients does not provide information on their cellular source within the intracranial space. A diffusion process from the brain tissue can be assumed for the passage of soluble molecules into the CSF through a pressure driven bulk flow into the ventricular system (Rosenberg *et al.* 1980). However, macrophages present in the choroid plexus or in the subarachnoid spaces may also release IL-6 directly into the CSF (Ohata *et al.* 1990). In order to clarify this issue, experimental models of TBI are required. It is widely accepted that animal models do not represent with fidelity the injury patterns occurring in humans (Laurer *et al.* 2000). However, the data derived from such studies have offered valuable information on molecular and cellular activation pathways after TBI. The key may be to examine identical processes using different models, such as focal versus diffuse injury, as well as to combine different types of lesions or to add clinical complications like hypoxia which are frequent in patients with severe TBI.

We tried to extend clinical findings using animal models, and studied the release of IL-6 into CSF in parallel to brain parenchyma expression in a rat model of traumatic axonal injury (Hans *et al.* 1999*b*). This impact acceleration injury model can be considered clinically relevant since it has been reported that axonal injury is very frequent in patients with fatal closed TBI, and has been associated with high morbidity and poor outcome (Gentleman *et al.* 1995). A second, fundamental aspect of the chosen model concerns the pathophysiology of traumatic axonal injury which still remains largely unexplored. In our study, an evident release of IL-6 into CSF was demonstrated in rats in the early hours after trauma which returned to the levels of sham operated animals within 24 h post-injury. Similarly to the study in humans, IL-6 concentrations in rat CSF always exceeded the levels in serum. Upregulation of IL-6 mRNA in the brain was localized predominantly on neurones in the cortex, thalamus, and macrophages within the subarachnoid spaces, whereas IL-6 protein expression was spread throughout the brain mainly in neurones (Hans *et al.* 1999*b*). In conclusion, these data strongly support the hypothesis that IL-6 measured in CSF may reflect the synthesis in brain parenchyma.

8.2.5 Tumour necrosis factor: a neurotoxic and neurotrophic cytokine

Tumour necrosis factor is produced in two forms, α (or cachectin) and β (or lymphotoxin), which are genetically related and share 30 per cent structural homology. TNF-α is secreted by macrophages which represent the major source of this mediator, as well as by T-cells, mast cells, microglia, and astrocytes, whereas TNF-β is produced predominantly by T-cells. It is assumed that TNF-α is the major mediator of endotoxic shock and tissue injury associated with endotoxaemia. Furthermore, passive immunization against TNF-α protects mice from normally lethal doses of LPS (Beutler *et al.* 1985). Much work has been dedicated to define the role played by TNF-α and -β in neuropathogenesis of a variety of CNS diseases. The cytotoxic effect of TNF on oligodendrocytes was believed to be the major cause of cell death and demyelination in the CNS of MS, experimental autoimmune encephalomyelitis (EAE) and AIDS-related dementia complex (Morganti-Kossmann *et al.* 1992; Morganti-Kossmann *et al.* 2000).

With regard to TBI, increased levels of TNF have been detected in human CSF exceeding the levels in serum (Csuka *et al.* 1999; Goodman *et al.* 1990; Ross *et al.* 1994). In experimental brain injury, cerebral upregulation of TNF has been described after fluid percussion injury, controlled cortical impact, closed head injury, and cerebral ischaemia (Fan *et al.* 1996; Liu *et al.* 1994; Shohami *et al.* 1994; Taupin *et al.* 1993). The early increase of TNF strongly suggested synthesis by resident CNS cells rather than by infiltrating leucocytes, TNF has been localized on neurones of the lesioned cortex by immunohistochemistry and was associated with neurological deficit as demonstrated by inhibition of its action by administration of the immunosuppressive mediator IL-10 (Knoblach and Faden 1998). More effective blockade of TNF was obtained by intraventricular injection of a soluble TNF receptor fusion protein or TNF binding protein corroborating the assumption of a cerebral synthesis and action of TNF (Knoblach *et al.* 1999; Shohami *et al.* 1996). Injection of TNF binding protein also resulted in attenuated brain oedema and BBB breakdown (Shohami et al. 1996).

Numerous studies have used inhibitors of TNF action in animal models of TBI (McIntosh et al. 1998; Shohami et al. 1999). Administration of general immunosuppressive agents such as pentoxifylline, HU-211 and IL-10 improve neuronal survival and neurological recovery of the animals (Knoblach and Faden 1998; Shohami et al. 1997).

Although TNF can induce the expression of intercellular adhesion molecule-1 (ICAM-1), BBB dysfunction and intrathecal infiltration of activated leucocytes—events considered detrimental for the injured brain—studies on TNF knockout animals, not only in TBI but also in EAE models, have revealed a dual role for TNF in neuropathology (Frohman et al. 1989; Kim et al. 1992; Morganti-Kossmann et al. 2000; Ramilo et al. 1990). Induction of NGF in astrocytes exposed to TNF as well as via the induction of the anti-inflammatory cytokine IL-10 may be at the basis of this neurotrophic activity (de Waal Malefyt et al. 1991; Gadient et al. 1990). TNF knockout mice subjected to controlled cortical impact injury revealed a deleterious effect of TNF early after trauma and beneficial function in the late phase with regard to neurological performance and tissue damage (Scherbel et al. 1999). We used TNF/LT-α double-knockout mice in a closed head injury model to show a higher post-traumatic mortality rate compared to wild type mice, suggesting a protective role for TNF as well as IL-6 after TBI. However, other parameters such as intrathecal leucocyte infiltration, BBB permeability and neurological impairment were not different between TNF/LT-α knockout and wild-type animals (Stahel et al. 2000b).

8.2.6 The adverseries: anti-inflammatory cytokines TGF-β and IL-10

Dysfunction of the immune system is one of the major complications observed in patients after TBI (Quattrocchi et al. 1992) and was initially attributed to the action of undefined tissue factors released by the injured brain. Anti-inflammatory cytokines are elevated after TBI and may be responsible for increased infection rate in these patients. Anti-inflammatory mediators may be important because cerebral immunoactivation could have deleterious consequences for the injured brain and contribute to secondary damage. This supports their potential therapeutic value. The most studied anti-inflammatory cytokines in neuropathology, TGF-β and IL-10, are induced by the classical pro-inflammatory cytokines and inhibit the production of IL-1, TNF, IFN-γ, oxygen radicals, MHC class II antigen expression, T-cell activation, adhesion of leucocytes and proliferation of various cells including astrocytes (de Waal Malefyt et al. 1991; Wahl 1994).

The beneficial role of anti-inflammatory cytokines has been suggested in various neurological diseases like bacterial meningitis, in which administration of TGF-β or IL-10 results in attenuated intracranial pressure, oedema and white blood cell count in CSF (Frei et al. 1993a; Frei et al. 1993b), while endogenous increases in IL-10 in EAE mice corresponded with decreased synthesis of inflammatory cytokines (Kennedy et al. 1992). Local administration of IL-10 following corticectomy reduces the number and the hypertrophic state of reactive astrocytes and microglia and diminished local expression of TNF mRNA (Balasingam and Yong 1996).

In TBI patients, IL-10 levels are higher in CSF than serum, whereas the opposite is true for TGF-β. Thus, due to differences in cytokine concentration, the passage of serum TGF-β to the CNS across the damaged BBB was hypothesized in response to trauma and supported by a strong correlation between TGF-β in CSF and the CSF-/serum-albumin quotient (Q_A) (Csuka *et al.* 1999; Morganti-Kossmann *et al.* 1999). Although TGF-β is a potent regulator of lymphocytic activities, the CD4/CD8 ratios in whole blood of head trauma patients remained within the normal range. Despite the advantageous effects of IL-10 described in animal models or *in vitro*, concentrations of IL-10 in CSF of children with TBI have been associated with higher mortality (Bell *et al.* 1997), and similarly in polytrauma patients highest IL-10 plasma measurements correlated with septical complications and multiple organ dysfunction syndrome (Neidhardt *et al.* 1997). Therefore, more experimental proof is needed to elucidate the exact functions of TGF-β and IL-10 in TBI.

8.2.7 ICAM-1 and IL-8: pivotal for the recruitment of neutrophils?

Tumour necrosis factor, together with IL-1 and IFN-γ, triggers the expression of chemotactic cytokines, also termed chemokines, and adhesion molecules. The presence of both agents is necessary for activation and accumulation of leucocytes into peripheral tissues. Chemokines are produced primarily by blood-derived leucocytes, however, there are several recent reports on their production by brain cells (Asensio and Campbell 1999; Glabinski and Ransohoff 1999; Ransohoff and Tani 1998). Most of these studies report regulation of IL-8, monocyte chemotactive protein-1 (MCP-1), macrophage inflammatory protein-1-α/β (MIP-1-α/β) *in vitro* by primary and transformed glial cells subjected to stimulation with pro- and anti-inflammatory cytokines and also after experimental brain injury (Hausmann *et al.* 1998).

In TBI, neutrophils recruitment is followed by activated monocyte/macrophages, microglial cells, and later astrocytes (Aihara *et al.* 1995). Due to their ability to release neurotoxic molecules, neutrophils are considered as potentially harmful cells for the injured brain, contributing to BBB dysfunction and neuronal damage, but reports are conflicting (Whalen *et al.* 1999b). Relevant for neutrophil action is the chemokine IL-8, which is a potent activator and chemotactic factor for these cells (Baggiolini *et al.* 1997). In parallel, the action of adhesion molecules (e.g. E-selectin and ICAM-1) triggered on endothelial cells by pro-inflammatory mediators, is fundamental for leucocyte transmigration which often occurs concomitant to BBB dysfunction (Carlos *et al.* 1997; Soares *et al.* 1995). ICAM-1 can be expressed in two forms, as a transmembrane as well as a released soluble protein deriving from either proteolytic cleavage or alternative RNA splicing (King *et al.* 1995). Expression of ICAM-1 in normal brain is low and increased in neuropathology. We showed that the concentrations of sICAM-1 in CSF of TBI patients correlates with cerebral contusion size assessed by CT after trauma (Pleines *et al.* 1998). The role of ICAM-1 and the recruitment of neutrophils in neurotrauma is quite controversial. Anti-ICAM-1 antibodies in TBI rats or ICAM-1 knockout mice exposed to stroke show reduced leucocyte infiltration, oedema, infarct size, neurological damage and improved survival (Bowes *et al.* 1993; Connolly *et al.* 1996). However, ICAM-1 knockout animals exposed to controlled cortical impact injury do not show differences in neutrophil infiltration, histological injury and functional outcome when compared to control animals (Whalen *et al.* 1999a). Thus, this study failed to support a role for ICAM-1 in the pathogenesis of TBI. Other adhesion molecules like E-selectin may have a stronger impact on cellular adhesion and migration since its maximal expression preceded neutrophil accumulation after cortical impact. However, both phenomena occurred with a significant delay (8 and 24 h, respectively for E-selectin and neutrophil infiltration) compared to the time of maximal BBB dysfunction (Whalen *et al.* 1998). Mechanical tear of the vessels in response to a traumatic impact may also cause a rapid damage of the cerebral endothelium in a fashion similar to that causing traumatic axonal damage. Stretching of vessels may activate cytokine expression as shown in an *in vitro* model of endothelial cell percussion injury resulting in increased TNF and IL-1 production. Therefore, enhanced ICAM-1 expression on cerebral endothelium may be due to upregulation by these pro-inflammatory mediators (Gourin and Shackford 1997). In accordance with these data, we have demonstrated a temporal upregulation of ICAM-1 in two models of TBI, one of experimental axonal injury and the other of focal closed head injury. ICAM-1 is increased at later time points compared to maximal neutrophil accumulation in the injured brain. After closed head injury, with peak infiltration of neutrophils at 24 h after trauma (Clark *et al.* 1994), maximal expression of ICAM-1 in brain homogenates appeared 7 days after injury, considerably later than cell migration (Otto *et al.* 2000). In addition, after moderate traumatic axonal injury, increased ICAM-1 expression detected histologically on cerebral microvessels also appeared at later time points and in complete absence of neutrophil accumulation, suggesting an alternative role for this molecule independent from the adhesion of neutrophils (Rancan *et al.* 2001). Dissociation of neutrophil infiltration from the expression of adhesion molecules was reported in ICAM-1/P-selectin double deficient mice subjected to experimental TBI in which the number of accumulated neutrophils did not change when compared to normal animals. In contrast, in these knockout animals brain oedema was reduced although neurological outcome was not affected (Whalen *et al.* 2000).

Release of the chemokine IL-8 into the CSF has been shown in both adults and children suffering severe TBI, and the latter group was associated with increased mortality (Kossmann *et al.* 1997*a*; Whalen *et al.* 2000). The relationship between the CSF levels of both IL-8 and soluble (s)ICAM-1 with BBB dysfunction was demonstrated previously in patients with severe TBI (Kossmann *et al.* 1997*a*; Pleines *et al.* 1998). Corroborating data have been reported (Bell *et al.* 1996), demonstrating that hippocampal injection of IL-8 or MIP-2 (the mouse homologue of IL-8) into rodent brain results in a dramatic recruitment of neutrophils and increased BBB permeability which was reduced by prior depletion of circulating leucocytes. We acknowledged the molecular interaction of TNF, ICAM, and IL-8 with regard to the function of the BBB on cultured microvascular endothelial cells and astrocytes isolated from mouse brain. We showed that (s)ICAM-1 is a strong stimulator of MIP-2 in astrocytes and endothelial cells. The kinetics of released MIP-2 differed considerably whether induced by (s)ICAM-1 or TNF, suggesting two different signalling pathways for the regulation of MIP-2. Confirmation of independent intracellular signals was given by the synergistic action obtained by costimulation using both factors (Otto *et al.* 2000). This potent and prolonged upregulation of MIP-2 by (s)ICAM-1 indicates an additional signalling action for this adhesion molecule which is consistent with the continuous elevation of (s)ICAM-1 and IL-8 found in human CSF after TBI.

8.2.8 Complement as a mediator of post-traumatic neuroinflammation: new challenge from an 'old' cascade

Activation of complement through either the classical, the alternative, or the lectin pathway plays a key role in innate immune responses aimed at protecting against infection or tissue injury. The generation of proteolytic complement fragments leads to pleiotropic inflammatory effects, such as opsonization of invading pathogens for phagocytosis, induction of increased vascular permeability, recruitment of phagocytic cells, augmentation of the acute-phase response, B-cell activation and cytolysis of pathogens by membrane pore formation through the terminal complement pathway. Resident brain cells (neurons, astrocytes and microglia), can synthesize all complement activation proteins, complement regulatory molecules and complement receptors (Barnum 1999; Gasque *et al.* 2000). Clinical and experimental studies have revealed potential pathophysiological mechanisms of complement-mediated secondary brain injury after TBI (Kaczorowski *et al.* 1995; Keeling *et al.* 2000; Stahel *et al.* 1998). These include the recruitment of inflammatory cells into the intrathecal compartment, induction of BBB dysfunction by the anaphylatoxins C3a and C5a, induction of neuronal apoptosis through the C5a receptor (C5aR) expressed on neurons and complement-mediated homologous cell lysis through the membrane attack complex (MAC/C5b-9), following inactivation of the physiological cellular protection mechanisms against complement attack (Morgan 1999; Singhrao *et al.* 2000; Stahel *et al.* 1998). Post-traumatic upregulation of neuronal expression of the C5aR was also detected in the brains of rats (Stahel *et al.* 1997*b*) and mice (Stahel *et al.* 2000*a*) after experimental TBI. Activated complement fragments were detected in injured rat brains by immunohistochemistry, demonstrating post-traumatic complement activation and deposition of the MAC in homologous tissue, suggesting that complement contributes to post-traumatic destruction of brain tissue (Bellander *et al.* 1996; Tornqvist *et al.* 1996). In severely head-injured patients, elevated levels of alternative pathway complement components C3 and factor B (Kossmann *et al.* 1997*b*) as well as activated soluble MAC (Stahel *et al.* 2001) were detected in the CSF and the extent of intrathecal complement activation was associated with a dysfunction of the BBB (Lindsberg *et al.* 1996; Stahel *et al.* 2001).

Complement C3 represents the most abundant complement component with high constitutive levels in serum. It plays a central role in the complement activation cascade, since all three activation pathways merge at the C3 activation step. Cleavage of C3 by C3 convertases of either activation pathway leads to formation of C3b, an activation product which acts as opsonin by covalent binding of pathogen surfaces, and to formation of a small peptide fragment, anaphylatoxin C3a, a potent inflammatory mediator implicated in cell activation and chemotaxis. Biological effects of C3a are mediated via binding of the C3a receptor (C3aR), a recently cloned member of a large superfamily of seven transmembrane domain-spanning receptors that are G protein-coupled (Ames *et al.* 1996). We and others have demonstrated that resident cells of the brain, such as astrocytes, microglia, and neurons express the C3aR constitutively (Davoust *et al.* 1999*a*; Gasque *et al.* 1998). Clinical and experimental studies have also reported upregulation of the C3aR within the influenced brain (Davoust *et al.* 1999*a*; Gasque *et al.* 1998; Van Beek *et al.* 2000). Recent *in vitro* studies have highlighted a potential neuroprotective role for C3a since recombinant C3a protects neurons in a dose-dependent fashion against N-Methy-D-Aspartate (NMDA)-induced excitotoxicity (van Beek *et al.* 2001). An important feature of C3 is the presence of a thioester bond in the native (inactivated) molecule, which is exposed upon activation by proteolytic cleavage of the C3 α-chain and thus allows the covalent binding of the activated C3b fragment to biological surfaces by interaction with amino and hydroxyl groups. Bound C3b initiates the alternative pathway and amplifies the effects of classical pathway of complement activation. Since formation of the C5 convertases requires binding of C3b, all activation pathways of the complement cascade are interrupted at the C3-level in the case of a genetic deficiency in C3, as described for the C3−/− mice (Circolo *et al.* 1999). Thus, these knockout mice provide a unique *in vivo* model for the analysis of the role of complement activation in neuroinflammatory diseases (Nataf *et al.* 2000).

The most potent inflammatory mediator derived from activation of the complement cascade is the anaphylatoxin C5a, generated by proteolytic cleavage of the amino-terminus of the α-chain of complement (C5) by C5 convertases. In peripheral tissues, the inflammatory functions of C5a include degranulation of mast cells and basophils leading to increased vascular permeability and oedema, activation of neutrophils and macrophages, neutrophil chemotaxis and induction of the respiratory burst, as well as the enhancement of the hepatic acute-phase response. Aside from these effects in blood and peripheral tissues, recent studies indicate a wide range of C5a-mediated responses in the CNS; for example recruitment of neutrophils across the BBB (Kaczorowski *et al.* 1995; Williams *et al.* 1985), glial cell chemotaxis (Armstrong *et al.* 1990; Yao *et al.* 1990), modulation of neuronal functions in the hypothalamus (Williams *et al.* 1985), and activation of signal transduction pathways in astrocytes (Osaka *et al.* 1999*a*) and neurones (Farkas *et al.* 1998*b*). A recent study provided evidence of C5a-mediated neuronal apoptosis *in vitro* (Farkas *et al.* 1998*a*). Contrary to these findings, C5a-mediated protection from apoptotic neuronal death was reported in a model of intraventricular kainic acid injection in mice (Osaka *et al.* 1999*b*). C5a may therefore also have neuroprotective effects as shown in a model of glutamate-induced neurotoxicity *in vivo* (Osaka *et al.* 1999*b*) and very recently in an *in vitro* model of β-amyloid-induced neurotoxicity (O'Barr *et al.* 2001). The functional responses to C5a are mediated by binding to the C5aR (CD88), a member of the rhodopsin family of G protein-coupled receptors with seven transmembrane segments (Gerard and Gerard 1994). Low constitutive expression of the C5aR by resident cells of the brain has been demonstrated in astrocytes (Gasque *et al.* 1995; Lacy *et al.* 1995), microglia (Lacy *et al.* 1995), oligodendrocytes (Nataf *et al.* 2001) and neurons (Nataf *et al.* 1999; O'Barr *et al.* 2001; Stahel *et al.* 1997*a*). Upregulation of C5aR expression on these cells occurs under various pathological conditions, such as experimental excitotoxic neurodegeneration (Osaka *et al.* 1999*a*), bacterial meningitis (Stahel *et al.* 1997*a*), MS (Gasque *et al.* 1997; Muller-Ladner *et al.* 1996), and EAE, the animal model for MS. We have also demonstrated recently enhanced post-traumatic C5aR gene expression on cortical neurons, cerebellar Purkinje cells, and intra-thecally infiltrating leucocytes in a model of experimental diffuse axonal injury in rats (Stahel *et al.* 1997*b*). In a mouse model of closed head injury, the neuronal C5aR expression was attenuated in TNF/LT-α−/− mice by 7 days after trauma, suggesting a regulation of the intracerebral C5aR through TNF receptor-dependent pathways (Stahel *et al.* 2000*a*).

There is a pressing need to develop pharmacological complement inhibitors which may prevent the adverse effects (Barnum 1999; McGeer and McGeer 1998; Pellas and Wennogle 1999). This therapeutic concept has received recent attention with regard to autoimmune CNS diseases, but to date there is only one report on complement inhibition in experimental neurotrauma (Kaczorowski *et al.* 1995). This study showed significant inhibition of complement-mediated intracerebral neutrophil accumulation in injured rat brains after systemic administration of soluble complement receptor type 1 (sCR1), a recombinant inhibitor of complement C3 convertases of the classical and alternative pathways. However, the study had technical limitations due to the use of human reagents (sCR1) in a head injury in rats, and additional parameters which reflect the extent of post-traumatic brain damage or the neurological recovery after treatment with sCR1 were not assessed (Kaczorowski *et al.* 1995). A severe limitation in experimental studies in the past was the lack in reagents for the mouse, since most murine complement inhibitors have only recently been cloned (Harris *et al.* 1999; Lener *et al.* 1998; Powell *et al.* 1997). Among these, a well-characterized complement regulatory protein in rodents is *Crry* (Complement receptor-related protein y) which represents a functional homologue of the human complement regulatory proteins DAF/CD55 and MCP/CD46 and exerts inhibitory activities for both the classical and alternative pathways of complement activation (Foley *et al.* 1993). The expression of murine *Crry* on resident cells in the murine brain was recently determined by *in vivo* and *in vitro* studies (Davoust *et al.* 1999*b*). Astrocytes and microglia were found to express *Crry* mRNA and protein constitutively as determined by RT-PCR, *in situ* hybridization, flow cytometry, Western blot analysis and immunohistochemistry. In addition, *Crry* mRNA expression was detected on cortical neurones and cerebellar Purkinje cells in the normal mouse brain (Davoust *et al.* 1999*b*). Transgenic mice with astrocyte-targeted overexpression of soluble *Crry* were shown to have a significantly attenuated extent of neuroinflammation and neurodegeneration in a model of autoimmune CNS disease (Davoust *et al.* 1999*c*). The cloning of the *Crry* gene, the availability of murine reagents such as monoclonal antibodies (Li *et al.* 1993), transgenic mice with systemic or CNS-specific overexpression of the *Crry* gene (Davoust *et al.* 1999*c*; Quigg *et al.* 1998) and the recent development of complement gene knockout mice (Botto *et al.* 1998; Circolo *et al.* 1999; Matsumoto *et al.* 1997; Miwa *et al.* 2001) now offer new tools for investigating the effects of complement inhibition in experimental TBI.

8.3 Conclusion

Although the pathophysiological mechanisms of TBI have not been fully elucidated yet, it is known that many different immunological processes are activated affecting primary as well as secondary brain injury and thus, influencing clinical outcome. Whereas most of the studies cited and discussed in this chapter were designed to investigate the potential role of single mediators involved in neuroinflammation, the cascades regulating cell activation, adhesion, and migration are complex and render this objective difficult to achieve. In addition, immune activation within the injured brain seems to play a dual role and great research effort has to be dedicated to clarify to what extent inflammation is detrimental or beneficial for the injured brain within the acute or the delayed post-traumatic period. Studies in various models of TBI using genetically manipulated mice either deficient in cytokines, cytokine receptors, adhesion molecules, and inducible nitric oxide synthase, which are potential mediators of cytotoxicity, or overexpressing anti-apoptotic factors or neuro-trophins, are in some cases disappointing and in particular those using knockout mice, possibly due to the fact that the absence of distinct genes may be compensated already during embryogenesis. In fact, it is most likely that the complex pathophysiology of TBI led to failure of most of the clinical trials in head trauma patients, since each focused on a single target (Reinert and Bullock 1999). Thus, combination of different approaches aimed at activating and inhibiting selected events at different stages of the post-injury cascades may offer a significant benefit for patients with severe TBI.

Acknowledgements

We would like to thank Mrs E. Ammann, Department of Surgery, Division of Research, University Hospital Zurich, for excellent technical support. The projects were kindly supported by the Swiss National Science Foundation (Nrs: 31-36375.92, 31-42490.94, 31-52482.97), Hartmann-Müller and Olga-Meyenfisch Foundations, Zurich, Switzerland and Bayer AG, Wuppertal, Germany.

References

Aihara, N., Hall, J. J., Pitts, L. H., Fukuda, K., and Noble, L. J. (1995). Altered immunoexpression of microglia and macrophages after mild head injury. *J Neurotrauma*, 12, 53–63.

Akira, S. and Kishimoto, T. (1992). IL-6 and NF-IL6 in acute-phase response and viral infection. *Immunol Rev*, 127, 25–50.

Allan, S. M. and Rothwell, N. J. (2001). Cytokines and acute neurodegeneration. *Nat Rev Neurosci*, 2, 734–44.

Ames, R. S., Li, Y., Sarau, H. M., Nuthulaganti, P., Foley, J. J., Ellis, C., *et al.* (1996). Molecular cloning and characterization of the human anaphylatoxin C3a receptor. *J Biol Chem*, 271, 20 231–4.

Armstrong, R. C., Harvath, L., and Dubois-Dalcq, M. E. (1990). Type 1 astrocytes and oligo-dendrocyte-type 2 astrocyte glial progenitors migrate toward distinct molecules. *J Neurosci Res*, 27, 400–7.

Asensio, V. C. and Campbell, I. L. (1999). Chemokines in the CNS: plurifunctional mediators in diverse states. *Trends Neurosci*, 22, 504–12.

Baethmann, A., Maier-Hauff, K., Kempski, O., Unterberg, A., Wahl, M., and Schurer, L. (1988). Mediators of brain edema and secondary brain damage. *Crit Care Med*, 16, 972–8.

Baggiolini, M., Dewald, B., and Moser, B. (1997). Human chemokines: an update. *Annu Rev Immunol*, 15, 675–705.

Balasingam, V. and Yong, V. W. (1996). Attenuation of astroglial reactivity by interleukin-10. *J Neurosci*, 16, 2945–55.

Barnum, S. R. (1999). Inhibition of complement as a therapeutic approach in inflammatory central nervous system (CNS) disease. *Mol Med*, 5, 569–82.

Beer, R., Franz, G., Schopf, M., Reindl, M., Zelger, B., Schmutzhard, E., *et al.* (2000). Expression of Fas and Fas ligand after experimental traumatic brain injury in the rat. *J Cereb Blood Flow Metab*, 20, 669–77.

Bell, M. D., Taub, D. D., and Perry, V. H. (1996). Overriding the brain's intrinsic resistance to leucocyte recruitment with intraparenchymal injections of recombinant chemokines. *Neuroscience*, 74, 283–92.

Bell, M. J., Kochanek, P. M., Doughty, L. A., Carcillo, J. A., Adelson, P. D., Clark, R. S., *et al.* (1997). Interleukin-6 and interleukin-10 in cerebrospinal fluid after severe traumatic brain injury in children. *J Neurotrauma*, 14, 451–7.

Bellander, B. M., von Holst, H., Fredman, P., and Svensson, M. (1996). Activation of the complement cascade and increase of clusterin in the brain following a cortical contusion in the adult rat. *J Neurosurg*, 85, 468–475.

Benveniste, E. N. (1995). The role of cytokines in multiple sclerosis/autoimmune encephalitis and other neurological disorders. In *Human cytokines, their role in research and therapy* (ed. B. Agarwal. and R. Puri), Blackwell Science, Boston, pp. 159–180.

Beutler, B., Milsark, I. W., and Cerami, A. C. (1985). Passive immunization against cachectin/tumor necrosis factor protects mice from lethal effect of endotoxin. *Science*, 229, 869–71.

Botto, M., Dell'Agnola, C., Bygrave, A. E., Thompson, E. M., Cook, H. T., Petry, F., *et al.* (1998). Homozygous C1q deficiency causes glomerulonephritis associated with multiple apoptotic bodies. *Nat Genet*, 19, 56–9.

Bowes, M. P., Zivin, J. A., and Rothlein, R. (1993). Monoclonal antibody to the ICAM-1 adhesion site reduces neurological damage in a rabbit cerebral embolism stroke model. *Exp Neurol*, 119, 215–19.

Buki, A., Okonkwo, D. O., and Povlishock, J. T. (1999). Postinjury cyclosporin A administration limits axonal damage and disconnection in traumatic brain injury. *J Neurotrauma*, **16**, 511–21.

Buki, A., Okonkwo, D. O., Wang, K. K., and Povlishock, J. T. (2000). Cytochrome c release and caspase activation in traumatic axonal injury. *J Neurosci*, **20**, 2825–34.

Campbell, I. L., Abraham, C. R., Masliah, E., Kemper, P., Inglis, J. D., Oldstone, M. B., and Mucke, L. (1993). Neurologic disease induced in transgenic mice by cerebral overexpression of interleukin 6. *Proc Natl Acad Sci USA*, **90**, 10 061–5.

Carlos, T. M., Clark, R. S., Franicola-Higgins, D., Schiding, J. K., and Kochanek, P. M. (1997). Expression of endothelial adhesion molecules and recruitment of neutrophils after traumatic brain injury in rats. *J Leukoc Biol*, **61**, 279–85.

Choi, C., Park, J. Y., Lee, J., Lim, J. H., Shin, E. C., Ahn, Y. S., *et al.* (1999). Fas ligand and Fas are expressed constitutively in human astrocytes and the expression increases with IL-1, IL-6, TNF-alpha, or IFN-gamma. *J Immunol*, **162**, 1889–95.

Circolo, A., Garnier, G., Fukuda, W., Wang, X., Hidvegi, T., Szalai, A. J., *et al.* (1999). Genetic disruption of the murine complement C3 promoter region generates deficient mice with extrahepatic expression of C3 mRNA. *Immunopharmacology*, **42**, 135–49.

Clark, R. S., Chen, J., Watkins, S. C., Kochanek, P. M., Chen, M., Stetler, R. A., *et al.* (1997). Apoptosis-suppressor gene Bcl-2 expression after traumatic brain injury in rats. *J Neurosci*, **17**, 9172–82.

Clark, R. S., Kochanek, P. M., Adelson, P. D., Bell, M. J., Carcillo, J. A., Chen, M., *et al.* (2000a). Increases in Bcl-2 protein in cerebrospinal fluid and evidence for programmed cell death in infants and children after severe traumatic brain injury. *J Pediatr*, **137**, 197–204.

Clark, R. S., Kochanek, P. M., Chen, M., Watkins, S. C., Marion, D. W., Chen, J., *et al.* (1999). Increases in Bcl-2 and cleavage of caspase-1 and caspase-3 in human brain after head injury. *FASEB J*, **13**, 813–21.

Clark, R. S., Kochanek, P. M., Watkins, S. C., Chen, M., Dixon, C. E., Seidberg, N. A., *et al.* (2000b). Caspase-3 mediated neuronal death after traumatic brain injury in rats. *J Neurochem*, **74**, 740–53.

Clark, R. S., Schiding, J. K., Kaczorowski, S. L., Marion, D. W., and Kochanek, P. M. (1994). Neutrophil accumulation after traumatic brain injury in rats: comparison of weight drop and controlled cortical impact models. *J Neurotrauma*, **11**, 499–506.

Connolly, E. S., Jr., Winfree, C. J., Springer, T. A., Naka, Y., Liao, H., Yan, S. D., *et al.* (1996). Cerebral protection in homozygous null ICAM-1 mice after middle cerebral artery occlusion. Role of neutrophil adhesion in the pathogenesis of stroke. *J Clin Invest*, **97**, 209–16.

Conti, A. C., Raghupathi, R., Trojanowski, J. Q., and McIntosh, T. K. (1998). Experimental brain injury induce regionally distinct apoptosis during the acute and delayed post-traumatic period. *J Neurosci*, **18**, 5663–72.

Csuka, E., Morganti-Kossmann, M. C., Lenzlinger, P. M., Joller, H., Trentz, O., and Kossmann, T. (1999). IL-10 levels in cerebrospinal fluid and serum of patients with severe traumatic brain injury: relationship to IL-6, TNF-alpha, TGF-beta1 and blood–brain barrier function. *J Neuroimmunol*, **101**, 211–21.

Davoust, N., Jones, J., Stahel, P. F., Ames, R. S., and Barnum, S. R. (1999a). Receptor for the C3a anaphylatoxin is expressed by neurones and glial cells. *Glia*, **26**, 201–11.

Davoust, N., Nataf, S., Holers, V. M., and Barnum, S. R. (1999b). Expression of the murine complement regulatory protein Crry by glial cells and neurones. *Glia*, **27**, 162–70.

Davoust, N., Nataf, S., Reiman, R., Holers, M. V., Campbell, I. L., and Barnum, S. R. (1999c). Central nervous system-targeted expression of the complement inhibitor sCrry prevents experimental allergic encephalomyelitis. *J Immunol*, **163**, 6551–6.

De Simoni, M. G., De Luigi, A., Gemma, L., Sironi, M., Manfridi, A., and Ghezzi, P. (1993). Modulation of systemic interleukin-6 induction by central interleukin-1. *Am J Physiol*, **265**, R739–42.

de Waal Malefyt, R., Abrams, J., Bennett, B., Figdor, C. G., and de Vries, J. E. (1991). Interleukin 10(IL-10) inhibits cytokine synthesis by human monocytes: an autoregulatory role of IL-10 produced by monocytes. *J Exp Med*, 174, 1209–20.

Ertel, W., Keel, M., Stocker, R., Imhof, H. G., Leist, M., Steckholzer, U., *et al.* (1997). Detectable concentrations of Fas ligand in cerebrospinal fluid after severe head injury. *J Neuroimmunol*, 80, 93–6.

Fan, L., Young, P. R., Barone, F. C., Feuerstein, G. Z., Smith, D. H., and McIntosh, T. K. (1996). Experimental brain injury induces differential expression of tumor necrosis factor-alpha mRNA in the CNS. *Brain Res Mol Brain Res*, 36, 287–91.

Farkas, I., Baranyi, L., Liposits, Z. S., Yamamoto, T., and Okada, H. (1998*a*). Complement C5a anaphylatoxin fragment causes apoptosis in TGW neuroblastoma cells. *Neuroscience*, 86, 903–11.

Farkas, I., Baranyi, L., Takahashi, M., Fukuda, A., Liposits, Z., Yamamoto, T., and Okada, H. (1998*b*). A neuronal C5a receptor and an associated apoptotic signal transduction pathway. *J Physiol*, 507, 679–87.

Fattori, E., Lazzaro, D., Musiani, P., Modesti, A., Alonzi, T., and Ciliberto, G. (1995). IL-6 expression in neurones of transgenic mice causes reactive astrocytosis and increase in ramified microglial cells but no neuronal damage. *Eur J Neurosci*, 7, 2441–9.

Foley, S., Li, B., Dehoff, M., Molina, H., and Holers, V. M. (1993). Mouse Crry/p65 is a regulator of the alternative pathway of complement activation. *Eur J Immunol*, 23, 1381–4.

Fox, G. B., Fan L., Levasseur, R. A., and Faden, A. I. (1998). Sustained sensory/motor and cognitive deficits with neuronal apoptosis following controlled cortical impact brain injury in the mouse. *J Neurotrauma*, 15, 599–614.

Frei, K., Malipiero, U. V., Leist, T. P., Zinkernagel, R. M., Schwab, M. E., and Fontana, A. (1989). On the cellular source and function of interleukin 6 produced in the central nervous system in viral diseases. *Eur J Immunol*, 19, 689–94.

Frei, K., Nadal, D., Pfister, H. W., and Fontana, A. (1993*a*). Listeria meningitis: identification of a cerebrospinal fluid inhibitor of macrophage listericidal function as interleukin 10. *J Exp Med*, 178, 1255–61.

Frei, K., Piani, D., Pfister, H. W., and Fontana, A. (1993*b*). Immune-mediated injury in bacterial meningitis. *Int Rev Exp Pathol*, 34 Pt B: 183–192.

Frohman, E. M., Frohman, T. C., Dustin, M. L., Vayuvegula, B., Choi, B., Gupta, A., *et al.* (1989). The induction of intercellular adhesion molecule 1 (ICAM-1) expression on human fetal astrocytes by interferon-gamma, tumor necrosis factor alpha, lymphotoxin, and interleukin-1: relevance to intracerebral antigen presentation. *J Neuroimmunol*, 23, 117–24.

Gadient, R. A., Cron, K. C., and Otten, U. (1990). Interleukin-1 beta and tumor necrosis factor-alpha synergistically stimulate nerve growth factor (NGF) release from cultured rat astrocytes. *Neurosci Lett*, 117, 335–40.

Gasque, P., Chan, P., Fontaine, M., Ischenko, A., Lamacz, M., Gotze, O., and Morgan, B. P. (1995). Identification and characterization of the complement C5a anaphylatoxin receptor on human astrocytes. *J Immunol*, 155, 4882–9.

Gasque, P., Dean, Y. D., McGreal, E. P., VanBeek, J., and Morgan, B. P. (2000). Complement components of the innate immune system in health and disease in the CNS. *Immunopharmacology*, 49, 171–86.

Gasque, P., Singhrao, S. K., Neal, J. W., Gotze, O., and Morgan, B. P. (1997). Expression of the receptor for complement C5a (CD88) is up-regulated on reactive astrocytes, microglia, and endothelial cells in the inflamed human central nervous system. *Am J Pathol*, 150, 31–41.

Gasque, P., Singhrao, S. K., Neal, J. W., Wang, P., Sayah, S., Fontaine, M., and Morgan, B. P. (1998). The receptor for complement anaphylatoxin C3a is expressed by myeloid cells and nonmyeloid cells in inflammed human central nervous system: analysis in multiple sclerosis and bacterial meningitis. *J Immunol*, 160, 3543–54.

Gentleman, S. W., Roberts, G. W., Gennarelli, T. A., Maxwell, W. L., Adams, J. H., Kerr, S., and Graham, D. I. (1995). Axonal Injury: A universal consequence of fatale closed head injury. *Acta Neuropathol*, **89**, 537–43.

Gerard, C. and Gerard, N. P. (1994). C5A anaphylatoxin and its seven transmembrane-segment receptor. *Annu Rev Immunol*, **12**, 775–808.

Glabinski, A. R. and Ransohoff, R. M. (1999). Chemokines and chemokine receptors in CNS pathology. *J Neurovirol*, **5**, 3–12.

Goodman, J. C., Robertson, C. S., Grossman, R. G., and Narayan, R. K. (1990). Elevation of tumor necrosis factor in head injury. *J Neuroimmunol*, **30**, 213–17.

Gourin, C. G. and Shackford, S. R. (1997). Production of tumor necrosis factor-alpha and interleukin-1beta by human cerebral microvascular endothelium after percussive trauma. *J Trauma*, **42**, 1101–7.

Graham, D. I., McIntosh, T. K., Maxwell, W. L., and Nicoll, J. A. (2000). Recent advances in neurotrauma. *J Neuropathol Exp Neurol*, **59**, 641–51.

Gruol, D. L. and Nelson, T. E. (1997). Physiological and pathological roles of interleukin-6 in the central nervous system. *Mol Neurobiol*, **15**, 307–39.

Hans, V. H., Kossmann, T., Joller, H., Otto, V., and Morganti-Kossmann, M. C. (1999*a*). Interleukin-6 and its soluble receptor in serum and cerebrospinal fluid after cerebral trauma. *Neuroreport*, **10**, 409–12.

Hans, V. H., Kossmann, T., Lenzlinger, P. M., Probstmeier, R., Imhof, H. G., Trentz, O., and Morganti-Kossmann, M. C. (1999*b*). Experimental axonal injury triggers interleukin-6 mRNA, protein synthesis and release into cerebrospinal fluid. *J Cereb Blood Flow Metab*, **19**, 184–94.

Harris, C. L., Rushmere, N. K., and Morgan, B. P. (1999). Molecular and functional analysis of mouse decay accelerating factor (CD55). *Biochem J*, **341**, 821–9.

Hausmann, E. H., Berman, N. E., Wang, Y. Y., Meara, J. B., Wood, G. W., and Klein, R. M. (1998). Selective chemokine mRNA expression following brain injury. *Brain Res*, **788**, 49–59.

Kaczorowski, S. L., Schiding, J. K., Toth, C. A., and Kochanek, P. M. (1995). Effect of soluble complement receptor-1 on neutrophil accumulation after traumatic brain injury in rats. *J Cereb Blood Flow Metab*, **15**, 860–4.

Kaya, S. S., Mahmood, A., Li, Y., Yavuz, E., Goksel, M., and Chopp, M. (1999). Apoptosis and expression of p53 response proteins and cyclin D1 after cortical impact in rat brain. *Brain Res*, **818**, 23–33.

Keeling, K. L., Hicks, R. R., Mahesh, J., Billings, B. B., and Kotwal, G. J. (2000). Local neutrophil influx following lateral fluid-percussion brain injury in rats is associated with accumulation of complement activation fragments of the third component (C3) of the complement system. *J Neuroimmunol*, **105**, 20–30.

Kennedy, M. K., Torrance, D. S., Picha, K. S., and Mohler, K. M. (1992). Analysis of cytokine mRNA expression in the central nervous system of mice with experimental autoimmune encephalomyelitis reveals that IL-10 mRNA expression correlates with recovery. *J Immunol*, **149**, 2496–505.

Kim, K. S., Wass, C. A., Cross, A. S., and Opal, S. M. (1992). Modulation of blood–brain barrier permeability by tumor necrosis factor and antibody to tumor necrosis factor in the rat. *Lymphokine Cytokine Res*, **11**, 293–8.

King, P. D., Sandberg, E. T., Selvakumar, A., Fang, P., Beaudet, A. L., and Dupont, B. (1995). Novel isoforms of murine intercellular adhesion molecule-1 generated by alternative RNA splicing. *J Immunol*, **154**, 6080–93.

Knoblach, S. M. and Faden, A. I. (1998). Interleukin-10 improves outcome and alters proinflammatory cytokine expression after experimental traumatic brain injury. *Exp Neurol*, **153**, 143–51.

Knoblach, S. M., Fan, L., and Faden, A. I. (1999). Early neuronal expression of tumor necrosis factor-alpha after experimental brain injury contributes to neurological impairment. *J Neuroimmunol*, **95**, 115–25.

Kossmann, T., Hans, V., Imhof, H. G., Trentz, O., and Morganti-Kossmann, M. C. (1996). Interleukin-6 released in human cerebrospinal fluid following traumatic brain injury may trigger nerve growth factor production in astrocytes. *Brain Res*, 713, 143–52.

Kossmann, T., Hans, V. H., Imhof, H. G., Stocker, R., Grob, P., Trentz, O., and Morganti-Kossmann, C. (1995). Intrathecal and serum interleukin-6 and the acute-phase response in patients with severe traumatic brain injuries. *Shock*, 4, 311–17.

Kossmann, T., Stahel, P. F., Lenzlinger, P. M., Redl, H., Dubs, R. W., Trentz, O., *et al.* (1997*a*). Interleukin-8 released into the cerebrospinal fluid after brain injury is associated with blood–brain barrier dysfunction and nerve growth factor production. *J Cereb Blood Flow Metab*, 17, 280–9.

Kossmann, T., Stahel, P. F., Morganti-Kossmann, M. C., Jones, J. L., and Barnum, S. R. (1997*b*). Elevated levels of the complement components C3 and factor B in ventricular cerebrospinal fluid of patients with traumatic brain injury. *J Neuroimmunol*, 73, 63–9.

Kraus, J. F., McArthur, D. L., Silverman, T. A., and Jayaraman, M. (1996). Epidemiology of brain injury. In: *Neurotrauma* (ed. R. K. Narayan, J. E. Wilberger, and J. T. Povlishock), McGrawn-Hill, New York, pp. 13–30.

Lacy, M., Jones, J., Whittemore, S. R., Haviland, D. L., Wetsel, R. A., and Barnum, S. R. (1995). Expression of the receptors for the C5a anaphylatoxin, interleukin-8 and FMLP by human astrocytes and microglia. *J Neuroimmunol*, 61, 71–8.

LaPlaca, M. C., Raghupathi, R., Verma, A., Pieper, A. A., Saatman, K. E., Snyder, S. H., and McIntosh, T. K. (1999). Temporal patterns of poly(ADP-ribose) polymerase activation in the cortex following experimental brain injury in the rat. *J Neurochem*, 73, 205–13.

Laurer, H. L., Lenzlinger, P. M., and McIntosh, T. K. (2000). Models of traumatic brain injury. *Eur J Trauma*, 26, 95–100.

Lener, M., Vinci, G., Duponchel, C., Meo, T., and Tosi, M. (1998). Molecular cloning, gene structure and expression profile of mouse C1 inhibitor. *Eur J Biochem*, 254, 117–22.

Li, B., Sallee, C., Dehoff, M., Foley, S., Molina, H., and Holers, V. M. (1993). Mouse Crry/p65. Characterization of monoclonal antibodies and the tissue distribution of a functional homologue of human MCP and DAF. *J Immunol*, 151, 4295–305.

Lindsberg, P. J., Ohman, J., Lehto, T., Karjalainen-Lindsberg, M. L., Paetau, A., Wuorimaa, T., *et al.* (1996). Complement activation in the central nervous system following blood–brain barrier damage in man. *Ann Neurol*, 40, 587–96.

Liu, T., Clark, R. K., McDonnell, P. C., Young, P. R., White, R. F., Barone, F. C., and Feuerstein, G. Z. (1994). Tumor necrosis factor-alpha expression in ischemic neurons. *Stroke*, 25, 1481–8.

Marz, P., Cheng, J. G., Gadient, R. A., Patterson, P. H., Stoyan, T., Otten, U., and Rose-John, S. (1998). Sympathetic neurons can produce and respond to interleukin 6. *Proc Natl Acad Sci USA*, 95, 3251–6.

Matsumoto, M., Fukuda, W., Circolo, A., Goellner, J., Strauss-Schoenberger, J., Wang, X., *et al.* (1997). Abrogation of the alternative complement pathway by targeted deletion of murine factor B. *Proc Natl Acad Sci USA*, 94, 8720–5.

Maxwell, W. L., Povlishock, J. T., and Graham, D. L. (1997). A mechanistic analysis of nondisruptive axonal injury: a review. *J Neurotrauma*, 14, 419–40.

McClain, C., Cohen, D., Phillips, R., Ott, L., and Young, B. (1991). Increased plasma and ventricular fluid interleukin-6 levels in patients with head injury [see comments]. *J Lab Clin Med*, 118, 225–31.

McGeer, E. G. and McGeer, P. L. (1998). The future use of complement inhibitors for the treatment of neurological diseases. *Drugs*, 55, 739–46.

McIntosh, T. K., Juhler, M., and Wieloch, T. (1998). Novel pharmacologic strategies in the treatment of experimental traumatic brain injury: 1998. *J Neurotrauma*, 15, 731–69.

McIntosh, T. K., Smith, D. H., Meaney, D. F., Kotapka, M. J., Gennarelli, T. A., and Graham, D. I. (1996). Neuropathological sequelae of traumatic brain injury: relationship to neurochemical and biomechanical mechanisms. *Lab Invest*, 74, 315–42.

Miwa, T., Sun, X., Ohta, R., Okada, N., Harris, C. L., Morgan, B. P., and Song, W. C. (2001). Characterization of glycosylphosphatidylinositol-anchored decay accelerating factor (GPI-DAF) and transmembrane DAF gene expression in wild-type and GPI-DAF gene knockout mice using polyclonal and monoclonal antibodies with dual or single specificity. *Immunology*, **104**, 207–14.

Morgan, B. P. (1999). Regulation of the complement membrane attack pathway. *Crit Rev Immunol*, **19**, 173–98.

Morganti-Kossmann, M. C., Hans, V. H. J., Lenzlinger, P. M., Dubs, R., Ludwig, E., Trentz, O., and Kossmann, T. (1999). TGF-beta is elevated in the CSF of patients with severe traumatic brain injuries and parallels blood–brain barrier function. *J Neurotrauma*, **16**, 617–28.

Morganti-Kossmann, M. C., and Kossmann, T. (1995). The immunology of brain injury. In *Immune responses in the nervous system* (ed. N. Rothwell), BIOS, Scientific Publisher Ltd., Oxford, pp. 159–87.

Morganti-Kossmann, M. C., Kossmann, T., and Wahl, S. M. (1992). Cytokines and neuropathology. *Trends Pharmacol Sci*, **13**, 286–91.

Morganti-Kossmann, M. C., Lenzlinger, P. M., Hans, V., Stahel, P., Csuka, E., Ammann, E., *et al.* (1997). Production of cytokines following brain injury: beneficial and deleterious for the damaged tissue. *Mol Psychiatry*, **2**, 133–6.

Morganti-Kossmann, M. C., Otto, V. I., Stahel, P. F., and Kossmann, T. (2000). The role of inflammation in neurologic disease. *Current Opin Crit Care*, **6**, 98–109.

Muller-Ladner, U., Jones, J. L., Wetsel, R. A., Gay, S., Raine, C. S., and Barnum, S. R. (1996). Enhanced expression of chemotactic receptors in multiple sclerosis lesions. *J Neurol Sci*, **144**, 135–41.

Napieralski, J. A., Raghupathi, R., and McIntosh, T. K. (1999). The tumor-suppressor gene, p53, is induced in injured brain regions following experimental traumatic brain injury. *Brain Res Mol Brain Res*, **71**, 78–86.

Nataf, S., Carroll, S. L., Wetsel, R. A., Szalai, A. J., and Barnum, S. R. (2000). Attenuation of experimental autoimmune demyelination in complement-deficient mice. *J Immunol*, **165**, 5867–73.

Nataf, S., Levison, S. W., and Barnum, S. R. (2001). Expression of the anaphylatoxin C5a receptor in the oligodendrocyte lineage. *Brain Res*, **894**, 321–6.

Nataf, S., Stahel, P. F., Davoust, N., and Barnum, S. R. (1999). Complement anaphylatoxin receptors on neurons: new tricks for old receptors? *Trends Neurosci*, **22**, 397–402.

Neidhardt, R., Keel, M., Steckholzer, U., Safret, A., Ungethuem, U., Trentz, O., and Ertel, W. (1997). Relationship of interleukin-10 plasma levels to severity of injury and clinical outcome in injured patients. *J Trauma*, **42**, 863–70; discussion 870–1.

Neugebauer, E., Hensler, T., Rose, S., Maier, B., Holanda, M., Raum, M., *et al.* (2000). Severe craniocerebral trauma in multiple trauma. An assessment of the interaction of local and systemic mediator responses. *Unfallchirurg*, **103**, 122–31.

Newcomb, J. K., Zhao, X., Pike, B. R., and Hayes, R. L. (1999). Temporal profile of apoptotic-like changes in neurons and astrocytes following controlled cortical impact injury in the rat. *Exp Neurol*, **158**, 76–88.

O'Barr, S. A., Caguioa, J., Gruol, D., Perkins, G., Ember, J. A., Hugli, T., and Cooper, N. R. (2001). Neuronal expression of a functional receptor for the C5a complement activation fragment. *J Immunol*, **166**, 4154–62.

Ohata, K., Marmarou, A., and Povlishock, J. T. (1990). An immunocytochemical study of protein clearance in brain infusion edema. *Acta Neuropathol (Berl)*, **81**, 162–77.

Osaka, H., McGinty, A., Hoepken, U. E., Lu, B., Gerard, C., and Pasinetti, G. M. (1999*a*). Expression of C5a receptor in mouse brain: role in signal transduction and neurodegeneration. *Neuroscience*, **88**, 1073–82.

Osaka, H., Mukherjee, P., Aisen, P. S., and Pasinetti, G. M. (1999*b*). Complement-derived anaphylatoxin C5a protects against glutamate-mediated neurotoxicity. *J Cell Biochem*, **73**, 303–11.

Otero, G. C. and Merrill, J. E. (1994). Cytokine receptors on glial cells. *Glia*, 11, 117–28.

Otto, V. I., Heinzel-Pleines, U. E., Gloor, S. M., Trentz, O., Kossmann, T., and Morganti-Kossmann, M. C. (2000). sICAM-1 and TNF-alpha induce MIP-2 with distinct kinetics in astrocytes and brain microvascular endothelial cells. *J Neurosci Res*, 60, 733–42.

Pellas, T. C. and Wennogle, L. P. (1999). C5a receptor antagonists. *Curr Pharm Des*, 5, 737–55.

Pleines, U. E., Stover, J. F., Kossmann, T., Trentz, O., and Morganti-Kossmann, M. C. (1998). Soluble ICAM-1 in CSF coincides with the extent of cerebral damage in patients with severe traumatic brain injury. *J Neurotrauma*, 15, 399–409.

Powell, M. B., Marchbank, K. J., Rushmere, N. K., van den Berg, C. W., and Morgan, B. P. (1997). Molecular cloning, chromosomal localization, expression, and functional characterization of the mouse analogue of human CD59. *J Immunol*, 158, 1692–702.

Quattrocchi, K. B., Issel, B. W., Miller, C. H., Frank, E. H., and Wagner, F. C., Jr. (1992). Impairment of helper T-cell function following severe head injury. *J Neurotrauma*, 9, 1–9.

Quigg, R. J., He, C., Lim, A., Berthiaume, D., Alexander, J. J., Kraus, D., and Holers, V. M. (1998). Transgenic mice overexpressing the complement inhibitor Crry as a soluble protein are protected from antibody-induced glomerular injury. *J Exp Med*, 188, 1321–31.

Raghupathi, R., Fernandez, S. C., Murai, H., Trusko, S. P., Scott, R. W., Nishioka, W. K., and McIntosh, T. K. (1998). BCL-2 overexpression attenuates cortical cell loss after traumatic brain injury in transgenic mice. *J Cereb Blood Flow Metab*, 18, 1259–69.

Ramilo, O., Saez-Llorens, X., Mertsola, J., Jafari, H., Olsen, K.D., Hansen, E. J., et al. (1990). Tumor necrosis factor alpha/cachectin and interleukin 1 beta initiate meningeal inflammation. *J Exp Med*, 172, 497–507.

Rancan, M., Otto, V., Hans, V. H., Gerlach, I., Jork, R., Trentz, O., et al. (2001). Upregulation of ICAM-1 and MCP-1 but not of MIP-2 and sensorimotor deficit in response to traumatic axonal injury in rats. *J Neurosci Res*, 63, 438–46.

Ransohoff, R. M. and Tani, M. (1998). Do chemokines mediate leucocyte recruitment in post-traumatic CNS inflammation? *Trends Neurosci*, 21, 154–9.

Reinert, M. M. and Bullock, R. (1999). Clinical trials in head injury. *Neurol Res*, 21, 330–8.

Rink, A., Fung, K. M., Trojanowski, J. Q., Lee, V. M., Neugebauer, E., and McIntosh, T. K. (1995). Evidence of apoptotic cell death after experimental traumatic brain injury in the rat. *Am J Pathol*, 147, 1575–83.

Rosenberg, G. A., Kyner, W. T., and Estrada, E. (1980). Bulk flow of brain interstitial fluid under normal and hyperosmolar conditions. *Am J Physiol*, 238, F42–9.

Ross, S. A., Halliday, M. I., Campbell, G. C., Byrnes, D. P., and Rowlands, B. J. (1994). The presence of tumour necrosis factor in CSF and plasma after severe head injury. *Br J Neurosurg*, 8, 419–25.

Rubin, L. L., and Staddon, J. M. (1999). The cell biology of the blood–brain barrier. *Annu Rev Neurosci*, 22, 11–28.

Scherbel, U., Raghupathi, R., Nakamura, M., Saatman, K. E., Trojanowski, J. Q., Neugebauer, E., et al. (1999). Differential acute and chronic responses of tumor necrosis factor-deficient mice to experimental brain injury. *Proc Natl Acad Sci USA*, 96, 8721–26.

Schobitz, B., Pezeshki, G., Pohl, T., Hemmann, U., Heinrich, P.C., Holsboer, F., and Reul, J. M. (1995). Soluble interleukin-6 (IL-6) receptor augments central effects of IL-6 *in vivo*. *FASEB J*, 9, 659–64.

Shohami, E., Bass, R., Wallach, D., Yamin, A., and Gallily, R. (1996). Inhibition of tumor necrosis factor alpha (TNF alpha) activity in rat brain is associated with cerebroprotection after closed head injury. *J Cereb Blood Flow Metab*, 16, 378–84.

Shohami, E., Gallily, R., Mechoulam, R., Bass, R., and Ben-Hur, T. (1997). Cytokine production in the brain following closed head injury: dexanabinol (HU-211) is a novel TNF-alpha inhibitor and an effective neuroprotectant. *J Neuroimmunol*, 72, 169–77.

Shohami, E., Ginis, I., and Hallenbeck, J. M. (1999). Dual role of tumor necrosis factor alpha in brain injury. *Cytokine Growth Factor Rev*, 10, 119–30.

Shohami, E., Novikov, M., Bass, R., Yamin, A., and Gallily, R. (1994). Closed head injury triggers early production of TNF alpha and IL-6 by brain tissue. *J Cereb Blood Flow Metab*, **14**, 615–19.

Singhrao, S. K., Neal, J. W., Rushmere, N. K., Morgan, B. P., and Gasque, P. (2000). Spontaneous classical pathway activation and deficiency of membrane regulators render human neurons susceptible to complement lysis. *Am J Pathol*, **157**, 905–18.

Smith, D. H., Chen, X. H., Pierce, J. E., Wolf, J. A., Trojanowski, J. Q., Graham, D. I., and McIntosh, T. K. (1997). Progressive atrophy and neuron death for one year following brain trauma in the rat. *J Neurotrauma*, **14**, 715–27.

Soares, H. D., Hicks, R. R., Smith, D., and McIntosh, T. K. (1995). Inflammatory leukocytic recruitment and diffuse neuronal degeneration are separate pathological processes resulting from traumatic brain injury. *J Neurosci*, **15**, 8223–33.

Sobel, R. A., Mitchell, M. E., and Fondren, G. (1990). Intercellular adhesion molecule-1 (ICAM-1) in cellular immune reactions in the human central nervous system. *Am J Pathol*, **136**, 1309–16.

Stahel, P. F., Frei, K., Eugster, H.P., Fontana, A., Hummel, K. M., Wetsel, R. A., *et al.* (1997*a*) TNF-alpha-mediated expression of the receptor for anaphylatoxin C5a on neurons in experimental Listeria meningoencephalitis. *J Immunol*, **159**, 861–9.

Stahel, P. F., Kariya, K., Shohami, E., Barnum, S. R., Eugster, H., Trentz, O., *et al.* (2000*a*). Intracerebral complement C5a receptor (CD88) expression is regulated by TNF and lymphotoxin-alpha following closed head injury in mice. *J Neuroimmunol*, **109**, 164–72.

Stahel, P. F., Kossmann, T., Morganti-Kossmann, M. C., Hans, V. H., and Barnum, S. R. (1997*b*). Experimental diffuse axonal injury induces enhanced neuronal C5a receptor mRNA expression in rats. *Brain Res Mol Brain Res*, **50**, 205–12.

Stahel, P. F., Morganti-Kossmann, M. C., and Kossmann, T. (1998). The role of the complement system in traumatic brain injury. *Brain Res Brain Res Rev*, **27**, 243–56.

Stahel, P. F., Morganti-Kossmann, M. C., Perez, D., Redaelli, C., Gloor, B., Trentz, O., and Kossmann, T. (2001). Intrathecal levels of complement-derived soluble membrane attack complex (sC5b-9) correlate with blood–brain barrier dysfunction in patients with traumatic brain injury. *J Neurotrauma*, **18**, 773–81.

Stahel, P. F., Shohami, E., Younis, F. M., Kariya, K., Otto, V. I., Lenzlinger, P. M., *et al.* (2000*b*). Experimental closed head injury: analysis of neurological outcome, blood-brain barrier dysfunction, intracranial neutrophil infiltration, and neuronal cell death in mice deficient in genes for pro-inflammatory cytokines. *J Cereb Blood Flow Metab*, **20**, 369–80.

Stocker, R., Bernays, R., Kossmann, T., and Imhof, H. G. (1995). Monitoring and treatment of acute head injury. In *The integrated approach to trauma care* (ed. R. J. A. Goris and O. Trentz), Springer Verlag, Berlin, pp. 196–210.

Taga, T. and Kishimoto, T. (1997). Gp130 and the interleukin-6 family of cytokines. *Annu Rev Immunol*, **15**, 797–819.

Taupin, V., Toulmond, S., Serrano, A., Benavides, J., and Zavala, F. (1993). Increase in IL-6, IL-1 and TNF levels in rat brain following traumatic lesion. Influence of pre- and post-traumatic treatment with Ro5 4864, a peripheral-type (p site) benzodiazepine ligand. *J Neuroimmunol*, **42**, 177–85.

Tornqvist, E., Liu, L., Aldskogius, H., Holst, H. V., and Svensson, M. (1996). Complement and clusterin in the injured nervous system. *Neurobiol Aging*, **17**, 695–705.

Van Beek, J., Bernaudin, M., Petit, E., Gasque, P., Nouvelot, A., MacKenzie, E. T., and Fontaine, M. (2000). Expression of receptors for complement anaphylatoxins C3a and C5a following permanent focal cerebral ischemia in the mouse. *Exp Neurol*, **161**, 373–82.

van Beek, J., Nicole, O., Ali, C., Ischenko, A., MacKenzie, E. T., Buisson, A., and Fontaine, M. (2001). Complement anaphylatoxin C3a is selectively protective against NMDA-induced neuronal cell death. *Neuroreport*, **12**, 289–93.

Wahl, S. M. (1994). Transforming growth factor beta: the good, the bad, and the ugly. *J Exp Med*, **180**, 1587–90.

Whalen, M. J., Carlos, T. M., Dixon, C. E., Schiding, J. K., Clark, R. S., Baum, E., *et al.* (1999*a*). Effect of traumatic brain injury in mice deficient in intercellular adhesion molecule-1: assessment of histopathologic and functional outcome. *J Neurotrauma*, 16, 299–309.

Whalen, M. J., Carlos, T. M., Kochanek, P. M., Clark, R. S., Heineman, S., Schiding, J. K., *et al.* (1999*b*). Neutrophils do not mediate blood–brain barrier permeability early after controlled cortical impact in rats. *J Neurotrauma*, 16, 583–94.

Whalen, M. J., Carlos, T. M., Kochanek, P. M., and Heineman, S. (1998). Blood–brain barrier permeability, neutrophil accumulation and vascular adhesion molecule expression after controlled cortical impact in rats: a preliminary study. *Acta Neurochir Suppl (Wien)*, 71, 212–14.

Whalen, M. J., Carlos, T. M., Kochanek, P. M., Wisniewski, S. R., Bell, M. J., Clark, R. S., *et al.* (2000). Interleukin-8 is increased in cerebrospinal fluid of children with severe head injury [see comments]. *Crit Care Med*, 28, 929–34.

Williams, C. A., Schupf, N., and Hugli, T. E. (1985). Anaphylatoxin C5a modulation of an alpha-adrenergic receptor system in the rat hypothalamus. *J Neuroimmunol*, 9, 29–40.

Woodroofe, M. N., Sarna, G. S., Wadhwa, M., Hayes, G. M., Loughlin, A. J., Tinker, A., and Cuzner, M. L. (1991). Detection of interleukin-1 and interleukin-6 in adult rat brain, following mechanical injury, by in vivo microdialysis: evidence of a role for microglia in cytokine production. *J Neuroimmunol*, 33, 227–36.

Yakovlev, A. G., Knoblach, S. M., Fan, L., Fox, G. B., Goodnight, R., and Faden, A. I. (1997). Activation of CPP32-like vcaspases contributes to neuronal apoptosis and neurological dysfunction after traumatic brain injury. *J Neurosci*, 17, 7415–24.

Yao, J., Harvath, L., Gilbert, D. L., and Colton, C. A. (1990). Chemotaxis by a CNS macrophage, the microglia. *J Neurosci Res*, 27, 36–42.

Chapter 9

Inflammatory demyelination and axonopathy in the central nervous system

M. L. Cuzner and M. N. Woodroofe

9.1 Introduction

An inflammatory response can be invoked in the central nervous system (CNS) by both innate and adaptive immunity leading to varying degrees of myelin and axonal damage. The innate response is represented by non-specific activation of microglia through, for example trauma or infection with focal, limited production of molecules toxic to myelin and axons. During an adaptive immune response, antigen-specific T lymphocytes are generated, the most potent immunogens in the CNS being located in white matter myelin (Wekerle 1997). In multiple sclerosis (MS) and experimental allergic encephalomyelitis (EAE), an auto-immune model of inflammatory demyelination, sustained cellular and humoral reactivity of T and B cells recruited to the CNS primes resident microglia and infiltrating macrophages to phagocytose and degrade myelin and secrete neurotoxins, pro-inflammatory cytokines, chemokines, and proteases (Gay et al. 1997; Luchinetti et al. 2001; Simpson et al. 1998; Gveric et al. 2001).

Central nervous system inflammation in EAE is induced through sensitization to the myelin antigens proteolipid protein (PLP), myelin oligodendrocyte glycoprotein (MOG) and most effectively myelin basic protein (MBP), with species differences accounting for varying degrees of demyelination and axonal pathology (Martin and McFarland 1997). Evidence of autoimmunity in MS is conjectural where demyelination is a more prominent feature accompanying its relapsing and remitting course, the result of recurring inflammation with macrophage enrichment at lesion sites (Li et al. 1993, Luchinetti et al. 2000). However it is clear that axonal loss is a concomitant event and can occur in the absence of myelinolysis (Bjartmar et al. 2001), although major axonal fallout occurs with demyelination (Bitsch et al. 2000).There is a general consensus that active MS foci are the culmination of widespread subtle changes in white matter over time reflecting low level dysregulated, genetically linked, inflammation.

9.2 The inflammatory lesion in MS and EAE

The cardinal feature of MS is focal primary demyelination for which an inflammatory reaction is considered a prerequisite. It is now clear that axons can also be damaged by inflammation per se (Bjartmar and Trapp 2001). The perivascular cuff of active lesions consists of macrophages, T lymphocytes with variable numbers of B lymphocytes and plasma cells with an extensive hypercellular zone of activated microglia and macrophages at the interface between normal and degenerating myelin (Prineas 1985). There is increased gene expression and protein synthesis of CD4[+] Th1 derived cytokines in the perivascular cuff, including interleukin (IL)-2, IL-12 and interferon γ (IFNγ) while CD8[+] T cells predominate at sites of active myelin destruction (Bitsch et al. 2001) where they have been shown, by single-cell polymerase chain reaction (PCR), to be clonally expanded (Babbe et al. 2000). The co-stimulatory molecules B7-1 and CD40, indicative of an adaptive immune response, are upregulated on B and T cells (Aloisi et al. 2000) although generally the T cell receptor Vα and Vβ repertoire is polyclonal (Wucherpfennig et al. 1992). However the immunodominant human T cell epitope, MBP 85-99, has recently been immunolocalized on antigen presenting macrophages/microglia in MS lesions with a monoclonal antibody specific for the peptide bound to the human leucocyte antigen (HLA)-DR-2, which is known to be associated with MS (Krogsgaard et al. 2000). Blood–brain barrier (BBB) permeability is apparent from visualization of fibrin(ogen) and plasminogen in active lesions, and leucocyte extravasation is evident from increased expression of chemokines and their receptors, urokinase plasminogen activator (uPA) complex, and matrix metalloproteases (MMPs) (Simpson et al. 1998, 2000a, 2000b; Gveric et al. 2001; Leppert et al. 2001). Effector properties of macrophages/microglia and astrocytes in lesions are represented by elevations in pro-inflammatory cytokines such as tumour necrosis factor (TNF) α and IL-1 (Woodroofe and Cuzner 1993; Cannella and Raine 1995), in serine and metalloproteases (Gveric et al. 2001) and in inducible nitric oxide synthase (iNOS) mRNA and protein (Liu et al. 2001; De Groot et al. 1997).

The evidence for primary autoimmunity in MS is as yet circumstantial, but this is not the case for EAE, which is induced by CD4[+] T cell sensitization in the context of HLA MHC class II to an expanding list of encephalitogenic brain autoantigens. These include the occluded and integral membrane proteins MBP and PLP, members of the immunoglobulin superfamily, that is, myelin-associated glycoprotein (MAG) and MOG and non-myelin antigens such as astrocyte S100-β (Wekerle 1997). However cytotoxic CD8[+] T cell clones specific for the MHC class I restricted fragment of MBP, peptide 79–87, have been found to induce severe EAE with paralysis and other neurological defects (Huseby et al. 2001). CD8[+] T cells reactive to MOG peptide 35–55 have also been found to induce inflammation and demyelination in the CNS (Sun et al. 2001). In both CD4[+] and CD8[+] T cell-induced EAE, perivascular cuffs and demyelination are present although pathology appears to be restricted to the brain in CD8[+] T cell-primed disease. Encephalitogenic T cells produce their effect within the CNS by a combination of mechanisms including direct cytotoxic attack and/or recruitment and activation of microglia and infiltrating macrophages (Wekerle 1997). Disease severity is closely associated with the concentration of macrophages in perivascular cuffs and surrounding white matter and in grey matter where inflammation is also prominent. In preclinical T cell transferred EAE, the TCR Vβ elements of the transferred T cell lines are detected by PCR but with the onset of disease the repertoire becomes more heterogeneous (Urban et al. 1998).

9.3 Pathophysiology

Axonal conduction block represents the central pathophysiological event in MS, which can be reversible under prevailing inflammatory conditions but becomes irreversible with an increasing load of demyelination.

9.3.1 Axonal pathology

The extent of axonal pathology correlates with inflammation and demyelination within the brain and spinal cord in MS (Ferguson *et al.* 1997; Trapp *et al.* 1998). Possible mechanisms of axonal damage include cell mediated cytotoxicity and the secreted effector molecules TNFα, MMPs, reactive oxygen intermediates (ROIs) and autoantibodies, all of which are also associated with inflammatory demyelination. Recent reports have suggested that glutamate released from microglia and activated leucocytes induces excitotoxicity as a mechanism of inducing both axonal damage and oligodendrocyte cell death (Smith *et al.* 2000; Pitt *et al.* 2000; Matute *et al.* 2001). Werner *et al.* (2001) demonstrated that microglia and macrophages in MS lesions express high levels of glutaminase, indicative of glutamine synthesis, in close association with damaged axons. Glutamate transporters (GLT) were robustly expressed on oligodendrocytes in control and MS white matter but the major one, GLT-1, was selectively lost from oligodendrocytes surrounding active MS lesions, implying deficiencies in glutamate detoxification. Glutamate synthetase and dehydrogenase expression was absent in active and chronic MS lesions, which was suggested to result in long lasting metabolic impairment. Oligodendrocytes are highly vulnerable to AMPA/kainate receptor mediated glutamate excitotoxicity. Thus failure of oligodendrocytes to remyelinate MS lesions may result from metabolic impairment (Werner *et al.* 2001). Glutamate levels in the CSF in MS are elevated in active versus chronic and silent disease and correlate with disease severity (Stover *et al.* 1997; Barkhatova *et al.* 1998). Whether the inflammatory autoimmune reaction occurs first followed by excitotoxic cell damage or vice versa is yet to be determined (Matute *et al.* 2001).

Axonal degeneration may also be a result of the action of nitric oxide (NO) as Smith and Hall (2001) have shown that in conducting axons, sustained impulses produce intermittent conduction failure in the presence of NO. They propose that the combination of normal electrical activity and NO at sites of inflammation may result in permanent disability in patients with neuroinflammatory conditions (Smith *et al.* 2001). In excitotoxic lesions, tissue type plasminogen activator (tPA) provokes neuronal damage through disruption of laminin–neuronal interactions (Chen and Strickland 1997). Localization of tPA in a subset of damaged axons with non-phosphorylated neurofilaments suggests a role in axonal damage (Gveric *et al.* 2001). However the co-localization on the same subset of damaged axons of tPA with fibrin deposition may represent a protective mechanism as reported in a study of sciatic nerve damage in tPA deficient mice in which exacerbation of axonal injury is associated with excessive accumulation of fibrin (Akassoglou *et al.* 2000).

9.3.2 Mechanisms of demyelination

The myelin sheath can be disrupted by serum factors and/or inflammatory cell secretory products including cytokines, ROIs and/or proteolytic enzymes, or by phagocytosis, generally preceded by permeabilization of the BBB (Cuzner 2001). Serum and plasma contain proenzymes which upon conversion have the capacity to cause disruption of the myelin sheath despite the presence in blood of proteinase inhibitors which inactivate neutral proteinases (Pescowitz *et al.* 1978). Myelin, with the capacity to activate the classical and alternative complement pathways, can be lysed through the formation of membrane attack complexes or by complement receptor-mediated opsonic phagocytosis (Silverman *et al.* 1984).

The predominant cellular route of myelin breakdown is via macrophages although polymorphonuclear leucocytes participate in acute haemorrhagic lesions. In EAE, mononuclear cell processes penetrate the myelin lamellae which are split at the intraperiod line and myelin is phagocytosed by what appears to be a receptor-mediated mechanism (Glynn and Linington 1989). Astrocytes may also contribute as they are observed with ingested myelin in chronic demyelinating MS plaques (Prineas 1985). Activated microglia and macrophages possess a wide range of receptors which can effect myelin uptake *in vitro* in the presence of antibody which is either antigen-specific or non-specific (Mosley and Cuzner 1996). These include Fc, lectin, scavenger and/or complement receptors, indicating the impressive scope for receptor-mediated phagocytosis. This is an important consideration in view of the search for the antigenic specificity of the intrathecally produced immunoglobulins in MS.

There are few reports of direct T cell-mediated demyelination and emphasis is placed on recruitment of effector cells by lymphocytes sensitized to brain antigens. However, MBP-specific T lymphocytes have been found capable of blocking action potentials in isolated rat optic nerve, providing the cells are HLA compatible (Yarom *et al.* 1983). The cytotoxic potential of MBP-specific T cells which is inseparably associated with the capacity to mediate clinical EAE is increasingly recognized, in particular through production of TNFα and β (Wekerle 1997).

Demyelination may also occur as the result of 'frustrated' phagocytosis or reverse endocytosis due to macrophages/microglia being unable to internalize myelin membrane, leading to discharge of lysosomal enzymes (Young and Zygas 1986). In a recent study of the immunopathology of secondary progressive MS many of the lesions in periplaque white matter exhibited evidence of low grade demyelination representative of frustrated phagocytosis (Prineas *et al.* 2001).

9.4 Effector processes in myelin and axon damage

The documented mediators of myelin and axon damage, products of activated microglia and primed T cells, include inflammatory cytokines and chemokines, acute response ROIs, and more chronically, proteolytic enzymes. The sequence, timing, and intensity of these responses govern the phenotypic nature of the CNS pathology.

9.4.1 Cytokines

The critical role of cytokines in the initiation, propagation and resolution of inflammatory demyelination is supported by their expression in MS and EAE lesions and from observations *in vivo* of raised levels in blood and CSF compartments. Most studies report an increase in Th1 pro-inflammatory cytokines with active disease and an increase in anti-inflammatory cytokines with recovery. For example, peripheral blood mononuclear cells (PBMCs) from MS patients have higher numbers of TNFα and IFNγ expressing cells and MBP-stimulated lymphocytes from MS patients express high levels of IFNγ (Olsson *et al.* 1992; Rieckmann *et al.* 1994). IL-12 expression by PBMCs is upregulated during active disease which may be critical in creating a pro-inflammatory Th1 mediated, destructive, autoimmune response (Ferrante *et al.* 1998). EAE can be prevented by treatment of SJL mice with anti-IL-12 neutralizing antibodies whereas the resistant BALB/c mice develop EAE when antibodies to IL-4, an anti-inflammatory cytokine, are administered (Constantinescu *et al.* 2001). Link *et al.* (1994) reported that patients with no or slight disability had significantly higher numbers of TGF-β[+]-cells and lower numbers of IFNγ[+]-cells, suggestive of a Th2 bias in quiescent disease. Th1 type cytokines were synthesized by CD4-, CD8- and CD14[+]-PBMCs from MS patients, following activation by MBP. During remission and in IFNβ-treated patients there was a decrease in expression of pro-inflammatory cytokines with a concomitant increase in Th2 anti-inflammatory cytokines IL-4 and IL-10. (Clerici *et al.* 2001). Furthermore, TNFα, IFNγ and IL-6 secreting PBMCs are augmented in MS compared to controls (Huang *et al.* 1999, 2001).

In some CSF studies, IL-1 and TNFα were identified as markers of relapse (Tsukada *et al.* 1991; Sharief and Hentges 1991), while others report no correlation with CSF or serum cytokine concentration (Peter *et al.* 1991). In a study from our laboratory, increased plasma levels of TNFα and IL-1β were detected at times of relapse (Zoukos *et al.* 1994).

Pro-inflammatory cytokines increase the expression of adhesion molecules on the endothelium as reported in active MS plaques (Sobel *et al.* 1990). During EAE upregulation of intercellular adhesion molecule (ICAM) is found on CNS endothelial cells prior to disease onset reaching maximal levels at peak disease (Cannella *et al.* 1991). Upregulation of VCAM expression was prevented by TNF neutralizing antibody treatment in EAE (Barten and Ruddle, 1994). Cytokine-induced expression of ROIs and NO by microglia and astrocytes (Section 9.4.3) and induction of MMPs (Section 9.4.4) also contributes to disease pathology. Although TNF neutralization was effective in treatment of EAE, it has proven ineffective in MS patients (The Lenercept Multiple Sclerosis Study Group and The University of British Columbia MS/MRI Analysis Group 1999). Indeed TNF neutralization therapy for juvenile rheumatoid arthritis has recently been reported to be associated with new onset MS in one patient (Sicotte and Voskuhl 2001). Kassiotis and Kollias (2001) shed some light on these apparently contradictory findings reporting a dual role for TNFα in a mouse model of EAE. In early disease stages TNFα is pro-inflammatory, however at late stages it induces apoptosis of autoreactive T cells and thus is immunosuppressive.

9.4.2 Chemokines

Expression of IFNγ, IL-1β and TNFα within the CNS induces chemoattractant cytokine (chemokine) expression by resident glial cells which then recruit T cells and macrophages into the CNS, amplifying the immune response (DeGroot and Woodroofe 2001). Chemokines have a crucial role in mediating cell migration as well as effector roles in influencing the differentiation of naïve T cells and inducing macrophages to produce ROIs and MMPs (De Groot and Woodroofe 2001; Baggiolini 1998). Within MS lesions, hypertrophic astrocytes predominantly express the CC chemokine, monocyte chemoattractant protein–1 (MCP-1) and the CXC chemokine, IFNγ inducible protein 10 (IP10) (Fig. 9.1A) whereas monokine induced by interferon-γ (Mig) was expressed by T cells and macrophages (Fig. 9.1B). Microglia express macrophage inflammatory protein (MIP) 1β and/or MIP1α, whereas RANTES is expressed by infiltrating cells, endothelial cells, and astrocytes (McManus *et al.* 1998; Simpson *et al.* 1998, 2000*a*; Van der Voorn *et al.* 1999; Boven *et al.* 2000). Endothelial cells express and present chemokines at the BBB and this is thought to be critical for inflammatory cell recruitment into the CNS (Andjelkovic *et al.* 1999). *In vitro* studies have demonstrated that glial cells synthesize and secrete chemokines in response to cytokine stimulation, for example, astroglial cells produce RANTES in response to Th1 cytokines (Li and Bever 2001). The chemokine receptor expression profile of Th1 and Th2 cells is characteristic, with Th1 cells expressing predominantly CCR2, CCR5, and CXCR3 whereas Th2 cells express CCR3 and CCR4 (Sallusto *et al.* 1998). The phenotype of T cells within the perivascular infiltrate is predominantly Th1 based on this chemokine receptor profile

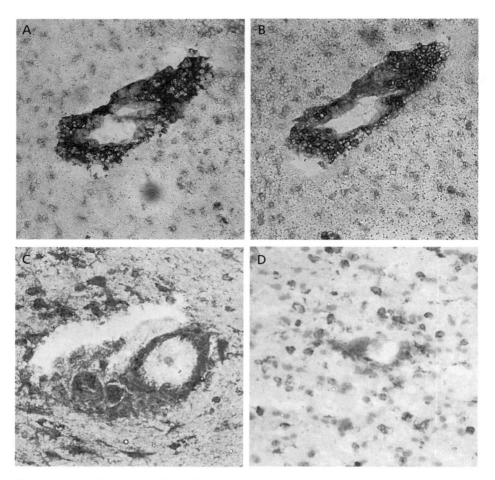

Fig. 9.1 Immunohistochemical investigation of actively demyelinating MS lesions demonstrates elevated expression of chemokines and their receptors. A. Within the perivascular cuff, infiltrating CD4 lymphocytes (brown) were CCR5 (red) positive, indicative of a Th1 phenotype. B. In contrast, few CD4 (brown), CCR3 (red) double immunopositive cells were detected. C. IP-10 immunoreactivity was associated with cells in the perivascular cuff and reactive astrocytes in the adjacent white matter. D. Mig immunoreactivity was associated with cells in the perivascular cuff and macrophages within the adjacent white matter. Magnifications A, B and D×400, C×800. For details of methodology see Simpson *et al.* 2000a, *b*. (Photographs kindly provided by Dr Julie Simpson, Sheffield Hallam University). See Plate 1.

(Fig. 9.1C and D). CCR2 and CCR5 are also present on foamy macrophages within lesions in MS (Simpson *et al.* 2000*b*).

In vivo studies assessing chemokine levels in the CSF of MS patients and controls have demonstrated that levels of IP10 are raised and those of MCP-1 decreased in MS patients compared to controls. T cells within the CSF and CNS express CXCR3, the IP10 receptor (Sørensen *et al.* 1999; Simpson *et al.* 2000*a*; Mahad *et al.* 2002). A role for CCR5 in MS

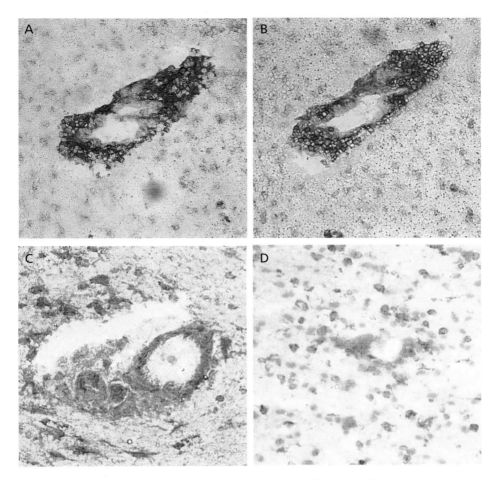

Plate 1 Immunohistochemical investigation of actively demyelinating MS lesions demonstrates elevated expression of chemokines and their receptors. A. Within the perivascular cuff, infiltrating CD4 lymphocytes (brown) were CCR5 (red) positive, indicative of a Th1 phenotype. B. In contrast, few CD4 (brown), CCR3 (red) double immunopositive cells were detected. C. IP-10 immunoreactivity was associated with cells in the perivascular cuff and reactive astrocytes in the adjacent white matter. D. Mig immunoreactivity was associated with cells in the perivascular cuff and macrophages within the adjacent white matter. Magnifications A, B and D×400, C×800. For details of methodology see Simpson *et al.* 2000*a, b*. (Photographs kindly provided by Dr Julie Simpson, Sheffield Hallam University).

pathogenesis is highlighted by the observation that delta 32, inactive, CCR5 allele is associated with a three year delay in onset of disease in families affected by MS (Barcellos *et al.* 2000).

The role of chemokines in inducing effector functions of glial cells has been less extensively researched. There are reports that chemokines induce MMP9 expression by microglia *in vitro*, suggesting a role in initiating demyelination as well as inducing the production of ROIs and NO by macrophages (Cross and Woodroofe 1999; Vaddi *et al.* 1997).

Studies on chemokine expression in EAE are generally in agreement with findings in MS. Astrocytes express MCP-1 and IP10 in EAE which correlates with clinical disease onset (Ransohoff 1997). In a chronic relapsing EAE model, MIP1α was associated with disease onset whereas MCP1 was associated with relapses (Karpus and Kennedy 1997). In studies using chemokine knockout mice or transgenic mice, there is some evidence that MCP-1 and its receptor CCR2 are required for induction of inflammation in the CNS in EAE (Gerard and Rollins 2001).

9.4.3 Reactive oxygen intermediates

A role for ROIs in disease pathogenesis has been demonstrated in studies of EAE and in MS based on histopathological studies and CSF and serum analyses. However the precise role is unclear as reports of NO as detrimental have now been tempered by more recent ones of beneficial effects. This is confirmed by studies in which therapies aimed at reducing NO have had variable outcomes, in some cases exacerbating disease (Smith *et al.* 1999). The outcome is most likely determined by the cell type producing NO, the time course and site of expression during the disease, or a combination of these factors (Licinio *et al.* 1999; Willenborg *et al.* 1999). Increased levels of NO are a result of induction of NOS in microglia and astrocytes (Smith *et al.* 1999), and NO has been found to upregulate IL-6 and TNFα production in a macrophage cell line (Deakin *et al.* 1995). However whether NO is produced by activated human monocytes/macrophages is controversial (Brosnan *et al.* 1995). Oligodendrocytes have been shown to be more susceptible to single stranded DNA breaks caused by NO than either microglia or astrocytes, possibly due to their diminished capacity for antioxidant defence (Smith *et al.* 1999).

Elevated levels of nitrite and nitrate have been demonstrated in the CSF during clinical exacerbations of MS, whereas raised serum levels correlated with clinical progression and were associated with fewer relapses and a non-progressive disease course, suggesting a beneficial effect of NO (Giovannoni *et al.* 1998, 2001; Brundin *et al.* 1999). Liu *et al.* (2001) reported expression of iNOS mRNA and protein in reactive astrocytes throughout lesions and in adjacent normal appearing white matter, while in chronic lesions it was restricted to astrocytes at the lesion edge. Macrophage and endothelial cell expression of iNOS was restricted to acute lesions. A protective effect of NO was demonstrated by downregulation of T cell proliferation in experiments on EAE in IFNγ knockout mice (Willenborg *et al.* 1999) as well as through induction of apoptosis and necrosis of T cells (Okuda *et al.* 1997). Genetic deletion of iNOS results in exacerbation of EAE, producing further evidence for a suppressive effect of NO in T cell mediated immunity (Van der Veen 2001). In DA rats with protracted relapsing EAE, TGF-β1 administration suppressed the disease through activation of PBMCs, which expressed high levels of iNOS and NO which then induced CD4$^+$ T cell apoptosis (Jin *et al.* 2000).

Superoxide radicals are involved in lipid peroxidation and can affect the lipid and protein content of myelin (Smith *et al.* 1999). Mouse or rat microglia release superoxide following PMA stimulation, which can be increased by pretreatment with pro-inflammatory cytokines to produce a strong respiratory burst (Woodroofe *et al.* 1989). Interaction of NO with superoxide to form peroxynitrite in response to cytokine activation of microglia diminishes the T cell regulatory activity of NO (Van der Veen 2001) as well as inducing cell death by causing strand breakage to DNA, lipid peroixidation and nitration of tyrosine residues affecting cell signalling (Smith *et al.* 1999). Peroxynitrite may also play a pathological role, by inducing the release of active MMPs from their proform by interaction with the cysteine switch mechanism in the propeptide autoinhibitory domain (Maeda *et al.* 1998). Neuronal cells, following hyperactivity of glutamate transmission, also produce peroxynitrite (Torreilles *et al.* 1999). *In vitro* studies have shown that myelin preparations exposed to peroxynitrite undergo lipid peroxidation, whereas NO inhibits lipid peroxidation (Van der Veen and Roberts 1999). The use of peroxynitrite scavengers, including uric acid, decreases disease severity in animals with EAE. MS patients with gout may be protected from relapses by hyperuricaemia due to its effects on peroxynitrite induced CNS cell damage (Hooper *et al.* 1998). Treatment of murine EAE with peroxynitrite scavengers delayed disease onset and the number of animals showing clinical signs was decreased, although disease progression was unaffected (Scott and Hooper 2001).

9.4.4 Proteolysis

In demyelinating MS lesions, myelin is broken down extracellularly by macrophage/microglial-derived serine and metalloproteases and/or following phagocytosis, by acid proteases such as cathepsin D (Cuzner 2001). The generation of plasmin by uPA is a rate-limiting step in the activation of MMPs which degrade the basement membrane and extracellular matrix (ECM), and promote extravasation of leucocytes. MMPs also have the capacity within the CNS to cleave MBP into fragments retaining encephalitogenicity (Proost *et al.* 1993; Chandler *et al.* 1995). In normal appearing white matter, increased expression of uPAR can initiate adhesion of mononuclear cells to blood vessel walls and migration of activated microglia from adjacent brain parenchyma during the formation of the primary MS lesion. Co-localization of uPAR with integrins on macrophages in the lesion further promotes adhesion to vitronectin which in turn leads to focal accumulation of PA activity (Gveric *et al.* 2001). Subsequent interference of the uPAR-vitronectin link by plasminogen activator inhibitor-1 promotes cell detachment and migration into the growing lesion.

Despite a quantitative increase in MMP-9 in the active MS lesion, enzyme activity is transient, localized and under stringent regulation by inhibitors which are present at high concentrations. Nonetheless, decreased immunostaining of tenascins C and R in the hypercellular zone of macrophages at the plaque edge points to a role for MMPs in remodelling the ECM (Gutowski *et al.* 1998). The cytokines documented as inducing MMP-9 expression are also readily detectable in active MS lesions both in perivascular cells and in activated microglia at the lesion edge (Woodroofe and Cuzner 1993; Cannella and Raine 1995).

The spectrum of MMPs appears to vary according to the cellular nature of the lesion in models of CNS inflammation, reflecting the proportion of neutrophils, lymphocytes, and macrophages in the perivasculature and the makeup of the ECM, although the majority of MMPs have a broad substrate specificity (Anthony *et al.* 1997). In general there is a correlation between mRNA levels and protein expression of MMPs, which are localized to the sites of inflammation (Cuzner and Opdenakker 1999). An increase in acid and neutral proteolytic activity in the CNS in EAE also appears to be primarily due to cellular infiltration and is greatest in the hyperacute lesions in primates.

In contrast to uPA there is significant constitutive tPA in normal human grey and white matter, in accord with its role in neuronal activity and synaptic remodelling. Although tPA is expressed on macrophages in MS lesions (Cuzner *et al.* 1996), it is predominantly concentrated on denuded axons in demyelinated zones. The decrease in concentration in the plaque contraindicates a major role for tPA in the transmigration of inflammatory cells but through activation by ECM proteins it may damage the BBB with leakage to the CSF. A specific increase in tPA in the CSF of patients in relapse is well documented (Akenami *et al.* 2000).

9.5 T cell responses in EAE and MS

The postulates for defining MS as a T cell-mediated autoimmune disease which are fulfilled in EAE include: (i) an association of disease susceptibility with MHC and TCR genes, (ii) recognition elements for T cell epitopes of autoantigens being disease associated MHC and TCR proteins, (iii) demonstration of *in vivo* activated and clonally expanded T cell populations specific for the target antigen in peripheral blood and brain of affected individuals and (iv) treatment of disease by tolerance induction to the target antigen or specific elimination of autoreactive T cells (Wucherpfennig *et al.* 1991). In studies of EAE in transgenic models of CNS-specific expression of cytokines and chemokines, induced by promotor regions of neural and glial cells, the $CD4^+$ Th1 cytokines, TNFα, IL-12 and IFNγ are found to synergize with a spectrum of chemokines in the induction of both inflammation and demyelination, while the $CD4^+$ Th2 anti-inflammatory cytokines IL-4 and IL-10 are associated with protection (Owens *et al.* 2001) (Section 9.4.1 and 9.4.2). The T cell response in rat and mouse EAE is governed by strict, although not absolute, epitope dominance in the early active phase of EAE with epitope spreading demonstrated at much later stages in the disease (Wekerle 1997). Restrictive usage of T cell receptor V-β genes by myelin antigen-specific T cells is also a feature of EAE, although selectivity varies fundamentally between epitopes on the same MBP molecule (Acha-Orbea *et al.* 1988, Urban *et al.* 1988).

The picture in EAE has been somewhat confounded by recent reports demonstrating a pathogenic role for MHC-class I restricted $CD8^+$ cytotoxic T cells in autoimmune demyelination in which the pathological features have a concordance with those of MS (Steinman 2001). The only major differences between the T cell $CD4^+$ and $CD8^+$ induced EAE appear to relate to the disease modulating effects of agents that block the cytokines TNFα and IFNγ. The immunodominant MHC class II restricted, $CD4^+$ T cell epitope, MBP 85–99, is immunolocalized in MS brain tissue (Krogsgaard *et al.* 2000) and longitudinal studies in individual MS patients of the T-cell response to MBP has confirmed long term persistence of individual clones (Hohlfeld and Wekerle 2001), however they have also been demonstrated in normal individuals. The role of PLP as another candidate autoantigen is highlighted by longitudinal studies demonstrating that MS patients have significantly elevated circulating PLP-reactive, IFNγ-producing $CD4^+$ Th1-like cells (Pelfrey *et al.* 2000). EAE has been found to develop spontaneously in triple transgenic animals humanized with components of the T cell response, MBP or PLP/MHC/TCR-specific clones derived from an MS patient (Madsen *et al.* 1999). Nonetheless the absolute and relative importance of autoimmunity in individual MS patients is still not established and antigen selective therapies have been largely ineffective.

9.6 **B cell responses in EAE and MS**

The first indicator of MS as an immune-mediated disease was the observation of selectively increased immunoglobulin levels in the CSF. The intrathecally synthesized IgG of individual patients displays an almost identical fingerprint oligoclonal pattern over time, suggestive of intermittent exposure to antigen and/or persistence of long lived plasma cells in a B-cell supporting environment (Glynn *et al*. 1982; Walsh and Tourtelotte 1986). Sequence analysis of complementarity-determining regions of antibodies from MS CSF and post-mortem tissue has revealed a high frequency of clonally expanded memory B cells with variable heavy chain sequences exhibiting extensive somatic mutations, indicative of antigen-driven B-cell selection (Qin *et al*. 1998). However the search for antigen specificity of the intrathecal IgG has not produced any clear candidates. Elevated antibody titres against viral and myelin antigens have been described and oligodendrocyte precursors have been identified as a target of the humoral response (Archelos *et al*. 2000). A pathogenic role for B cells in the pathogenesis of MS stems from the detection of IgG and complement, in particular the C9 neoantigen of the terminal lytic complex, deposited on phagocytic macrophages engaged in demyelination (Gay *et al*. 1997). The only EAE model with substantial focal demyelination resembling MS is that in which disease is induced with MOG, the protein which is expressed on the outermost lamellae of myelin. Autoantibodies to MOG enhance clinical severity, activate the complement cascade and augment demyelination in MBP T cell-induced inflammatory EAE (Piddlesden *et al*. 1993). Despite the demonstration of MOG auto-antibodies in MS lesions the involvement in the pathogenesis of MS is unproven.

9.7 **Normal-appearing white matter: indictment of microglia in priming inflammation**

Biochemical and immunocytochemical analysis of post-mortem MS normal appearing white matter demonstrates that there are subtle but significant diffuse abnormalities in myelin, axonal, and astrocytic proteins and an increased cellular activation status of microglia and astrocytes (Cuzner and Norton 1996). There is a consensus that the primary MS lesion may consist of focal areas of activated microglia, positive for the histochemical marker nucleoside diphosphatase (Li *et al*. 1996), strongly HLA DQ- and DR- positive and with detectable phagocytosed MBP, but no obvious myelin loss around the cells. (Cuzner 1997; Gay *et al*. 1997; Sriram and Rodriguez 1997). The co-localization of oxidized low density lipoprotein and MBP peptides in these macrophage-like cells is indicative of local pro-duction of ROIs in response to BBB damage (Newcombe *et al*. 1994). Release of peptides from these sites exposing neoepitopes could then lead to activation of specific immune responses. With an increasing degree of demyelination perivenular macrophages with non-specific esterase activity, a marker for monocytes which is absent in microglia, become the major cell in the growing lesion. Remarkably the primary lesion shows little evidence of fibrinogen leakage with parenchymal $CD4^+$ T cells detectable only occasionally and in very small numbers (Gay *et al*. 1997). Reactive microglia have increased expression of FcRI, II and III receptors for IgG, providing routes of uptake for IgG in both monomeric and complexed forms and IgG is co-localized with C3d on microglia closely associated with intact myelin sheaths (Ulvestad *et al.* 1994).

Microglia activated by infective agents or non-specific events in individuals with a pre-disposing immunogenetic profile may release factors which damage the BBB leading to ingress of plasma proteins. Oxidation and uptake of these proteins may trigger differenti-ation of microglia into macrophages which phagocytose and proteolytically degrade myelin and release inflammatory mediators attracting circulating lymphocytes and monocytes through upregulation of adhesion molecules and chemokine expression. The resulting antigen presentation generates a T cell response resulting in frank demyelination.

Axonal dysfunction as detected by magnetic resonance spectroscopy also appears to be a pathological feature of normal appearing white matter (Bjartmar *et al.* 2001). Resolution of the signal over time reflects its putative inflammatory nature. Although the vulnerable axons show relative histological preservation of myelin sheaths, they are surrounded by MHC Class II$^+$-microglia with internalized myelin.

9.8 Neuroprotective effects of inflammation

In the context of inflammatory demyelination, neuroprotection must be focused upon axon preservation/repair, glial scar limitation, and remyelination. It has been proposed that cells of the immune system have a neuroprotective function (Hohlfeld *et al.* 2000). Activated T cells specific for MBP or non-CNS antigen injected intraperitoneally immediately after nerve crush have a substantial neuroprotective effect, evident from electrophysiological studies (Moalem *et al.* 1999). Cells accumulated at the site of injury but only MBP-specific T cells had a substantial effect on limiting secondary degeneration. Injection of macrophages into transected spinal cord also stimulates tissue repair and partial recovery of motor function (Rapalino *et al.* 1998). A probable mechanism of repair is through the antigen stimulated production of growth factors, in particular brain derived (BDNF) and glial cell line derived neurotrophic factors by T cells and macrophages. BDNF-positive mononuclear cells are localized throughout demyelinating MS lesions (Hohlfeld *et al.* 2000).

Macrophages, which are prominent in the inflammatory cell environment of the lesion and the principal source of chemical mediators driving inflammatory demyelination, also secrete growth factors promoting proliferation and differentiation of oligodendrocyte pro-genitors (Diemel *et al.* 1998). Oligodendrocyte precursors are present in active MS lesions and limited but incomplete remyelination is apparent at sites of ongoing demyelination (Wolswijk 1998). Enhanced myelinogenesis is observed in macrophage-supplemented CNS aggregate cell cultures and appears to result from increased synthesis of TGF-β1 and fibroblast growth factor (FGF)-2, which stimulate oligodendrocyte proliferation and dif-ferentiation (Diemel *et al.* 2001). Addition of TGF-β1 to cultures upregulates FGF-2 pro-duction which stimulates oligodendrocyte progenitors to divide, leading to increased myelin synthesis. These results have implications for MS in which macrophages with abundant immunostaining for TGF-β isoforms have been demonstrated in active lesions (DeGroot *et al.* 1999).

The extracellular proteolytic system appears also to have a dual role in neurodegeneration and repair (Section 3.1). In excitotoxin-induced neuronal death in which BBB breakdown is not a contributory factor the tPA/plasmin proteolytic cascade promotes neuronal degenera-tion (Tsirka *et al.* 1995), also in acute monophasic EAE it is considered pro-inflammatory, promoting vascular permeability. However in chronic, relapsing remitting EAE it may have a protective role in removing fibrin deposits which exacerbate axonal damage (Koh et al. 1993).

References

Acha-Orbea, H., Mitchell, D. J., Timmermann, L., et al. (1988). Limited heterogeneity of T cell receptors from lymphocytes mediating autoimmune encephalomyelitis allows specific immune intervention. Cell, 54, 263–27.

Akassoglou, K., Kombrinck, K. W., Degen, J., and Stricklan, S. (2000). Tissue plasminogen Activator-mediated fibrinolysis protects against axonal degeneration and demyelination after sciatic nerve injury. J Cell Biol, 149, 1157–66.

Akenami, F. O. T., Koskiniemi, M., and Vaheri, A. (2000). Plasminogen activation in multiple sclerosis and other neurological disorders. Fibrinolysis and Proteal., 14, 1–14.

Aloisi, F., Ria, F., and Adorini, L. (2000). Regulation of T cell responses by CNS antigen presenting cells: different roles for microglia and astrocytes. Immunol Today, 21, 141–7.

Andjelkovic, A. V., Spencer, D. D., and Pachter, J. S. (1999). Visulization of chemokine binding sites on human brain microvessels. J Cell Biol, 145, 403–12.

Anthony, D. C., Ferguson, B., Matyzak, M. K., Miller, K. M., Esiri, M. M., and Perry, V. H. (1997). Differential matrix metalloproteinase expression in cases of multiple sclerosis and stroke. Neuropathology and Appl Neurobiol, 23, 406–15.

Archelos, J. J., Storch, M. K., and Hartung, H-P. (2000). The role of B cells and autoantibodies in multiple sclerosis. Ann Neurol, 47, 694–706.

Babbe, H., Roers, A., Waisman, A., et al. (2000). Clonal expansion of CD8 T cells dominate the T cell infiltrate in active multiple sclerosis lesions as shown by micromanipulation and single cell polymerase chain reaction. J Exp Med, 192, 393–404.

Baggiolini, M. (1998). Chemokines and leukocyte traffic. Nature, 392, 565–8.

Barcellos, L. F., Schito, A. M., Rimmler, J. B., et al. (2000). CC-chemokine receptor 5 polymorphism and age of onset in familial multiple sclerosis. Immunogenetics, 51, 281–8.

Barkhatova, V. P., Zavalishin, I. A., Askarova, L. Sh., Shavratskii, V. Kh., and Demina, E. G. (1998). Changes in neurotransmitters in multiple sclerosis. Neuroscience and Behavioral Physiology, 28, 341–4.

Barten, D. M. and Ruddle, N. H. (1994). Vascular cell adhesion molecule-1 modulation by tumor necrosis factor in experimental allergic encephalomyelitis. J Neuroimmunol, 51, 123–33.

Bitsch, A., Kuhlmann, T., Stadelmann, C., Lassmann, H., Lucchinetti, C., and Brück, W. (2001). A longitudinal MRI study of histopathologically defined hypointense multiple sclerosis lesions. Ann Neurol, 49, 793–6.

Bitsch, A., Schuchardt, J., Bunkowski, S., et al. (2000). Acute axonal injury in multiple scelrosis: correlation with demyelination and inflammation. Brain, 123, 1174–83.

Bjartmar, C., Kinkel, R. P., Kidd, G., Rudick, R. A., and Trapp, B. D. (2001). Axonal loss in normal-appearing white matter in a patient with acute MS. Neurology, 157, 1248–52.

Bjartmar, C. and Trapp, B. D. (2001). Axonal and neuronal degeneration in multiple sclerosis: mechanisms and functional consequences. Curr Opin Neurol, 14, 271–8.

Boven, L. A., Montagne, L., Nottet, H. S. L. M., and De Groot, C. J. A. (2000). MIP-1α, MIP-1β and RANTES mRNA semi-quantification and protein expression in active demyelinating multiple sclerosis lesions. Clin Exp Immunol, 122, 257–63.

Brosnan, C. F., Cannella, B., Battistini, L., and Raine, C. (1995). Cytokine localization in multiple sclerosis lesions: correlation with adhesion molecule expression and reactive nitrogen species. Neurology, 45, S16–21.

Brundin, L., Morcos, E., Olsson, T., Wiklund, N. P., and Andersson, M. (1999). Increased intrathecal nitric oxide formation in multiple sclerosis; cerebrospinal fluid nitrite as activity marker. Eur J Neurol, 6, 585–90.

Cannella, B., Cross, A., and Raine, C. (1991). Adhesion molecules in the central nervous system. Upregulation correlates with inflammatory cell influx during relapsing experimental autoimmune encephalomyelitis. *Lab Invest*, **65**, 23–31.

Cannella, B. and Raine, C. (1995). The adhesion molecule and cytokine profile of multiple sclerosis lesions. *Ann Neurol*, **37**, 424–35.

Chandler, S., Coates, R., Gearing, A., Lury, J., Wells, G., and Bone, E. (1995). Bone metalloproteinases degrade myelin basic protein. *Neurosci Lett*, **201**, 223–26.

Chen, Z. L. and Strickland, S. (1997). Neuronal death in the hippocampus is promoted by plasmin-catalyzed degradation of laminin. *Cell*, **91**, 917–25.

Clerici, M., Saresella, M., Trabattoni, D., *et al.* (2001). Single-cell analysis of cytokine production shows different immune profiles in multiple sclerosis patients with active or quiescent disease. *J Neuroimmunol*, **121**, 88–101.

Constantinescu, C. S., Hilliard, B., Ventura, E., *et al.* (2001). Modulation of susceptibility and resistance to an autoimmune model of multiple sclerosis in prototypically susceptible and resistant strains by neutralization of interleukin-12 and interleukin-4, respectively. *Clin Immunol*, **98**, 23–30.

Cross, A. K. and Woodroofe, M. N. (1999). Chemokine modulation of matrix metalloproteinase and TIMP production in adult rat brain microglia and a human microglial cell line *in vitro*. *Glia*, **28**, 183–9.

Cuzner, M. L. (1997). Molecular Biology of Microglia. In *Molecular biology of multiple sclerosis* (ed. W. C. Russell), John Wiley & Sons, New York, pp. 97–120.

Cuzner, M. L. (2001). Proteases in demyelination. In *Role of proteases in the pathophysiology of neurodegenerative diseases* (ed. A. Lajtha and N. L. Banik), Kluwer Academic/Plenum Publishers, New York, London. pp. 5–23.

Cuzner, M. L., Gveric, D., and Strand, C., *et al.* (1996). The expression of tissue-type plasminogen activator, matrix metalloproteases and endogenous inhibitors in the central nervous system in multiple sclerosis: comparison of stages in lesion evolution. *J. Neuropathol Exp Neurol*, **55**, 1194–1204.

Cuzner, M. L. and Norton, W. T. (1996). Biochemistry of demyelination. In M. L. Cuzner, H. Wekerle, Eds. Immunopathology of Demyelinating Disease (Symposium). *Brain Pathol*, 231–42.

Cuzner, M. L. and Opdenakker, G. (1999). Plasminogen activators and matrix metalloproteases, mediators of extracellular proteolysis in inflammatory demyelination of the central nervous system. *J Neuroimmunol*, **94**, 1–14.

Deakin, A. M., Payne, A. N., Whittle, B. J., and Moncada, S. (1995). The modulation of IL-6 and TNF-alpha release by nitric oxide following stimulation of J774 cells with LPS and IFN-gamma. *Cytokine*, **7**, 408–16.

DeGroot, C. J. A., Montagne, L., Barten, A. D., Sminia, P., and Van der Valk, P. (1999). Expression of transforming growth factor (TGF)-beta 1, -beta 2, and -beta 3 isoforms and TGF-beta type I and type II receptors in multiple sclerosis lesions and human adult astrocyte cultures. *J Neuropathol Exp Neurol*, **58**, 174–87.

De Groot, C. J., Ruuls, S. R., Theeuwes, J. W., Dijkstra, C. D., and Van der Valk, P. (1997). Immunocytochemical characterization of the expression of inducible and constitutive isoforms of nitric oxide synthase in demyelinating multiple sclerosis lesions. *J Neuropathol Exp Neurol*, **56**, 10–20.

DeGroot, C. J. A. and Woodroofe, M. N. (2001). The role of chemokines and chemokine receptors in CNS inflammation. *Prog Brain Res*, **132**, 543–54.

Diemel, L. T., Copelman, C. A., and Cuzner, M. L. (1998). Macrophages in CNS remyelination: Friend or Foe? *Neurochem Res*, **23**, 341–47.

Diemel, L. T., Jackson, S. J., Copelman, C. A., and Cuzner, M. L. (2001). TGF-β1 induction of FGF-2 protein is associated with increased MBP synthesis in CNS aggregate cultures. *Soc Neurosci Abstr* 157.12.

Ferguson, B., Matyszak, M. K., Esiri, M. M., and Perry, V. H. (1997). Axonal damage in acute multiple sclerosis lesions. *Brain*, 120, 393–9.

Ferrante, P., Fusi, M. L., and Saresella, M., *et al.* (1998). Cytokine production and surface marker expression in acute and stable multiple sclerosis: altered IL-12 production and augmented signaling lymphocytic activation molecule (SLAM)-expressing lymphocytes in acute multiple sclerosis. *J Immunol*, 160, 1514–21.

Gay, F. W., Drye, T. J., Dick, G. W. A., and Esiri, M. M. (1997). The application of multifactorial cluster analysis in the staging of plaques in early multiple sclerosis. Identification and characterization of the primary demyelinating lesion. *Brain*, 120, 1461–83.

Gerard, C., and Rollins, B. J. (2001). Chemokines and disease. *Nature Immunology*, 2, 108–115.

Giovannoni, G., Heales, S. J., Land, J. M., and Thompson, E. J. (1998). The potential role of nitric oxide in multiple sclerosis. *Multiple Sclerosis*, 4, 212–16.

Giovannoni, G., Miller, D. H., and Losseff, N. A. (2001). Serum inflammatory markers and clinical/MRI markers of disease progression in multiple sclerosis. *J Neurol*, 248, 487–95.

Glynn, P., Gilbert, G. P., Newcombe, J., and Cuzner, M. L. (1982). Analysis of immunoglobulin G in multiple sclerosis brain: quantitative and isoelectric focusing studies. *Clin Exp Immunol*, 48, 102–110.

Glynn, P. and Linington, C. (1989). Cellular and molecular mechanisms of autoimmune demyelination in the central nervous system. *CRC Crit Rev Neurobiol*, 4, 367–85.

Gutowski, N. J., Newcombe, J., and Cuzner, M. L. (1998). Changes in extracellular matrix tenascins during glial scar formation in MS plaques. *Neuropathol Appl Neurobiol*, 24, 155.

Gveric, D., Hanemaaijer, R., Newcombe, J., Van Lent, N. A., Sier, C. F. M, and Cuzner, M. L. (2001). Plasminogen activators in multiple sclerosis lesions: Implications for the inflammatory response and axonal damage. *Brain*, 124, 1978–88.

Hohlfeld, R., Kerschensteiner, M., Stadelmann, C., Lassmann, H., and Wekerle, H. (2000). The neuroprotective effect of inflammation: implications for the therapy of multiple sclerosis. *J Neuroimmunol*, 107, 161–6.

Hohlfeld, R., and Wekerle, H. (2001). Immunological update of multiple sclerosis. *Curr Opin Neurol*, 14, 299–304.

Hooper, D. C., Spitsin, S., Kean, R. B., *et al.* (1998). Uric acid, a natural scavenger of peroxynitrite, in experimental allergic encephalomyelitis and multiple sclerosis. *Proc Natl Acad Sci USA*, 95, 675–80.

Huang, W. X., Huang, P., Link, H., and Hillert, J. (1999). Cytokine analysis in multiple sclerosis by competitive RT - PCR: A decreased expression of IL-10 and an increased expression of TNF-alpha in chronic progression. *Multiple Sclerosis*, 5, 342–8.

Huang, Y. M., Stoyanova, N., and Jin, Y. P., *et al.* (2001). Altered phenotype and function of blood dendritic cells in multiple sclerosis are modulated by IFN-beta and IL-10. *Clin Exp Immunol*, 124, 306–14.

Huseby, E. D., Liggitt, T., Brabb, B., Schnabel, C., Ohlen, and Goverman, J. (2001). A pathogenic role for CD8[+] T cells in a model for multiple sclerosis. *J Exp Med*, 194, 669–76.

Jin, Y. X., Xu, L. Y., Guo, H., Ishikawa, M., Link, H., and Xiao, B. G. (2000). TGF-beta1 inhibits protracted-relapsing experimental autoimmune encephalomyelitis by activating dendritic cells. *J Autoimmunity*, 14, 213–20.

Karpus, W. J., and Kennedy, K. J. (1997). MIP-1α and MCP-1 differentially regulate acute and relapsing autoimmune encephalomyelitis as well s Th1/Th2 lymphocyte differentiation. *J leukocyte Biol*, 62, 681–7.

Kassiotis, G., and Kollias, G. (2001). Uncoupling the proinflammatory from the immunosuppressive properties of tumor necrosis factor (TNF) at the p55 TNF receptor level: implications for pathogenesis and therapy of autoimmune demyelination. *J Exp Med*, 193, 427–34.

Koh, C. S., Gausas, J., and Paterson, P. Y. (1993). Neurovascular permeability and fibrin deposition in the central neuraxis of Lewis rats with cell-transferred experimental allergic encephalomylitis in relationship to clinical and histopathological features of the disease. *J Neuroimmunol*, 47, 141–5.

Krogsgaard, M., Wucherpfennig, K. W., and Canella, B. (2000). Visualization of myelin basic protein (MBP) T cell epitopes in multiple sclerosis using a monoclonal antibody specific for the human histocampatibility leukocyte antigen. *J Exp Med*, 191, 1395–12.

Leppert, D., Raija, L. P., and Lindberg., *et al.* (2001). Matrix metalloproteinases: multifunctional effectors of inflammation in multiple sclerosis and bacterial meningitis. *Brain Res Rev*, 36, 249–57.

Li, Q. Q. and Bever, C.T. (2001). Th1 cytokines stimulate RANTES chemokine secretion by human astroglial cells depending on de novo transcription. *Neurochem Res*, 26, 125–33.

Li, H., Cuzner, M. L., and Newcombe, J. (1996). Microglia-derived macrophages in early multiple sclerosis plaques. *Neuropathol and Appl Neurobiol.* 22, 207–15.

Li, H., Newcombe, J., and Cuzner, M. L. (1993). Characterisation and distribution of phagocytic macrophages in MS plaques. *Neuropathol Appl Neurobiol*, 19, 214–23.

Licinio, J., Prolo, P., McCann, S. M., and Wong, M. L. (1999). Brain iNOS: current understanding and clinical implications. *Mol Med Today*, 5, 225–32.

Link, J., Söderström, M., Olsson, T., *et al.*(1994). Increased transforming growth factor-beta, interleukin-4, and interferon-gamma in multiple sclerosis. *Ann Neurol*, 36, 379–86.

Liu, J. S., John, G. R., Sikora, A., Lee, S. C., and Brosnan, C. F. (2000). Modulation of interleukin-1beta and tumor necrosis factor alpha signaling by P2 purinergic receptors in human fetal astrocytes. *J Neurosci*, 20, 5292–9.

Liu, J. S., Zhao, M. L., Brosnan, C. F., and Lee, S. C. (2001). Expression of inducible nitric oxide synthase and nitrotyrosine in multiple sclerosis lesions. *Amer J Pathol*, 158, 2057–66.

Lucchinetti, C., Bruck, W., and Parisi, J.*et al.* (2000). Heterogeneity of multiple sclerosis lesions: implication for the paghogenesis of demyelination. *Ann Neurol*, 47, 707–17.

Lucchinetti, C., Brück, W., Noseworthy, J. (2001). Multiple sclerosis: recent developments in neuropathology, pathogenesis, magnetic resonance imaging studies and treatment. *Curr Opin Neurolol*, 14, 259–69.

Madsen, L. S., Andersson, E. C., and Jansson, L., *et al.* (1999). A humanized model for multiple sclerosis using HLA DR2 and a human T cell receptor. *Nat Genet*, 23, 343–7.

Maeda, H., Okamoto, T., and Akaike, T. (1998). Human matrix metalloprotease activation by insults of bacterial infection involving proteases and free radicals. *Biol Chem*, 379, 193–200.

Mahad, D. J., Howell, S., and Woodroofe, M. N. (2002). Expression of chemokines in the CSF and correlation with clinical disease activity in patients with multiple sclerosis. *J Neurol Neurosurg and Psychiatr*, 72, 498–502.

Martin, R. and McFarland, H. F. (1997). Immunology of multiple sclerosis and experimental allergic encephalomyelitis. In *Multiple sclerosis clinical and pathogenetic basis*. Chapman & Hall, London, pp. 221–39. (Eds. Cedric S. Raine, Henry, F. McFarland, and Wallace, W. Tourtellotte.)

Matute, C., Alberdi, E., Domercq, M., Pérez-Cerdá, F., Pérez-Samartín, A., and Sánchez-Gmez, M. V. (2001). The link between excitotoxic oligodendroglial death and demyelinating diseases. *Trends Neurosci*, 24, 224–30.

McManus, C., Berman, J. W., Brett, F. M., Staunton, H., Ferrell, M., and Brosnan, C. (1998). MCP-1, MCP-2 and MCP-3 expression in multiple sclerosis lesions: an immunohistochemical and in situ hybridization study. *J Neuroimmunol*, 86, 20–9.

Moalem, G., Leibowitz-Amit, R., Yoles, E., Mor, F., Cohen, I. R., Schwartz, M. (1999). Autoimmune T cells protect neurons from secondary degeneration after central nervous system axotomy. *Nat Med*, 5, 49–55.

Mosley, K., and Cuzner, M. L. (1996). Receptor-mediated phagocytosis of myelin by macrophages and microglia: effect of opsonization and receptor blocking agents. *Neurochem Res*, 21, 479–85.

Newcombe, J., Li, H., and Cuzner, M. L. (1994). Low density lipoprotein uptake by macrophages in multiple sclerosis plaques: Implications for pathogenesis. *Neuropathol Appl Neurobiol*, 20, 152–62.

Okuda, M., Sakoda, S., Fujimura, H., and Yanagihara, T. (1997). Nitric oxide via an inducible isoform of nitric oxide synthase is a possible factor to eliminate inflammatory cells from the central nervous system of mice with experimental allergic encephalomyelitis, *J Neuroimmunol*, 73, 107–16.

Olsson, T., Sun, J., Hillert, J., *et al.* (1992). Increased numbers of T cells recognizing multiple myelin basic protein epitopes in multiple sclerosis. *European Journal of Immunology*, 22, 1083–87.

Owens, T., Wekerle, H., and Antel, J. (2001). Genetic models for CNS inflammation. *Nature*, 7, 161–67.

Pelfrey, C. M., Rudick, R. A., Cotleur, A. C., *et al.* (2000). Quantification of self-recognition in multiple sclerosis by single-cell analysis of cytokine production. *J Immunol*, 165, 1641–51.

Pescovitz, M. D., Paterson, P. Y., and Lorand, L. (1978). Serum degradation of myelin basic protein with loss of encephalitogenic activity: evidence for an enzymatic process. *Cell Immunol*, 39, 355–65.

Peter, J. B., Boctor, F. N., and Tourtellotte, W. W. (1991) Serum and CSF levels of IL-2, sIL-2R. TNF-α, and IL-1β in chronic progressive multiple sclerosis: expected lack of clinical utility. *Neurology*, 41, 121–3.

Piddlesden, S. J., Lassmann, H., Zimprich, F., Morgan, B. P., and Linington, C. (1993). The demyelinating potential of antibodies to myelin oligodendrocyte glycoprotein is related to their ability to fix complement. *Amer J Pathol*, 143, 555–64.

Pitt, D; Werner, P., and Raine, C. S. (2000). Glutamate excitotoxicity in a model of multiple sclerosis, *Nat Med*, 6, 67–70.

Prineas, J. W. (1985). The neuropathology of multiple sclerosis. In *Handbook of clinical neurology* (ed. Koetsier, J. C.) Elsevier Science Publishing, Amsterdam, New York, pp. 213–57.

Prineas, J. W., Kwon, E. E., Cho, E. S., *et al.* (2001). Immunopathology of secondary MS. *Ann Neurol*, 50, 646–57.

Proost, P., Van Damme, J., Opdenakker, G. (1993). Leukocyte gelatinase B cleavage releases encephalitogens from human myelin basic protein. *Biochem Biophys Res Commun*, 192, 1175–81.

Qin, Y. F., Duquett, P., Zhang, Y. P., Talbot, P., Poole, R., and Antel, J. (1998). Clonal expansion and somatic hypermutation of V-H genes of B cells from cerebrospinal fluid in multiple sclerosis. *J Clin Invest*, 102, 1045–50.

Ransohoff, R. M. (1997) Chemokines in neurological disease models: correlation between chemokine expression patterns and inflammatory pathology. *J Leukocyte Biol*, 82, 845–52.

Rapalino, O., Lazarov-Spiegler, O., Agranov, E., *et al.* (1998). Implantation of stimulated homologous macrophages results in partial recovery of paraplegic rats. *Nat Med*, 4: 814–21.

Rieckmann, P., Albrecht, M., and Kitze, B., *et al.* (1994). Cytokine mRNA levels in mononuclear blood cells from patients with multiple sclerosis. *Neurology*, 44, 1523–6.

Sallusto, F., Lanzavecchia, A., and Mackay, C. R. (1998). Chemokines and chemokine receptors in T cell priming and Th1/Th2 mediated responses. *Immunol Today*, 19, 568–74.

Scott, G. S., and Hooper, D. C. (2001). The role of uric acid in protection against peroxynitrite-mediated pathology. *Med Hypotheses*, 56, 95–100.

Sharief, M. K., and Hentges, R. (1991). Association between tumor necrosis factor-alpha and disease progression in patients with multiple sclerosis. *N Engl J Med*, 325, 467–72.

Sicotte, N. L., and Voskuhl, R. R. (2001). Onset of multiple sclerosis associated with anti-TNF therapy, *Neurology*, 57, 1885–88.

Silverman, B. A., Carney, D. F., Johnston, C. A., Vanguri, P., and Shin, M. L. (1984). Isolation of membrane attack complex of complement from myelin membranes treated with serum complement. *J Neurochem*, 42, 1024–30.

Simpson, J. E., Newcombe, J., Cuzner, M. L., and Woodroofe, M. N. (1998). Expression of monocyte chemoattractant protein-1 and other β-chemokines by resident glia and inflammatory cells in multiple sclerosis lesions. *J Neuroimmunol*, **84**, 238–49.

Simpson, J. E; Newcombe, J., Cuzner, M. L., and Woodroofe, M. N. (2000*a*). Expression of the interferon-gamma-inducible chemokines IP-10 and Mig and their receptor, CXCR3, in multiple sclerosis lesions. *Neuropathol Appl Neurobiol*, **26**, 133–42.

Simpson, J. E., Rezaie, P., Newcombe, J., Cuzner, M. L., Male, D., and Woodroofe, M. N. (2000*b*). Expression of the β-chemokine receptors CCR2, CCR3 and CCR5 in multiple sclerosis central nervous system tissue. *J Neuroimmunol*, **108**, 192–200.

Smith, K. J., and Hall, S. M. (2001). Factors directly affecting impulse transmission in inflammatory demyelinating disease: recent advances in our understanding, *Curr Opin Neurol*, **14**, 289–98.

Smith, K. J., Kapoor, R., Hall, S. M., and Davies, M. (2001). Electrically active axons degenerate when exposed to nitric oxide, *Ann Neurol*, **49**, 470–6.

Smith, K. J., Kapoor, R., and Felts, P. A. (1999). Demyelination: the role of reactive oxygen and nitrogen species. *Brain Pathol*, **9**, 69–92.

Smith, T., Groom, A., Zhu, B., and Turski, L. (2000). Autoimmune encephalomyelitis ameliorated by AMPA antagonists. *Nat Med*, **6**, 62–6.

Sobel, R. A., Mitchell, M. E., and Fondren, G. (1990). Intercellular adhesion molecule-1 (ICAM-1) in cellular immune reactions in the human central nervous system. *Amer J Pathol*, **136**, 1309–16.

Sørensen, T. L., Tani, M., Jensen, J., *et al.* (1999). Expression of specific chemokines and chemokine receptors in the central nervous system of multiple sclerosis patients. *J Clin Invest*, **103**, 807–15.

Sriram, S., and Rodriguez, M. (1997). Indictment of the microglia as the villain in multiple sclerosis. *Neurology*, **48**, 464–70.

Steinman, L. (2001). Myelin-specific CD8 T cells in the pathogenesis of experimental allergic encephalitis and multiple sclerosis. *J Exp Med*, **194**, F27–30.

Stover, J.F., Lowitzsch, K., and Kempski, O. S. (1997). Cerebrospinal fluid hypoxanthine, xanthine and uric acid levels may reflect glutamate-mediated excitotoxicity in different neurological diseases. *Neurosc Lett*, **238**, 25–8.

Sun, D., Whitaker, J. N., Huang, Z., *et al.* (2001). Myelin antigen-specific CD8 T cells are encephalitogenic and produce severe disease in C57BL/6 mice. *J Immunol*, **166**, 7579–87.

The Lenercept Multiple Sclerosis Study Group and The University of British Columbia MS/MRI Analysis Group (1999). TNF neutralization in MS: results of a randomized, placebo-controlled multicenter study. *Neurology*, **53**, 457–65.

Torreilles, F., Salman-Tabcheh, S., Guérin, M., and Torreilles, J. (1999). Neurodegenerative disorders: the role of peroxynitrite, *Brain Res. Brain Res Rev*, **30**, 153–63.

Trapp, B. D., Peterson, J., Ransohoff, R. M., Rudick, R., Mörk, S., and Bö, L. (1998). Axonal transection in the lesions of multiple sclerosis. *N Engl J Med*, **338**, 278–85.

Tsirka, S. E., Gualandris, A., Amaral, D. G., and Strickland, S. (1995). Excitotoxin-induced neuronal degeneration and seizure are mediated by tissue-plasminogen activator. *Nature*, **377**, 340–44.

Tsukada, N., Miyagi, K., Matsuda, M., Yanagisawa, N., Yonne, K. (1991). Tumor necrosis factor and interleukin-1 in the CSF and sera of patients with multiple sclerosis. *J Neurol Sci*, **102**, 230–34.

Ulvestad, E., Williams, K., Vedeler, C., *et al.* (1994). Reactive microglia in multiple sclerosis lesions have an increased expression of receptors for the Fc part of IgG. *J Neurol Sci*, **121**, 125–31.

Urban, J. L., Kumar, V., Kono, D., *et al.* (1988). Restricted use of T cell receptor V genes in murine autoimmune encephalomyelitis raises possibilities for antibody therapy. *Cell*, **54**, 577–92.

Vaddi, K., Keller, M., and Newton, R. C. (1997). In *The Chemokine Facts Book.*, (ed. K. Vaddi, M. Keller, and R. C., Newton), Academic Press, California, p. 95.

Van der Veen, R. C. (2001). Nitric oxide and T helper cell immunity. *Int Immunopharmacol*, **1**, 1491–500.

Van der Veen, R. C., and Roberts, L. J. (1999). Contrasting roles for nitric oxide and peroxynitrite in the peroxidation of myelin lipids. *J Neuroimmunol*, **95**, 1–7.

Van der Voorn, J. P., Tekstra, J., Beelen, R. H. J., Tensen, C. P., Van der Valk, P., and De Groot, C. J. A. (1999). Expression of MCP-1 by reactive astrocytes in demyelinating multiple sclerosis lesions. *Amer J Pathol*, 154, 45–51.

Walsh, M. J., and Tourtellotte, W. W. (1986). Temporal invariance and clonal uniformity of brain and cerebrospinal IgG, IgA and IgM in multiple sclerosis. *J Exp Med*, 163, 41–53.

Wekerle, H. (1997). CD4 effector cells in autoimmune diseases of the central nervous system. In Immunology of the Nervous System. Oxford University Press, New York, pp. 460–92. (ed. Robert, W. Keane, and William, F. Hickey).

Werner, P., Pitt, D., and Raine, C. S. (2001). Multiple sclerosis: altered glutamate homeostasis in lesions correlates with oligodendrocyte and axonal damage. *Ann Neurol*, 50, 169–80.

Willenborg, D. O., Fordham, S. A., Staykova, M. A., Ramshaw, I. A., and Cowden, W. B. (1999). IFN-gamma is critical to the control of murine autoimmune encephalomyelitis and regulates both in the periphery and in the target tissue: a possible role for nitric oxide, *J Immunol*, 163, 5278–86.

Wolswijk, G. (1998). Chronic stage multiple sclerosis lesions contain a relatively quiescent population of oligodendrocyte precursor cells. *J Neurosci*, 18, 601–9.

Woodroofe, M. N., and Cuzner, M. L. (1993). Cytokine mRNA expression in inflammatory multiple sclerosis lesions: detection by non-radioactive ISH. *Cytokine*, 5, 583–8.

Woodroofe, M. N., Hayes, G. M., and Cuzner, M. L. (1989). Fc receptor density, MHC antigen expression and superoxide production are increased in interferon-gamma-treated microglia isolated from adult rat brain, *Immunology*, 68, 421–6.

Wucherpfennig, K. W., Newcombe, J., Li, H., Keddy, C., Cuzner, M. L., and Hafler, D. A. (1992). T cell receptor Vα-Vβ repertoire and cytokine gene expression in active multiple sclerosis lesions. *J Exp Med*, 175, 993–1002.

Wucherpfennig, K. W., Weiner, H. L., and Hafler, D. A. (1991). T-cell recognition of myelin basic protein. *Immunol Today*, 12, 277–82.

Yarom, Y., Naparstek, Y., Lev-Ram, V., Holoshitz, J., Ben-Nun, A., Cohen, I. R. (1983). Immunospecific inhibition of nerve conduction by T lymphocytes reactive to basic protein of myelin. *Nature*, 303, 246–7.

Young, P. R., and Zygas, A. P. (1986). Secretion of lactic acid by peritoneal macrophages during extracellular phagocytosis - The possible role of local hyperacidity in inflammatory demyelination. *J Neuroimmunol*, 15, 295–308.

Zoukos, Y., Kidd, D., Woodroofe, M. N., Kendall, B. E., Thompson, A., Cuzner, M. L. (1994). Increased expression of high affinity IL-2 receptors and β-adrenoceptors on peripheral blood mononuclear cells is associated with clinical and MRI activity in MS. *Brain*, 117, 307–15.

Chapter 10

CNS immune reactions in Alzheimer's disease: microglia mediated mechanisms of inflammation in the Alzheimer's disease brain and their relevance to new therapeutic strategies

Joseph Rogers, Carl J. Kovelowski, and Ron Strohmeyer

From the discovery, nearly two decades ago, that microglia are activated to express major histocompatibility complex (MHC) cell surface glycoproteins in the Alzheimer's disease (AD) cortex (Luber-Narod and Rogers 1988; McGeer *et al.* 1989; Tooyama *et al.* 1990; Perlmutter *et al.* 1992; Itagaki *et al.* 1988), hundreds of studies have confirmed that brain inflammation is a characteristic pathological process in AD (reviewed in Rogers and O'Barr 1996; McGeer and McGeer 1998; Rogers *et al.* 1996; Strohmeyer and Rogers 2001; Akiyama *et al.* 2000). When one considers classic stimulants for inflammation that have been studied in the periphery for nearly a century, AD inflammation is not wholly unexpected. That is, the presence of dead and damaged cells and the chronic accumulation of highly inert, insoluble deposits engenders inflammation virtually anywhere in the body (Rosenberg and Gallin 1999). The AD brain is no exception. It features a loss of neurones and neurites that is universally accepted as the underlying cause of AD dementia. The AD brain also shows chronic accumulation of aggregated, highly insoluble amyloid β (Aβ) deposits and paired helical filaments—the type of material that drives inflammatory cells into heightened states of activation. The fact that AD inflammation occurs is not surprising. What is surprising is that it took so long to notice it.

Initially, chronic and acute phase inflammatory reactions were regarded as epiphenomena in AD, secondary responses to clear the damage caused by other mechanisms such as Aβ peptide deposition and neurofibrillary tangle formation. However, this view began to change rapidly as more and more cytotoxic inflammatory responses were documented, and as novel interactions of inflammatory mediators with AD pathology were discovered. Today, inflammation has come to be understood as a secondary, but pathogenic event in AD: it may arise as a consequence of more primary pathologies in the AD brain, but it nonetheless causes significant damage. This is especially true because inflammation is chronic throughout the disease process, from the earliest, preclinical stages to death. Alternatively, as is equally well documented in the periphery, some aspects of inflammation are devoted to rebuilding damaged tissue, and these mechanisms, too, may also come into play in AD. Inflammation is a very complicated business, whatever the organ that is impacted.

Microglia are widely viewed as a pivotal cellular element in AD inflammation. They comprise approximately 10–15 per cent of the cellular population in the brain (McGeer and McGeer 1995; Chao et al. 1999; Barron 1995), but likely have a monocyte origin (Perry et al. 1985; Perry et al. 1999; Barron 1995). In the resting state, microglia normally subserve neuro-trophic roles (reviewed in Streit et al. 1999; Barron 1995), and exhibit ramified morpho-logies, few or no macrophage-like characteristics, and very low turnover rates (Lawson et al. 1994; Krall et al. 1994; Barron 1995). By numerous criteria, however, microglia in the AD brain, like microglia in a variety of other neuropathological conditions (Gehrmann et al. 1993; Morioka et al. 1992; Morioka et al. 1993; Streit and Sparks 1997; Streit et al. 1999), are appropriately considered to be activated (Barron 1995). They assume an amoeboid mor-phology, become phagocytic, and increase their expression of MHCII, cytokines, chemokines, complement, and other acute phase proteins (reviewed in Walker 1998; Kreutzberg 1996; Akiyama et al. 2000; Giulian 1987; Barron 1995).

Activated microglia cluster at sites of aggregated Aβ deposition, assuming central, intra-plaque positions (Luber-Narod and Rogers 1988; Haga et al. 1989). They are present in virtually all diffuse (noncongophilic) plaques, have their far greatest densities in neuritic plaques, and are seldom associated with dense core, non-neuritic ('burned out') plaques (Griffin et al. 1995; Griffin et al. 1997). By contrast, astrocytes take up peri-plaque positions encircling Aβ deposits. This co-localization of microglia and astrocytes with Aβ deposits may provide opportunities for intercellular inflammatory signalling. IL-1β secreted by microglia, for example, induces astrocyte expression of S100β protein (Sheng et al. 1997).

The clustering of microglia within plaques is readily explained by chemotactic signalling by Aβ itself (Davis et al. 1992) and by several inflammatory mediators that are associated with Aβ in senile plaques, including complement activation fragments, cytokines, and chemokines (reviewed in Akiyama et al. 2000). In addition, AD microglia reportedly upregulate their expression of the macrophage scavenger receptor (MSR) (Christie et al. 1996; El Khoury et al. 1996) and the receptor for advanced glycation end products (RAGE) (Yan et al. 1996), both of which appear to have Aβ as ligands (El Khoury et al. 1996; Yan et al. 1996). Stimulation of the RAGE receptor with Aβ induces M-CSF in microglia (Yan et al. 1997), just as it does in macrophages. Similarly, adhesion of microglia to Aβ fibrils via class A scavenger receptors leads to immobilization of the cells and induces production of reactive oxygen species (El Khoury et al. 1996, 1998). It has also been demonstrated recently that the chemotactic formyl peptide receptor (FPR) binds Aβ, triggering G protein-dependent calcium mobil-ization and activation of chemokine signal transduction pathways (Lorton et al. 2000).

Beyond their chemotaxis and physical proximity to Aβ deposits, the role of microglia in plaque evolution is still incompletely understood. Although microglia have been suggested to play a direct role in the synthesis of Aβ precursor protein (AβPP), and cultured microglia can secrete Aβ and metabolize AβPP in a manner that might favour Aβ deposition (Bauer et al. 1991; Bitting et al. 1996), microglial AβPP mRNA expression is yet to be demonstrated (Scott et al. 1993). By contrast, neurones in vivo and neurones in culture exhibit abundant expression of AβPP (LeBlanc, 1995), and are therefore believed by most investigators to be a more likely source of brain Aβ than microglia.

A potential role for microglia in processing AβPP and Aβ is more tenable. Microglial aggregation within Aβ-containing neuritic plaques is nearly universal, whereas it is substantially less in diffuse plaques in AD, normal aging (Coria *et al.* 1993; Itagaki *et al.* 1994; Mackenzie 2000; Rozemuller *et al.* 1989), and AβPP-overexpressing transgenic mice (Frautschy *et al.* 1998; Stalder *et al.* 1999). This association of microglia with aggregated, congophilic Aβ deposits suggests that they, like peripheral macrophages in systemic amyloidosis (Shirahama *et al.* 1990), may be involved in the conversion of nonfibrillar Aβ into amyloid fibrils. Such a possibility is supported by many studies (Cotman and Tenner 1996; Griffin *et al.* 1994; Mackenzie and Munoz 1998; Sasaki *et al.* 1997; Walker 1998), including ultrastructural observations (Wisniewski *et al.* 1989).

Finally, microglial clearance of Aβ via phagocytosis is another plausible prospect, in keeping with the emerging view that Aβ burden in the AD brain reflects a dynamic balance or imbalance between deposition and removal (Hyman *et al.* 1993). Many laboratories have shown that microglia actively phagocytose exogenous fibrillar Aβ *in vivo* and in culture (Ard *et al.* 1996; Frautschy *et al.* 1992; Oliver *et al.* 1997; Paresce *et al.* 1996, 1997; Shaffer *et al.* 1995; Shago *et al.* 1997; Shen *et al.* 1999; Shigematsu *et al.* 1992; DeWitt *et al.* 1998). Such mechanisms have been particularly highlighted by recent reports that immunization with Aβ or passive immunization with anti-Aβ antibodies results in clearance of Aβ deposits from AβPP-overexpressing transgenic mice (Schenk *et al.* 1999, 2000). Here, it is hypothesized that the Aβ antibodies opsonize the Aβ deposits, facilitating microglial removal, a view that has been supported in culture models (Bard *et al.* 2000). One also notes that complement opsonins are readily demonstrated on Aβ deposits even without immunization (e.g. Rogers *et al.* 1992). In this sense, this one particular facet of AD inflammation, Aβ opsonization by Igs or by complement, might be considered beneficial in the disease process. Alternatively, other mechanisms of AD inflammation are likely to contribute to Aβ deposition by increasing AβPP synthesis (Griffin *et al.* 1994, 1995, 1997), increasing aggregation of Aβ (Webster *et al.* 1994, 1995, 1997*a*), and hindering microglial phagocytosis of Aβ (Webster *et al.* 1999).

To study microglial responses to Aβ, our laboratory has developed a model system based on microglia cultures derived from rapid autopsies of AD and elderly control patients (Lue *et al.* 1996*a*). These cultures replicate many of the physiological processes observed in the AD brain. For example, if we dry down a spot of Aβ to the culture well floor and then seed it with microglia, we see a pronounced migration of the cells to the perimeter of the Aβ spot. Within 3–10 days the microglia enter and carpet the spot and phagocytosis of the Aβ ensues (Rogers and Lue 2001; Kovelowski *et al.* 2001; Lue *et al.* 2001*b*; Shen *et al.* 1999; Lue *et al.* 1997). Opsonization with anti-Aβ Igs enhances both chemotaxis and phagocytosis (Kovelowski, Strohmeyer, Lue, and Rogers, unpublished observations). RAGE appears to play an important role in these processes. As noted previously, RAGE binds Aβ, and activated microglia of the AD cortex profusely express RAGE (Lue *et al.* 2001*b*; Mackic *et al.* 1998; Yan *et al.* 1996; Yan *et al.* 1997). Blockade of RAGE with anti-RAGE Fab fragments in our culture model significantly inhibits microglial chemotaxis to Aβ (Lue *et al.* 2001*b*).

In addition to direct actions on Aβ clearance, the activation of microglia in AD must also be considered in the context of altered secretory activities by these cells. Some of the inflammatory products expressed by activated microglia are likely to be neurotrophic and beneficial (e.g. S-100 protein) (Griffin *et al.* 1997), whereas a great many others are likely to signal a neurocytopathic state (Adams and Hamilton 1992; Chao *et al.* 1994; van der Laan *et al.* 1996; Kopec and Carroll 1998; Dawson and Dawson 1996; Dickson *et al.* 1993; Multhaup *et al.* 1997).

Aβ activates numerous signalling cascades within microglia (Combs *et al.* 1999; McDonald *et al.* 1998) that are common to peripheral inflammatory responses. Among these are the tyrosine kinase-based cascades (McDonald *et al.* 1997; Wood and Zinsmeister 1991), calcium-dependent activation of Pyk2 and PKC pathways (Combs *et al.* 1999), and p38 and ERKs/MAP kinase cascades (Combs *et al.* 1999; McDonald *et al.* 1997). These, and certainly others, lead to the activation of transcription factors responsible for subsequent pro-inflammatory gene expression. In addition, Aβ-stimulated activation of intracellular signalling pathways in microglia leads to production of reactive oxygen species through NADPH oxidase, and to the synthesis and secretion of neurotoxins (Della-Bianca *et al.* 1999; Combs *et al.* 2000; McDonald *et al.* 1998) and excitotoxins. Excitotoxins released by activated microglia—for example, glutamate (Piani *et al.* 1992) and quinolinic acid (Espey *et al.* 1997)—can cause significant dendritic pruning, as these molecules act preferentially on vulnerable subcellular synaptic and dendritic compartments (Mattson *et al.* 1993). Notably, synapse loss is one of the most consistent correlates of AD cognitive impairment (Masliah *et al.* 1994; Terry *et al.* 1991).

At the level of the secretory products themselves, continued microglial exposure to Aβ in culture yields progressive activation, as well as elevated expression of a wide range of inflammatory mediators. The classic pro-inflammatory cytokines, IL-1, IL-6, and TNF-α, for example, are significantly increased after exposure to Aβ (Lue *et al.* 1996*b*; Shen *et al.* 1999; Kovelowski *et al.* 2001; Rogers and Lue 2001) just as they are in the AD brain. So too are the chemokines IL-8, MCP-1, and MIP-1α; the complement component C1q; the growth factor M-CSF; and reactive nitrogen intermediates (Lue *et al.* 2001*a,b*). Interestingly, C1q and M-CSF are constitutively overexpressed by AD microglia compared to normal elderly microglia, even without Aβ stimulation (Lue *et al.* 2001*a*). All of these inflammation products, and many others, are reported to be increased significantly in pathologically-vulnerable regions of the AD brain (reviewed in Akiyama *et al.* 2000).

The inflammatory mediators secreted by glia in the AD brain have a high potential for causing cytotoxic damage. We have shown, for example, that C1q is activated by Aβ, leading to full activation of the classical complement pathway (Jiang *et al.* 1994; Webster *et al.* 1994, 1995; Webster and Rogers, 1996; Bergamaschini *et al.* 1999; Cribbs *et al.* 1997; Daly and Kotwal 1998; Webster *et al.* 1997). Microglia may also express alternative pathway complement components (Strohmeyer *et al.* 2000; Lemercier *et al.* 1992; Gasque *et al.* 1992; Schwaeble *et al.* 1994; Whaley 1980). The endpoint of complement activation is formation of the membrane attack complex (MAC), C5b–9. The MAC is formed on cellular membranes targeted by complement attack. If sufficient MAC deposition occurs, the cell is lysed. As with peripheral cells, neurones in the AD brain attempt to defend themselves from complement attack by endocytosis and blebbing of that part of their membranes where complement is fixed (Webster *et al.* 1997*b*; Webster *et al.* 1992). Electron micrographs of this response in peri-plaque areas of AD cortex clearly demonstrate that inflammatory mechanisms such as complement are not limited to clearing already dead cells, but cause significant damage to living neurones and their neurites (Webster *et al.* 1997*b*; Webster *et al.* 1992).

At the pathological level, we have shown that patients who have profuse AD pathology at autopsy, but without overt dementia ante-mortem, fail to exhibit signs of inflammation such as enhanced MHCII or complement expression (Lue *et al.* 1996, 1999). IL-1 polymorphisms appear to be a risk factor for AD in several independent studies (Nicoll *et al.* 2000; Grimaldi *et al.* 2000; Griffin *et al.* 2000; Du *et al.* 2000), and other inflammation-related genes may prove to be important as well (reviewed in Akiyama *et al.* 2000; Strohmeyer and Rogers 2001; Griffin *et al.* 2000; Urakami *et al.* 2001; Tanzi and Bertram 2001; Mori 2001; Kovacs 2000).

Finally, at the clinical level, nearly two-dozen studies suggest that nonsteroidal anti-inflammatory drugs (NSAIDs) may delay the onset or slow the progression of AD (Gottlieb 2001; Ferencik *et al.* 2001; Bennett 2001; Akiyama *et al.* 2000; Breitner *et al.* 1995; Andersen *et al.* 1995; Breitner *et al.* 1994; Strohmeyer and Rogers 2001; Mackenzie 2000; Mackenzie and Munoz 1998; McGeer *et al.* 1996; Pasinetti, 1998; Rich *et al.* 1995; Stewart *et al.* 1997; Vane and Botting 1998; Cutler and Sramek 2001; In't Veldt *et al.* 1998). Definitive trials, especially those using prevention rather than intervention strategies, are still underway.

From the research conducted it can be seen that the activation of microglia potentially can have both beneficial and cytotoxic effects. On the one hand, the activation of microglia in the process of Aβ phagocytosis leads to secretion of cytotoxic inflammatory mediators, a pathogenic outcome that harms nearby cells. On the other hand, activated microglia may secrete neurotrophic products and remove Aβ. We must therefore ask what the balance of these forces may be in AD. At one pole, a few prominent investigators have suggested that anti-inflammatory drugs should not be given to AD patients because such drugs could dampen microglial removal of Aβ. Alternatively, as already noted, several dozen clinical reports have suggested that NSAIDs may delay the onset and slow the progression of AD. Because the clinical findings in a sense integrate both the positive and negative influences of inflammation in AD, the most parsimonious conclusion is that, on balance, inflammation is more deleterious than helpful in the disorder, and that NSAIDs may be useful therapeutically. Indeed, by more clearly understanding the role of various AD inflammatory mechanisms, we may be able to do even better. We note, for example, that microglial chemotaxis and phagocytosis of Aβ may be pharmacologically distinguishable from microglial secretion of cytotoxic inflammatory mediators. The doses of NSAIDs required to inhibit scavenger cell migration and phagocytosis in the periphery are typically supraphysiologic by an order of magnitude or more—and this is with unopsonized targets. Inhibition of migration and phagocytosis of an Ig-opsonized target, as in the Aβ immunization approach, would require even higher NSAID doses, if they could be effective at all. Thus, far from being contra-indicated in AD, NSAIDs could prove to be an ideal therapeutic adjunct to Aβ removal approaches: at physiologic concentrations they are unlikely to hinder phagocytosis of Aβ, but they are well known, at such concentrations, to inhibit the expression of potentially toxic inflammatory intermediates.

References

Adams, D. O. and Hamilton, T. A. (1992). Molecular basis of macrophage activation. In *The macrophage*, (ed. C. E. Lewis and J. O. McGee) IRL, Oxford, UK, pp. 75–114.

Aguado, F., Ballabriga, J., Pozas, E., and Ferrer, I. (1998). TrkA immunoreactivity in reactive astrocytes in human neurodegenerative diseases and colchicine-treated rats. *Acta Neuropathol*, **96**, 495–501.

Akiyama, H., Barger, S., Barnum, S., Bradt, B., Bauer, J., Cole, *et al.* (2000). Inflammation and Alzheimer's disease. *Neurobiol Aging*, **21**, 383–421.

Andersen, K., Launer, L. J., Ott, A., Hoes, A. W., Breteler, M. M., and Hofman, A. (1995). Do nonsteroidal anti-inflammatory drugs decrease the risk for Alzheimer's disease? The Rotterdam Study. *Neurology*, **45**, 1441–5.

Ard, M. D., Cole, G. M., Wei, J., Mehrle, A. P., and Fratkin, J. D. (1996). Scavenging of Alzheimer's Amyloid β-protein by microglia in culture. *J Neurosci Res*, **43**, 190–202.

Bard, F., Cannon, C., Barbour, R., Burke, R. L., Games, D., Grajeda, H. *et al.* (2000). Peripherally administered antibodies against amyloid β peptide enter the central nervous system and reduce pathology in a mouse model of Alzheimer's disease. *Nat Med*, **6**, 916–9.

Barron, K. D. (1995). The microglial cell. A historical review. *J Neurol Sci*, **134**, 57–68.

Bauer, J., Konig, G., Strauss, S., Jonas, U., Ganter, U., Weidemann, A., (1991). *In vitro* matured human macrophages express Alzheimer's beta A4-amyloid precursor protein indicating synthesis in microglial cells. *FEBS Lett*, **282**, 335–40.

Bennett, A. (2001). Anti-inflammatory drugs, cyclooxygenases and other factors. *Expert Opin Pharmacother*, **2**, 1–2.

Bergamaschini, L., Canziani, S., Bottasso, B., Cugno, M., Braidotti, P., and Agostoni, A. (1999). Alzheimer's beta-amyloid peptides can activate the early components of complement classical pathway in a C1q-independent manner. *Clin Exp Immunol*, **115**, 526–33.

Bitting, L., Naidu, A., Cordell, B., and Murphy, G. M. J. (1996). β-amyloid peptide secretion by a microglial cell line is induced by b-amyloid (25–35) and lipopolysaccharide. *J Biol Chem*, **271**, 16 084–9.

Boissiere, F., Hunot, S., Faucheux, B., Duyckaerts, C., Hauw, J. J., Agid, Y., and Hirsch, E. C. (1997). Nuclear translocation of NF-kappaB in cholinergic neurons of patients with Alzheimer's disease. *Neuroreport*, **8**, 2849–52.

Breitner, J. C., Gau, B. A., Welsh, K. A., Plassman, B. L., McDonald, W. M., Helms, M. J., and Anthony, J. C. (1994). Inverse association of anti-inflammatory treatments and Alzheimer's disease: initial results of a co-twin control study. *Neurology*, **44**, 227–32.

Breitner, J. C., Welsh, K. A., Helms, M. J., Gaskell, P. C., Gau, B. A., Roses, A. D., *et al.* (1995). Delayed onset of Alzheimer's disease with nonsteroidal anti-inflammatory and histamine H2 blocking drugs. *Neurobiol Aging*, **16**, 523–30.

Breitner, J. C., Hu, S., Frey, W. H., Ala, T. A., Tourtellotte, W. W., and Peterson, P. K. (1994). Transforming growth factor beta in Alzheimer's disease. *Clin Diagn Lab Immunol*, **1**, 109–110.

Breitner, J. C., Hu, S., W. S., Kravitz, F. H., and Peterson, P. K. (1999). Inflammation-mediated neuronal cell injury. In *Inflammatory cells and mediators in CNS diseases*, (ed. R. R. Ruffolo, G. Z. Feuerstain, A. J. Hunter, G. Poste, and B. W. Metcalf), Harwood Academic Publishers, Canada pp. 483–95.

Christie, R. H., Freeman, M., and Hyman, B. T. (1996). Expression of the macrophage scavenger receptor, a multifunctional lipoprotein receptor, in microglia associated with senile plaques in Alzheimer's disease. *Am J Pathol*, **148**, 399–403.

Combs, C. K., Johnson, D. E., Cannady, S. B., Lehman, T. M., and Landreth, G. E. (1999). Identification of microglial signal transduction pathways mediating a neurotoxic response to amyloidogenic fragments of beta-amyloid and prion proteins. *J Neurosci*, **19**, 928–39.

Combs, C. K., Johnson, D. E., Karlo, J. C., Cannady, S. B.., and Landerth, G. E. (2000). Inflammatory mechanisms in Alzheimer's disease: inhibition of beta-amyloid-stimulated proinflammatory responses and neurotoxicity by PPARgamma agonists. *J Neurosci*, **20**, 558–67.

Coria, F., Moreno, A., Rubio, I., Garcia, M. A., Morato, E., and Mayor, F. J. (1993). The cellular pathology associated with Alzheimer beta-amyloid deposits in non-demented aged individuals. *Neuropathol Appl Neurobiol*, **19**, 261–8.

Cotman, C. W. and Tenner, A. J. (1996). β-amyloid converts an acute phase injury response to chronic injury response. *Neurobiol Aging*, **17**, 723–31.

Cribbs, D. H., Velazquez, P., Soreghan, B., Glabe, C. G., and Tenner, A. J. (1997). Complement activation by cross-linked truncated and chimeric full-length beta-amyloid. *Neuroreport*, **8**, 3457–62.

Cutler, N. R. and Sramek, J. J. (2001). Review of the next generation of Alzheimer's disease therapeutics: challenges for drug development. *Prog Neuropsychopharmacol Biol Psychiatry*, **25**, 27–57.

Daly, J. and Kotwal, G. J. (1998). Pro-inflammatory complement activation by the A beta peptide of Alzheimer's disease is biologically significant and can be blocked by vaccinia virus complement control protein [In Process Citation]. *Neurobiol Aging*, **19**, 619–27.

Davis, J. B., McMurray, H. F., and Schubert, D. (1992). The amyloid beta-protein of Alzheimer's disease is chemotactic for mononuclear phagocytes. *Biochem Biophys Res Commun*, **189**, 1096–1100.

Dawson, V. L. and Dawson, T. M. (1996). Nitric oxide neurotoxicity. *J Chem Neuroanat*, **10**, 179–90.

Della-Bianca, V., Dusi, S., Bianchini, E., Dal-Pra, I., and Rossi, F. (1999). β amyloid activates the O_2 forming NADPH oxidase in microglia, monocytes and neutrophils. A possible inflammatory mechanism of neuronal damage in Alzheimer's disease. *J Biol Chem*, **274**, 15 493–9.

DeWitt, D.A., Perry, G., Cohen, M., Doller, C., and Silver, J. (1998). Astrocytes regulate microglial phagocytosis of senile plaque cores of Alzheimer's disease. *Exp Neurol*, **149**, 329–40.

Dickson, D. W., Lee, S. C., Mattiace, L. A., Yen, S. H., and Brosnan, C. (1993). Microglia and cytokines in neurological disease, with special reference to AIDS and Alzheimer's disease. *Glia*, **7**, 75–83.

Du, Y., Dodel, R. C., Eastwood, B. J., Bales, K. R., Gao, F., Lohmuller, F., *et al.* (2000). Association of an interleukin 1 alpha polymorphism with Alzheimer's disease. *Neurology*, **55**, 480–3.

El Khoury, J., Hickman, S. E., Thomas, C. A., Cao, L., Silverstein, S. C., and Loike, J. D. (1996). Scavenger receptor-mediated adhesion of microglia to beta-amyloid fibrils. *Nature*, **382**, 716–19.

El Khoury, J., Hickman, S. E., Thomas, C. A., Loike, J. D., and Silverstein, S. C. (1998). Microglia, scavenger receptors, and the pathogenesis of Alzheimer's disease. *Neurobiol Aging*, **19**, S81–4.

Espey, M. G., Chernyshev, O. N., Reinhard, J. F. J., Namboodiri, M. A., and Colton, C. A. (1997). Activated human microglia produce the excitotoxin quinolinic acid. *Neuroreport*, **8**, 431–4.

Ferencik, M., Novak, M., Rovensky, J., and Rybar, I. (2001). Alzheimer's disease, inflammation and non-steroidal anti-inflammatory drugs. *Bratisl Lek Listy*, **102**, 123–32.

Ferrer, I., Marti, E., Lopez, E. and Tortosa, A. (1998). NF-kB immunoreactivity is observed in association with beta A4 diffuse plaques in patients with Alzheimer's disease. *Neuropathol Appl Neurobiol*, **24**, 271–7.

Frautschy, S. A., Cole, G. M., and Baird, A. (1992). Phagocytosis and deposition of vascular beta-amyloid in rat brains injected with Alzheimer beta-amyloid. *Am J Pathol*, **140**, 1389–99.

Frautschy, S. A., Yang, F., Irrizarry, M., Hyman, B., Saido, T. C., Hsiao, K., and Cole, G.M. (1998). Microglial response to amyloid plaques in APPsw transgenic mice. *Am J Pathol*, **152**, 307–17.

Gasque, P., Julen, N., Ischenko, A. M., Picot, C., Mauger, C., Chauzy, C., Ripoche, J., and Fontaine, M. (1992). Expression of complement components of the alternative pathway by glioma cell lines. *J Immunol*, **149**, 1381–7.

Gehrmann, J., Mies, G., Bonnekoh, P., Banati, R., Iijima, T., Kreutzberg, G. W., and Hossmann, K. A. (1993). Microglial reaction in the rat cerebral cortex induced by cortical spreading depression. *Brain Pathol*, **3**, 11–17.

Giulian, D. (1987). Ameboid microglia as effectors of inflammation in the central nervous system. *J Neurosci Res*, **18**, 155–71, 132–3.

Gottlieb, S. (2001). NSAIDs can lower risk of Alzheimer's. *BMJ*, **323**, 1269A.

Griffin, W. S., Nicoll, J. A., Grimaldi, L. M., Sheng, J. G., and Mrak, R. E. (2000). The pervasiveness of interleukin-1 in Alzheimer pathogenesis: a role for specific polymorphisms in disease risk. *Exp Gerontol*, **35**, 481–7.

Griffin, W. S., Sheng, J. G., Gentleman, S. M., Graham, D. I., Mrak, R. E., and Roberts, G. W. (1994). Microglial interleukin-1 alpha expression in human head injury: correlations with neuronal and neuritic beta-amyloid precursor protein expression. *Neurosci Lett*, **176**, 133–6.

Griffin, W. S., Sheng, J. G., Roberts, G. W., and Mrak, R. E. (1995). Interleukin-1 expression in different plaque types in Alzheimer's disease: significance in plaque evolution. *J Neuropathol Exp Neurol*, **54**, 276–81.

Griffin, W. S. T., Sheng, J. G., and Mrak, R. E. (1997). Inflammatory pathways. Implications in Alzheimer's disease. In *Molecular mechanisms of dementia*, (ed. W. Wasco and R. E. Tanzi), Humana Press Inc., Totowa, NJ, pp. 169–76.

Grimaldi, L. M., Casadei, V. M., Ferri, C., Veglia, F., Licastro, F., Annoni, G., (2000). Association of early-onset Alzheimer's disease with an interleukin-1alpha gene polymorphism. *Ann Neurol*, **47**, 361–5.

Haga, S., Akai, K., and Ishii, T. (1989). Demonstration of microglial cells in and around senile (neuritic) plaques in the Alzheimer brain. An immunohistochemical study using a novel monoclonal antibody. *Acta Neuropathol (Berl)*, **77**, 569–75.

Hyman, B. T., Marzloff, K., and Arriagada, P. V. (1993). The lack of accumulation of senile plaques or amyloid burden Alzheimer's disease suggests a dynamic balance between amyloid deposition and resolution. *J Neuropathol Exp Neurol*, **52**, 594–600.

In't Veldt, V., Launer, L. J., Hoes, A. W., Ott, A., Hofman, A., Breteler, M. M., and Stricker, B. H. (1998). NSAIDs and incident Alzheimer's disease. The Rotterdam Study. *Neurobiol Aging*, **19**, 607–11.

Itagaki, S., Akiyama, H., Saito, H., and McGeer, P. L. (1994). Ultrastructural localization of complement membrane attack complex (MAC)-like immunoreactivity in brains of patients with Alzheimer's disease. *Brain Res*, **645**, 78–84.

Itagaki, S., McGeer, P. L., and Akiyama, H. (1988). Presence of T-cytotoxic suppressor and leucocyte common antigen positive cells in Alzheimer's disease brain tissue. *Neurosci Lett*, **91**, 259–64.

Jiang, H., Burdick, D., Glabe, C. G., Cotman, C. W., and Tenner, A. J. (1994). β-Amyloid activates complement by binding to a specific region of the collagen-like domain of the C1q A chain. *J Immunol*, **152**, 5050–9.

Kopec, K. K. and Carroll, R. T. (1998). Alzheimer's beta-amyloid peptide 1-42 induces a phagocytic response in murine microglia. *J Neurochem*, **71**, 2123–31.

Kovacs, D. M. (2000). Alpha2-macroglobulin in late-onset Alzheimer's disease. *Exp Gerontol*, **35**, 473–9.

Kovelowski, C. J., Lue, L.-F., Walker, D., Mueller, K., Seetharaman, R., and Rogers, J. (2001). Opsonization and anti-inflammatory drug effects on microglial chemotaxis, phagocytosis, and cytokine secretion in vitro after amyloid-beta peptide exposure. *Neuroscience Abstracts*, **27**, 890.11

Krall, W. J., Challita, P. M., Perlmutter, L. S., Skelton, D. C., and Kohn, D. B. (1994). Cells expressing human glucocerebrosidase from a retroviral vector repopulate macrophages and central nervous system microglia after murine bone marrow transplantation. *Blood*, **83**, 2737–48.

Kreutzberg, G. W. (1996). Microglia: a sensor for pathological events in the CNS. *Trends Neurosci*, **19**, 312–18.

Lawson, L. J., Frost, L., Risbridger, J., Fearn, S., and Perry, V.H. (1994). Quantification of the mononuclear phagocyte response to Wallerian degeneration of the optic nerve. *J Neurocytol*, **23**, 729–44.

LeBlanc, A. (1995). Increased production of 4 kDa amyloid beta peptide in serum deprived human primary neuron cultures: possible involvement of apoptosis. *J Neurosci*, **15**, 7837–46.

Lemercier, C., Julen, N., Coulpier, M., Dauchel, H., Ozanne, D., Fontaine, M., and Ripoche, J. (1992). Differential modulation by glucocorticoids of alternative complement protein secretion in cells of the monocyte/macrophage lineage. *Eur J Immunol*, **22**, 909–15.

Lorton, D., Schaller, J., Lala, A., and De Nardin, E. (2000). Chemotactic-like receptors and Abeta peptide induced responses in Alzheimer's Disease. *Neurobiol Aging*, **21**, 463–73.

Luber-Narod, J. and Rogers, J. (1988). Immune system associated antigens expressed by cells of the human central nervous system. *Neurosci Lett*, **94**, 17–22.

Lue, L.F., Brachova, L., Civin, W. H. and Rogers, J. (1996). Inflammation, Aβ deposition, and neurofibrillary tangle formation as correlates of Alzheimer's disease neurodegeneration. *J Neuropathol Exp Neurol*, **55**, 1083–8.

Lue, L. F., Brachova, L., and Rogers, J. (1997). Modeling Aβ deposition in cultures of Alzheimer's glia and hnt neurons. *Neuroscience Abstracts*, **23**, 533.

Lue, L. F., Brachova, L., Walker, D. G. and Rogers, J. (1996a). Characterization of glial cultures from rapid autopsies of Alzheimer's and control patients. *Neurobiol Aging*, 17, 421–9.

Lue, L. -F., Brachova, L., Walker, D. G. and Royer, S. M. (1996b). Alzheimer's disease and nondemented elderly glial cultures: constitutive and stimulated expression of complement, cytokines, and apolipoprotein E. *Neurobiology of Aging Supplement*, 17, 520.

Lue, L. F., Kuo, Y. M., Roher, A. E., Brachova, L., Shen, Y., Sue, L., *et al.* (1999). Soluble amyloid beta peptide concentration as a predictor of synaptic change in Alzheimer's disease. *Am J Pathol*, 155, 853–62.

Lue, L. F., Rydel, R., Brigham, E. F., Yang, L.B., Hampel, H., Murphy, G.M. Jr., *et al.* (2001a). Inflammatory repertoire of Alzheimer's disease and nondemented elderly microglia in vitro. *Glia*, 35, 72–9.

Lue, L. F., Walker, D. G., Brachova, L., Beach, T. G., Rogers, J., Schmidt, A. M., *et al.* (2001b). Involvement of microglial receptor for advanced glycation endproducts (rage) in Alzheimer's disease: identification of a cellular activation mechanism. *Exp Neurol*, 171, 29–45.

Mackenzie, I. R. (2000). Anti-inflammatory drugs and Alzheimer type pathology in aging. *Neurology*, 54, 732–4

Mackenzie, I. R. and Munoz, D. G. (1998). Nonsteroidal anti-inflammatory drug use and Alzheimer-type pathology in aging. *Neurology*, 50, 986–90.

Mackic, J. B., Stins, M., McComb, J. G., Calero, M., Ghiso, J., Kim, K. S., *et al.* (1998). Human blood–brain barrier receptors for Alzheimer's amyloid-beta 1-40. Asymmetrical binding, endocytosis, and transcytosis at the apical side of brain microvascular endothelial cell monolayer. *J Clin Invest*, 102, 734–43.

Masliah, E., Mallory, M., Hansen, L., DeTeresa, R., Alford, M., and Terry, R. (1994). Synaptic and neuritic alterations during the progression of Alzheimer's disease. *Neurosci Lett*, 174, 67–72.

Mattson, M. P., Cheng, B., Culwell, A.R., Esch, F.S., Lieberburg, I., and Rydel, R. E. (1993). Evidence for excitoprotective and intraneuronal calcium-regulating roles for secreted forms of the beta-amyloid precursor protein. *Neuron*, 10, 243–54.

McDonald, D. R., Bamberger, M. E., Combs, C. K., and Landreth, G. E. (1998). Beta-Amyloid fibrils activate parallel mitogen-activated protein kinase pathways in microglia and THP1 monocytes. *J Neurosci*, 18, 4451–60.

McDonald, D. R., Brunden, K. R., and Landreth, G. E. (1997). Amyloid fibrils activate tyrosine kinase-dependent signalling and superoxide production in microglia. *J Neurosci*, 17, 2284–94.

McGeer, E. G. and McGeer, P. L. (1998). The importance of inflammatory mechanisms in Alzheimer disease. *Exp Gerontol*, 33, 371–8.

McGeer, P. L., Akiyama, H., Itagaki, S., and McGeer, E. G. (1989). Immune system response in Alzheimer's disease. *Can J Neurol Sci*, 16, 516–27.

McGeer, P. L. and McGeer, E. G. (1995). Central nervous system immune reactions in Alzheimer's disease. In *Immune responses in the nervous system*, (ed. N. J. Rothwell) Bios Scientific Publishers Manchester, UK, pp. 143–57.

McGeer, P. L., Schulzer, M., and McGeer, E. G. (1996). Arthritis and anti-inflammatory agents as possible protective factors for Alzheimer's disease: a review of 17 epidemiologic studies. *Neurology*, 47, 425–32.

Mori, S. (2001). [Apolipoprotein E4 and Alzheimer's disease]. *Nippon Rinsho*, 59 Suppl 3, 812–17.

Morioka, T., Baba, T., Black, K. L., and Streit, W. J. (1992). Immunophenotypic analysis of infiltrating leukocytes and microglia in an experimental rat glioma. *Acta Neuropathol (Berl)*, 83, 590–7.

Morioka, T., Kalehua, A. N., and Streit, W. J. (1993). Characterization of microglial reaction after middle cerebral artery occlusion in rat brain. *J Comp Neurol*, 327, 123–32.

Multhaup, G., Ruppert, T., Schlicksupp, A., Hesse, L., Beher, D., Masters, C. L., and Beyreuther, K. (1997). Reactive oxygen species and Alzheimer's disease. *Biochem Pharmacol*, 54, 533–9.

Nicoll, J. A., Mrak, R. E., Graham, D. I., Stewart, J., Wilcock, G., MacGowan, S., *et al.* (2000). Association of interleukin-1 gene polymorphisms with Alzheimer's disease. *Ann Neurol*, 47, 365–8.

Oliver, J. D., Van der Wal, F. J., Bulleid, N. J., and High, S. (1997). Interaction of the thiol-dependent reductase ERp57 with nascent glycoproteins. *Science*, 275, 86–8.

Paresce, D. M., Chung, H., and Maxfield, F. R. (1997). Slow degradation of aggregates of the Alzheimer's disease amyloid beta-protein by microglial cells. *J Biol Chem*, 272, 29 390–7.

Paresce, D. M., Ghosh, R. N., and Maxfield, F. R. (1996). Microglial cells internalize aggregates of the Alzheimer's disease amyloid beta-protein via a scavenger receptor. *Neuron*, 17, 553–65.

Pasinetti, G. M. (1998). Cyclooxygenase and inflammation in Alzheimer's disease: experimental approaches and clinical interventions. *J Neurosci Res*, 54, 1–6.

Perlmutter, L. S., Scott, S. A., Barron, E., and Chui, H. C. (1992). MHC class II-positive microglia in human brain: association with Alzheimer lesions. *J Neurosci Res*, 33, 549–58.

Perry, V. H., Bell, M. D., and Anthony, D. C. (1999). Unique aspects of inflammation in the central nervous system. In *Inflammatory cells and mediators in CNS diseases*, (ed. R. R. Ruffolo, G. Z. Feuerstain, A. J. Hunter, G. Poste, and B. W. Metcalf), Harwood Academic Publishers, Canada, pp. 21–38.

Perry, V. H., Hume, D. A., and Gordon, S. (1985). Immunohistochemical localization of macrophages and microglia in the adult and developing mouse brain. *Neuroscience*, 15, 313–26.

Piani, D., Spranger, M., Frei, K., Schaffner, A., and Fontana, A. (1992). Macrophage-induced cytotoxicity of N-methyl-D-aspartate receptor positive neurons involves excitatory amino acids rather than reactive oxygen intermediates and cytokines. *Eur J Immunol*, 22, 2429–36.

Rich, J. B., Rasmusson, D. X., Folstein, M. F., Carson, K. A., Kawas, C., and Brandt, J. (1995). Nonsteroidal anti-inflammatory drugs in Alzheimer's disease. *Neurology*, 45, 51–5.

Rogers, J., Cooper, N. R., Webster, S., Schultz, J., McGeer, P. L., Styren, S. D., *et al.* (1992). Complement activation by beta-amyloid in Alzheimer's disease. *Proc Natl Acad Sci USA*, 89, 10016–20.

Rogers, J. and Lue, L. (2001). Microglial chemotaxis, activation, and phagocytosis of amyloid beta-peptide as linked phenomena in Alzheimer's disease. *Neurochem Int*, 39, 333–40.

Rogers, J. and O'Barr S. (1996). Inflammatory Mediators in Alzheimer's Disease. In *Molecular Approaches to Alzheimer's Disease*, (ed. R. Tanzi and W. Wasco), Humana Press, Totowa, NJ pp. 177–97.

Rogers, J., Webster, S., Lue, L. F., Brachova, L., Civin, W. H., Emmerling, M., (1996). Inflammation and Alzheimer's disease pathogenesis. *Neurobiol Aging*, 17, 681–6.

Rosenberg, H. F., and Gallin, J. I. (1999). Inflammation. In *Fundamental Immunology*, 4th edn. (ed. W. E. Paul), Lippincott-Raven Publishers, Philadelphia pp. 1051–66.

Rozemuller, J. M., Eikelenboom, P., Stam, F. C., Beyreuther, K., and Masters, C. L. (1989). A4 protein in Alzheimer's disease: primary and secondary cellular events in extracellular amyloid deposition. *J Neuropathol Exp Neurol*, 48, 674–91.

Sasaki, A., Yamaguchi, H., Ogawa, A., Sugihara, S., and Nakazato, Y. (1997). Microglial activation in early stages of amyloid beta protein deposition. *Acta Neuropathol (Berl)*, 94, 316–22.

Schenk, D., Barbour, R., Dunn, W., Gordon, G., Grajeda, H., Guido, T., *et al.* (1999). Immunization with amyloid-beta attenuates Alzheimer-disease-like pathology in the PDAPP mouse. *Nature*, 400, 173–7.

Schenk, D. B., Seubert, P., Lieberburg, I., and Wallace, J. (2000). Beta-peptide immunization: a possible new treatment for Alzheimer disease. *Arch Neurol*, 57, 934–6.

Schwaeble, W., Huemer, H. P., Most, J., Dierich, M. P., Strobel, M., Claus, C., *et al.* (1994). Expression of properdin in human monocytes. *Eur J Biochem*, 219, 759–64.

Scott, S. A., Johnson, S. A., Zarow, C., and Perlmutter, L. S. (1993). Inability to detect β-amyloid protein precursor mRNA in Alzheimer plaque-associated microglia. *Exp Neurol*, 121, 113–8.

Shaffer, L. M., Dority, M. D., Gupta-Bansal, R., Frederickson, R. C., Younkin, S. G., and Brunden, K. R. (1995). Amyloid beta protein (Aβ) removal by neuroglial cells in culture. *Neurobiol Aging*, 16, 737–45.

Shago, M., Flock, G., Leung-Hagesteijn, C. Y., Woodside, M., Grinstein, S., Giguere, V., and Dedhar, S. (1997). Modulation of the retinoic acid and retinoid X receptor signalling pathways in P19 embryonal carcinoma cells by calreticulin. *Exp Cell Res*, 230, 50–60.

Shen, Y., Lue, L. -F., Brachova, L., Yang, L. -B., Hampel, H., Rydel, R. E., Sahagan, B., and Rogers, J. (1999). Responses of Alzheimer's disease and normal elderly microglia to amyloid β peptide exposure in culture. *Neuroscience Abstracts*, 25, 1107

Sheng, J. G., Mrak, R. E., and Griffin, W. S. (1997). Glial-neuronal interactions in Alzheimer disease: progressive association of IL-1alpha+ microglia and S100beta+ astrocytes with neurofibrillary tangle stages. *J Neuropathol Exp Neurol*, 56, 285–90.

Shigematsu, K., McGeer, P. L., Walker, D. G., Ishii, T., and McGeer, E. G. (1992). Reactive microglia/ macrophages phagocytose amyloid precursor protein produced by neurons following neural damage. *J Neurosci Res*, 31, 443–53.

Shirahama, T., Miura, K., Ju, S. T., Kisilevsky, R., Gruys, E., and Cohen, A. S. (1990). Amyloid enhancing factor-loaded macrophages in amyloid fibril formation. *Lab Invest*, 62, 61–8.

Stalder, M., Phinney, A., Probst, A., Sommer, B., Staufenbiel, M., and Jucker, M. (1999). Association of microglia with amyloid plaques in brains of APP23 transgenic mice. *Am J Pathol*, 154, 1673–84.

Stewart, W. F., Kawas, C., Corrada, M., and Metter, E. J. (1997). Risk of Alzheimer's disease and duration of NSAID use. *Neurology*, 48, 626–32.

Streit, W. J. and Sparks, D. L. (1997). Activation of microglia in the brains of humans with heart disease and hypercholesterolemic rabbits. *J Mol Med*, 75, 130–8.

Streit, W. J., Walter, S. A., and Pennell, N. A. (1999). Reactive microgliosis. *Prog Neurobiol*, 57, 563–81.

Strohmeyer, R., Li, R., Liang Z., and Rogers, J. (2001). Upregulation of the transcription factor C/EBP-β in Alzheimer's disease compared to non-demented elderly cortex. *Neuroscience Abstracts*, 27, 652.3.

Strohmeyer, R., Shen, Y., and Rogers, J. (2000). Detection of complement alternative pathway mRNA and proteins in the Alzheimer's disease brain. *Brain Res Mol Brain Res*, 81, 7–18.

Strohmeyer, R. and Rogers, J. (2001). Molecular and cellular mediators of Alzheimer's disease inflammation. *J Alzheimer's Dis*, 3, 131–57.

Tanzi, R. E., and Bertram, L. (2001). New frontiers in Alzheimer's disease genetics. *Neuron*, 32, 181–4.

Terry, R. D., Masliah, E., Salmon, D. P., Butters, N., DeTeresa, R., Hill, R., *et al.* (1991). Physical basis of cognitive alterations in Alzheimer's disease: synapse loss is the major correlate of cognitive impairment. *Ann Neurol*, 30, 572–80.

Tooyama, I., Kimura, H., Akiyama, H., and McGeer, P. L. (1990). Reactive microglia express class I and class II major histocompatibility complex antigens in Alzheimer's disease. *Brain Res*, 523, 273–80.

Urakami, K., Wakutani, Y., Wada-Isoe, K., Yamagata, K., Adachi, Y., and Nakashima, K. (2001). Causative genes in Alzheimer's disease. *Nippon Ronen Igakkai Zasshi*, 38, 117–20.

van der Laan, L. J., Ruuls, S. R., Weber, K. S., Lodder, I. J., Dopp, E. A., and Dijkstra, C. D. (1996). Macrophage phagocytosis of myelin in vitro determined by flow cytometry: phagocytosis is mediated by CR3 and induces production of tumor necrosis factor-alpha and nitric oxide. *J Neuroimmunol*, 70, 145–52.

Vane, J. R. and Botting, R. M. (1998). Anti-inflammatory drugs and their mechanism of action. *Inflamm Res*, 47 Suppl 2, S78–87.

Walker, D. G. (1998). Inflammatory markers in chronic neurodegenerative disorders, with emphasis on Alzheimer's Disease. In: *Neuroinflammation: Mechanisms and Management*, Wood, P. L., (ed.) Totowa, New Jersey: Humana Press, pp. 61–90.

Webster, S., Bonnell, B., and Rogers, J. (1997*a*). Charge-based binding of complement component C1q to the Alzheimer amyloid beta-peptide. *Am J Pathol*, **150**, 1531–6.

Webster, S., Glabe, C., and Rogers, J. (1995). Multivalent binding of complement protein C1Q to the amyloid beta-peptide (A beta) promotes the nucleation phase of A beta aggregation. *Biochem Biophys Res Commun*, **217**, 869–75.

Webster, S., Lue, L. F., Brachova, L., Tenner, A. J., McGeer, P. L., Terai, K., Walker, D. G., Bradt, B., Cooper, N.R., and Rogers, J. (1997*b*). Molecular and cellular characterization of the membrane attack complex, C5b-9, in Alzheimer's disease. *Neurobiol Aging*, **18**, 415–21.

Webster, S., O'Barr, S., and Rogers, J. (1994). Enhanced aggregation and beta structure of amyloid beta peptide after coincubation with C1q. *J Neurosci Res*, **39**, 448–56.

Webster, S. and Rogers, J. (1996). Relative efficacies of amyloid beta peptide (Aβ) binding proteins in A beta aggregation. *J Neurosci Res*, **46**, 58–66.

Webster, S., Tenner, A. J., Poulos, T. L., and Cribbs, D. The mouse C1q A chain sequence alters beta-amyloid induced complement activation. *Neurobiol Aging*, **20**, 297–304.

Webster, S. D., Lue, L. F., McKinley, M., and Rogers, J. (1992) Ultrastructural localization of complement proteins to neuronal membranes and β-amyloid peptide containing Alzheimer's disease pathology. *Neuroscienc Abstract*, **18**, 765.

Whaley, K. (1980). Biosynthesis of the complement components and the regulatory proteins of the alternative complement pathway by human peripheral blood monocytes. *J Exp Med*, **151**, 501–16.

Wisniewski, H. M., Wegiel, J., Wang, K. C., Kujawa, M., and Lach, B. (1989). Ultrastructural studies of the cells forming amyloid fibers in classical plaques. *Can J Neurol Sci*, **16**, 535–42.

Wood, J. G. and Zinsmeister, P. (1991). Tyrosine phosphorylation systems in Alzheimer's disease pathology. *Neurosci Lett*, **121**, 12–6.

Yan, S. D., Chen, X., Fu, J., Chen, M., Zhu, H., Roher, A., *et al.* (1996). RAGE and amyloid-beta peptide neurotoxicity in Alzheimer's disease. *Nature*, **382**, 685–91.

Yan, S. D., Zhu, H., Fu, J., Yan, S. F., Roher, A., Tourtellotte, W. W., *et al.* (1997). Amyloid-beta peptide-receptor for advanced glycation endproduct interaction elicits neuronal expression of macrophage-colony stimulating factor: a proinflammatory pathway in Alzheimer disease. *Proc Natl Acad Sci USA*, **94**, 5296–301.

Chapter 11

Transplantation of neuronal and non-neuronal cells into the brain

Håkan Widner

11.1 The brain as a transplantation site

Neurosurgical attempts to reconstruct the damaged central nervous system by transplantation of various cells and tissues have revived the interest of the immunological status of brain as a transplantation site. In 1953 the term 'immunologically privileged site' was coined, denoting a prolongation of graft survival in comparison with the outcome in another non-privileged site (Billingham and Boswell 1953) and the brain was recognized as one along with several other sites (Barker and Billingham 1977). The factors responsible for the prolonged graft survival in the different sites are not uniform. Under certain circumstances, immune reactions occur in the brain as effectively as in other sites, for example in multiple sclerosis or viral infections. The privileged status of the brain is thus not absolute but rather regulated and result from the the the net balance of factors contribute to immune privilege or responses (Widner and Brundin 1988; Hickey 2001).

Transplantation to the brain and the central nervous system is rapidly becoming a therapeutic and clinically relevant alternative, with a potential to reverse many serious conditions. There are currently clinical trials in Parkinson's disease, Hungtington's disease, multiple sclerosis, retinal diseases, stroke, epilepsy, and for deafness (Björklund and Lindvall 2000). There are also strategies for supplementation of essential growth factors that rely on grafting procedures and the stem cell paradigm involves transfer of cells accross immunological barriers (Dunnett and Björklund 1999). In all cases, immunological factors are of importance and interventions are needed to secure successful outcome.

This chapter reviews some of the factors involved in this regulation of relevance for transplantations of neuronal and non-neuronal tissue into the brain parenchyma for repair and neuroprotective purposes.

11.1.1 Transplantation biology

Several factors determine when and if a graft will be rejected, that is, the type of graft, degree of disparity between donor and recipient and to what implantation site the graft is made. Table 11.1 lists some definitions and examples of diferent types of grafts.

The immunological identity of an individual and a species are defined by surface molecules, the highly polymorphic major histocompatibility complex antigens (MHC), encoded by genes of the MHC gene locus, and by peptides bound in the MHC molecule (Auchincloss and Sultan 1996). Minor transplantation antigens are polymorphic peptides

Table 11.1 Definitions and classifications

Autologous graft, autograft	Grafts taken from and returned to the same individual
Syngeneic graft, isogeneic	Graft between genetically identical members of a species
Allogeneic graft, allograft (homograft)	Graft to a genetically different member of the same species
Xenogeneic graft, xenograft (heterogeneic graft; heterograft)	Graft to a member of a different species
Concordant xenograft	Arbitrary distance between how closely related species are; refers to when no hyperacute rejection occurs of primarily vascularized organ xenograft
Discordant xenograft	Refers to when hyperacute rejection occurs of primarily vascularized organ xenograft
Orthotopic	Graft to a site normal for that tissue/organ
Heterotopic	Graft to another site not normal for that tissue/organ
Orthologous	Derived from an identical source
Heterologous	Derived from a different source
Primary vascularized grafts (organ graft)	For example, heart, lung, kidney, liver, exocrine pancreas
Secondarily vascularlized tissue grafts:	For example, solid neural tissue grafts, cornea, islets, thyroid gland, free skin, bone
Secondarily vascularlized cellular grafts: Avascular cellular grafts	Suspension neural tissue grafts, non-neural tissue Blood transfusion, bone marrow, hematogenic stem cell
MHC	Major histocompatibility complex antigens
Major transplantation antigen	Allogeneic MHC + allogeneic peptides
Minor transplantation antigen	Syngeneic MHC + allogeneic peptides
ABO-system	Donor blood group antigens and recipient natural antibodies
First set rejection	Acute rejection
Second set rejection Chronic rejection	Acute rejection, occuring faster after a sequential graft Slow rejection occuring over prolonged period
Innate immune system	Inflammatory responses involved in control and regulation of immune responses; complement system
APC	Natural Killer cells, NK-T cells; phagocytes; natural antibodies antigen presenting cell

(sometimes tissue specific), which are processed and presented within the variable portions of MHC I or II molecules. Lipids and carbohydrates may be presented via CD1 and similar molecules and may be important for cellular immune responses as well (Hong *et al.* 1999). Blood group antigens (ABO-system), and the presence of natural antibodies against many of the blood group antigens that an individual do not express, are important also for host responses against grafted tissue.

The immune responses against xenogeneic tissue (grafting across species) are more complex and encompass not only the specific, induced immune reactions, but also several of the innate immune responses, such as the complement system, NK and NKT-cells, natural antibodies and the coagulation cascade systems (Cascalho and Platt 2001). When cells, tissue, or organs are grafted between relatively closely related species (condordant xeno-grafts), the immune reactions are dominated by cellular reactions against a xenogeneic MHC plus xenogeneic peptides, and resemble allograft responses one more distantly related species (discordant xenografts), the immune responses involve also innate responses and may result in hyperacute rejection. Humans, and the non-human primates, have a deletional mutation for the α-1,3 galactosyl tranferase enzyme, and these species do not express the Gal-α-1,3Gal polysaccharide epitopes on lipids and proteins. The epitope is expressed on bacteria in the normal gut flora, and all humans have high titers (1 : 2500 or higher) of anti-Gal 'natural antibodies' (Galili 1993). Grafts between humans and non-human primates consitute concordant xenografts, and human and any other species would be 'discordant', with a risk for hyperacte rejection. Even if species both have the α-1,3 galactosyl transferase, there may be preformed antibodies against other antigens, along with complement incompatibilities. These species combinations are also discordant.

In addition to the immunological differences, the type of graft, and how the cells, tissue or organs are implanted are important. The most vigourous graft resposes are against primarily vascularized discordant organ xenografts, when the donor organ is immediately exposed to the host circulation, whereas the least are against secondarily vascularized cellular allografts, for which the vascualrization may take several days.

The implantation site is also important with a cellular graft in the brain being quite favourable compared with, for example in the portal vein.

11.1.2 Afferent pathways from the brain to the immune system

The brain was long thought to be devoid of any lymphatic drainage, and indeed the brain parenchyma lack conventional lymphatic vessels. In most species investigated, ranging from mice, rats, rabbits, cats, sheep and goat, a large proportion of the extracellular fluid rapidly drain into the deep cervical lymph nodes in the neck, via an anatomical passage across the lamina cribosa, and via the nose lymph vessels (Cserr and Knopf 1992; Widner *et al.* 1987). Direct injection of antigens in the brain parenchyma has been shown to lead to a specific immune response in these lymph nodes, as well as in the spleen (Widner *et al.* 1988; Lynch *et al.* 1989). There is direct evidence for donor tissue derived cells in the lymph nodes, and spleen of the recipients have been found after neural tissue grafting in rats (Broadwell *et al.* 1994).

In non-human primates and humans, the extent of the extracellular fluid drainage to the lymphatic system is quantitatively small, but there are indications that some direct passage of antigens is possible also in humans, since arachnoidal bodies in direct connection with the subrachnoid space, can be observed in the nasal cavity, draining into the extravascular space (Lövhagen *et al.* 1994).

The perivascular spaces are probably more important for the presentation of intracerebral antigens in humans. The perivascular microglia cells (pericyte) are specialized bone marrow derived cells that can have APC function (Hickey 2001). These perivascular spaces can also be transformed into organized tissue, resembling of lymphoid tissue in chronic immune mediated disorders such as multiple sclerosis (Prineas 1979).

11.1.3 Antigen presenting cells

The cells within the brain that are mainly responsible for the antigen presentation (AP) from the brain is still under active investigations. The previously held notion that the brain lacked not only lymphactic vessels, but also efficient antigen presenting cells, such as the dendritic cells (DC) (Hart and Fabre 1981), has been replaced by a view of a dynamic interplay between various cells within the brain parenchyma.

There are two populations of bone marrow derived microglia cells; one resting, permanent type scattered throughout the parenchyma, which enters the brain under fetal period (Perry *et al.* 1985), and another that is periodically exchanged in the perivascular spaces (Graeber and Streit 1990; Hickey and Kimura 1988). These cells differ mainly in the level of expression of CD45, co-stimulatory factors and MHC class II, with the latter cell type expressing higher levels. The resident micrgoglia are considered to be relatively immature and can mature into macrophages and DC, the most efficient antigen presenting cell type (Banchereau and Steinman 1998; Santambrogio *et al.* 2001). In slice cultures, parenchymal microglia can migrate to the vascular space and form round, macrophage like cells in response to injury (Czapiga and Colton 2001).

Isolated, brain derived DCs and activated microglia cells can activate naive T-cells whereas astocytes are unable (Aloisi *et al.* 1999). Within the brain there is close interaction between various cells via cytokines and growth factors, such as astrocyte derived GM-CSF and M-CSF. These substances contribute to the maturation of immature microglia cells into DC and fully effective AP cells (APC) (Fisher and Bielinsky 1999).

In the context of transplantation, APC are very important. The strongest stimulus for an allogeneic response is donor derived APC. The donor tissue content of APC and their drainage route determine largely how efficient the recipient is immunized agains the graft tissue. Allogeneic APC can directly activate host lymphocytes, so called direct presentation. Host APC can also take up donor antigens, either intact MHC molecules or allo- or xenogeneic fragments of proteins, and present these in the context of host MHC, as an indirect presentation (Gould and Auchincloss 1999).

For xenogeneic grafts, this latter mode of presentation is more important than the direct route which requires very specific interaction between the T-cell receptor and the xenogeneic MHC (Murphy *et al.* 1996).

When grafting allogeneic or xenogeneic neural tissue, there is activation of host microglia, and to some extent donor derived migroglia cells. Their role in iniating immune responses is outlined in Fig. 11.1 along with further interconnections between the brain and the immune system.

11.1.4 Lympoid tissue

In lymphoid tissue the conditions for activation of specific lymphocytes are optimized. The complex binding of the TCR-MHC + antigen, re-enforced by the CD/8 molecules, and the co-stimulatory signal ligands such as CD80/86 with CTLA4 and CD28, CD40-CD40L and

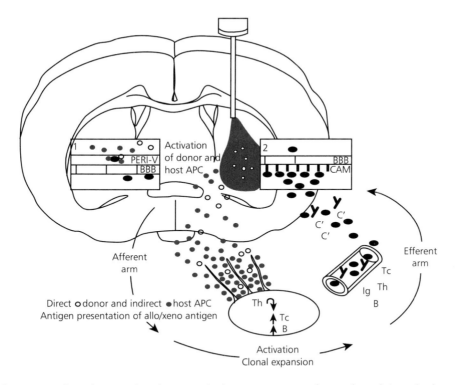

Fig. 11.1 Outline of connections between the immune system and transplanted tissue in the brain of rodents. The afferent pathway consists of activated host (filled circles) and donor (open circles) antigen presenting cells, which migrate to regional lymphatic organ, such as a the deep cervical lymph nodes via the lamina cribriformis and the nasal lymphatic vessels, or remain inside of the brain in the peri-vascular spaces. Donor APC present allogeneic or xenogeneic MHC in a direct way to host T-cells, and host APC can take up and partially process allogeneic and xenogeneic structures and present in the context of self-MHC in an indirect process. Inserted box 1: Schematic drawing of the peri-vascular space where antigen presentation may occur. APC from the host and the donor tissue migrate to the space, and interact with lymphocytes that have migrated across the endothelium. The efferent pathway consists of migration of activated lymphocytes to the graft region, across an activated blood–brain barrier. Resident microglia cells and invading macrophages contribute to the inflammatory response and participate in delayed type hypersensitivity reactions. Complement factors, and immunoglobulins enter mainly through passive mechanisms, or are produced locally after entry of macrophages and plasma cells. Inserted box 2: Schematic passage across the blood–brain barrier. Activated endothelia cells express adhesion molecules that allow for homing of activated lymphocytes to accumulate and enter the peri-vascular space and the parenchyma. Bar lines indicate 1 mm. APC: antigen presenting cell; BBB: blood–brain barrier; B: B-cells; C: complement factors; CAM: cell adhesion molecules; Th: T-helper cells; Tc: T-cytotxic cells; Ig: immunoglobulin.

the additional binding of LFA (1/3) with ICAM-1 and CD2 are all occurring at the correct sequence and in sufficient strength, activation of the T-cell takes place. If this sequence is not fulfilled, and no co-stimulatory activation signal is provided, this can lead to an anergic state of the T-cells (Waldmann and Cobbald 2001), or the development of regulatory T-cells that further modify the host reponses (Maloy and Poiwre 2001). Immunosuppressive drugs and immunomodulatory interventions aim at these functions.

11.1.5 Efferent arm from the lympoid tissue to the brain

The brain is ensheathed by a series of barriers, effectively isolating brain metabolism and electric activity from the surrounding, less well regulated homeostasis, as reviewed in this book. The meningeal-brain barrier complex, the brain-choroidal plexus, the pial vessel-extracellular space, and the capillary blood–brain barrier are each components of this insulation of the brain. The capillary barrier consists of tight junction between the endothelial cells, a low pinocytotic capacity, presence of distinct enzymatic functions an electrostatic potential difference across the lumen lack of response to a number of agents normally acting on the endothelium, such as histamine and bradykinins, and a complex of active transporters such as G-proteins. Immunoglobulins, complement and other plasma factors not usually present in the brain parenchyma in high concentrations (1 : 200 or less compared with that in plasma). Cells normally have a very restricted passage. After activation, alloreactive lymphocytes proliferate and enter the blood circulation. These cells 'home' to the graft, directed by cues present on the endothelium of the vessels in and around the graft. The brain endothelium can express a number of homing signals, under the control of transcription factors that respond to inflammatory stimulus. Pro-inflammatory cytokines such as tumor necrosis factor-α (TNF-α), γ-interferon (γ-IFN), interleukin-1 (IL-1) and nirtic oxide can induce expression of intercellular cell nitric adhesion molecules (ICAM-1) and vascular cell adhesion molecules (VCAM-1), the latter being crucial for the entry of cells (Baron et al. 1993; Merill and Murphy 1997). Once accross the barrier, further migration is mediated by chemokines such as IL-8, IP-10, RANTES and MIP-1 and MCP-1 (reviewed in Merill and Murphy 1997).

11.1.6 Graft vessels and the blood–brain barrier

The origin of blood vessels in a graft depend on the type of tissue grafted and whether the donor tissue is processed into a cellular cell suspension. A non-neural tissue such as skin or adrenal medullary tissue grafted to the brain does not form a blood–brain barrier (Stewart et al. 1984). Suspension neural grafts are revascularized mainly by host vessels and after implantation into the parenchyma, a blood–brain barrier for macromolecules are reformed within about a week (Brundin et al. 1989; Barker-Cairns et al. 1996). Solid pieces of neural tissue grafts carry with them donor derived blood vessels, which interconnect with the host vessels. A barrier complex is usually formed, at least when the graft is placed in the ventricular system or in the brain parenchyma (Broadwell et al. 1994).

11.1.7 Internal millieu of the brain parenchyma

It has been suggested that the brain contain locally immunosuppressive factors (Barker and Billingham 1977). TGF-β is a family of locally acting anti-inflammatory, anti-mitotic, down regulatory cytokines, and TGF-β is the endogeneous ligand for the immunophilins, which are the intracellular targets for the immunosuppressive drugs FK506 and cyclosporin A (Wang et al. 1994). TGF-β has also been implicted in reducing the immune responses in the eye (Streilein 1993). The internal mileiu of the brain has been suggested to favour tolerance development or anergia, but that the conditions may change after local trauma and inflammation (Brabb *et al.* 2000). Other factors have been implicated such as FAS/FAS-L expression in the brain (Bechmann *et al.* 1999).

11.2 Immunological responses against intracerebral neural allografts

Experimentally, various levels of MHC incompatibility have been addressed, and allograft rejection episodes have been observed in all settings, however under certain conditions, prolonged graft survival is possible in spite of complete MHC incompatibility (Mason *et al.* 1986; Widner *et al.* 1989), in particular after suspension graft implanted stereotaxically with an atraumatic technique. The strain combinations may also influence the outcome with good survival in low responder combinations between donor and host, versus high responders matters as well (Poltorak and Freed 1991).

In a model of parkinsonism in the rat, and well defined donor tissue properties, with a standardized aturamtic technique it is possible to achieve long-term graft survival without any immunosuppression, at the same time as there are evidence for host immunization (Widner and Brundin 1993). When challenged with a second intracerebral graft, the first established graft is not affected, nor is the second graft necessarily rejected, but there is evidence for increased host responses around the latter graft (Duan *et al.* 1994). In strongly pre-immunized animals, the subsequent brain tissue grafts are promptly rejected, but established grafts are not always rejected after a challenge of a skin graft albeit a slow, chronic rejection may be operative (Duan *et al.* 1997). Grafting to a site where microglia and astrocytes have been activated by a toxin to stimulate inflammation, resulted in a better graft survival of an allograft, in comparison with a normal site, and the non-neuronal part of the graft increased in volume. This is probably due to the production of growth factors in the area (Duan *et al.* 1998).

If rejection occurs in the brain, there may be 'innocent by-stander' damage, which has been tested experimentally in one study with mixed allogeneic and xenogeneic grafts. In the group with rejection of the xenograft, there was a reduced syngeneic or allogeneic graft survival, compared to immunosuppressed controls without any signs of xenograft rejections (Schwarz *et al.* 1996).

There are few studies on the effects and need for immunosuppression in allogeneic neural grafts. Wood *et al.* (1993) have used a monoclonal antibody against the IL-2 receptor to increase the survival of grafted neural tissue in the ventricles and it has been demonstrated that this treatment may induce long-term and in high proportion of grafts, specific immunological tolerance to a subsequent allograft in the periphery. So far there are no studies in non-human primates published, but our own data in squirrel monkeys indicate favourable effcts with systemic immunosuppression for allografts, in particular to allow for sequential grafting sessions.

11.3 Clinical allogeneic neural tissue transplantation

Embryonic allogeneic neural tissue grafts have been performed in more than 300 patients with PD, and this procedure has been shown to be effective in ameliorating many of the symptoms in PD. In the best cases, patients have been able to return to full time employment, and have been able to tolerate withdrawal of all anti-parkinsonism and immunosuppressive drug treatment.

The status of the transplantation technique is now such that there is proof-of-principle regarding the possibilites to repair the brain with embryonic primary neural tissue and that the neuronal circuitries are reformed (Björklund and Lindvall 2000; Lindvall and Hagell 2000). There are ongoing attempts to broaden this to a wider use and studies to the efficacy has been initiated (Freed *et al.* 2001), with various success and failures. However, the technique is far from standardized, and several studies have failed to obtain the same results. The critical factors for graft induced functional recovery to occur are that sufficient number of grafted cells survive the implantation process and that the host brain is effectively rein-nervated with reformation of a neuronal circuitry. The donor tissue must be embryonic. There is a very narrow time limit when the tissue can be grafted, between 5–7 weeks post-gestation for human tissue, and only 5–40 per cent survive the implantation process. Better survival rates are achieved with pretreatment of the donor tissue with factors which inhibit processes such as apoptotic cell death and free radicals (Hagell and Brundin 2001). Multiple donors are needed to achieve sufficient graft effects. The embryonic donor tissue can be stored under cool conditions for some period of time, but cryo-preservation has not been possible (redmond). Short term culture may reduce the number of donor APC, but the survival rate of the dopaminergic neurones is decreased in turn. In the Freed study, tissue was cultured prior to implantation for up to 4 weeks, and no immunosuppression was used. There was poor survival compared with non-cultured tissue and immunosuppressed recipi-ents (about 1/3 of other studies) (Hagell and Brundin 2001; Freed *et al.* 2001; Kordower *et al.* 1995).

Implantation is made stereotaxically, with patient lightly sedated. Twenty microliters of cell suspension is deposited in each track, about 15 mm long, and each patient receives 5–7 implants in each putamen, and 1–2 implants in each caudate nucleus. In most cases, a patient is grafted unilaterally, but in sequence with a minimum of 2 weeks interval. In the Freed study (Freed *et al.* 2001), the implantation procedure failed to reach the whole putamen, and created a gradient, which may account for the developent of the abnormal movements observed in 15 per cent of the patients.

Patients in the Swedish programme received a slightly modified traditional protocol for kidney grafting, with cyclosporin A, at 8–5 mg/kg starting 2 days prior to implantation aiming at a concentration of 200–250 ng/mL at time of surgery, and a maintenance level of about 100–150 ng/mL. In addition 2 mg azathioprine, and an iv dose of 500 mg methyl-prednisolone at the time of implantation, with oral 100 mg prednisolone being reduced to a maintenance dose of 10 mg/day after 2–3 months are given. The treatment is maintained for 12 months after the last surgery, and is then slowly tapered. A majority of patients have been on immunosuppressive treatment about 18 months, some 5 years. In all cases, withdrawal has not resulted in any rejection episodes. In the Kordower case II, T cells have been observed after sessation of CSA in a case that came to autopsy 12 months after immunosuppression was stopped, and 18 months after grafting but the were very good graft survival and clinical effects (Kordower *et al.* 1995, 1997).

Positron emission tomography (PET) can directly visualize the pre-synaptic and the post-synaptic receptors, as objective measurements of dopamine production that correlate directly with the clinical effects. This is an objective measurement of the graft surival rate and a significant increase should be observed for robust clinical effects. Tracers specific for inflammatory responses, particularly microglia, PK11195 can be used to detect massive infiltration around the grafts.

11.4 Immunological responses against experimental intracerebral neural xenografts

The main impetus has been to replace human donor tissue, as reviewed in (Pakzaban and Isacson 1994; Pedersen and Widner 2000). Several biological differences need to be known: that is, the number of cells in the ventral mesencephalic region, the developmental phase and the optimal time window for when good graft survival can be achieved. Pigs have been chosen as the source animal for clinical xenografts. Pigs have a long life span, (at least 25 years in captivity), short breeding span, and multiple off-spring. In addition they can be trans-genically modified, cloned and targeted gene deletions have recently been successful (GAL-KO). The species has been domesticated for millennia and ethically commercial breeding has been accepted for a long period. There are about 2 00 000 dopaminergic neuroblasts in the pig, and the optimal age is E 26–27. Allogeneic pig grafts have been made in to parkinsonian mini-pigs with functional recovery and PET signal improvement demonstrating that the same principles apply to this tissue as for human tissue in the absence of major immunological differences (Cummings *et al.* 2001).

The immune responses against discordant embryonic porcine tissue has been addressed in mice and rats, and the critical factors for graft rejection determined, as reviewed in (Brevig *et al.* 2000) and outlined in Fig. 11.2.

When grafting porcine neural tissue to mice lacking immunoglobulins there was a pro-longation of the survival of the grafted cells, and a shift from CD4 to CD8 dependent lymphocyte infiltration, and they were eventually rejected by 6 weeks (Larsson *et al.* 1999). Rats depleted transiently of complement function by cobra venom factor (CVF), reject porcine grafts (Barker *et al.* 2000) and complement deficient mice (C3−/−) rejected porcine grafts as fast as wild-type animals indicating only a minor role of complement *in vivo* (Larsson *et al.* 2002*b*). Resting human NK cells are not directly damaging the porcine ventral mesencephalic cells *in vitro*, but can function as mediators of ADCC if human AB serum is added. Activated NK cells, by IL-2, are directly lytic (Sumitran *et al.* 1999). In mice depleted of NK cells, porcine grafts were not protected from rejection. In mice lacking the CD1d1 molecule, and thus NK-T cells, grafts were present at higher numbers at 2 weeks compared with control, but all grafts were rejected by 5 weeks (Larsson *et al.* 2001). Con-ventional immunosuppressive drugs in monotherapy, CSA or tacrolimus did not protect grafts effectively in a long study, only after combination with, for example prednisolone (Wennberg *et al.* 2001). Functional assessment also indicates that CSA offers 50 per cent protection for porcine neural tissue in rats (Galpern *et al.* 1996; Larsson *et al.* 2000). Porcine neural tissue can restore neural functions in immunosuppressed rats, but there are very few examples of any functional recovery in non-human primates, despite several attempts. Short treatment co-stimulation blockade has resulted in very good graft survival in mice blocking CD40L, LFA1, and CTLA4Ig (Larsson *et al.* 2002).

The relative selective expression of GAL epitopes on the endothelial and microglia cells has been the basis for purging experiments, using human serum and complement as reviewed in (Brevig *et al.* 2000). Non-purged tissue activates human T-cells *in vitro* after culture. After purging GAL-antibody reactivity and T-cell responses have been drastically reduced and partial protection against rejection in rats has been observed.

Another mode of interfering with the first signal has been to block MHC class I molecules in the donor tissue by immunomasking with F(ab)$_2$ antibody-fragments. Fetal neural

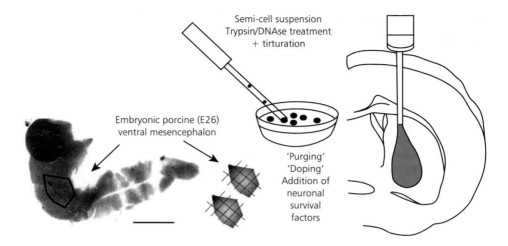

Fig. 11.2 Schematic intracerebral transplantation of xenogeneic tissue. The ventral mesencephalon is dissected from the mid-brain region of an embryonic porcine donor, aged E26, and cut in several small pieces. These are incubated in 0.1 per cent trypsin for 20 min and then washed several times in buffered salt solutions in 0.05 per cent DNAse to facilitate gentle tirturation in a Pasteur pipette to generate a semi-cell suspension. This is further processed, by for example 'purging' of endothelia cells and microglia cells, or 'doped' by addition of for example, liposomes laden with cell surface factors such as complement inhibitors or co-stimulation inhibitors. In order to improve the survival rate of the neurones, survival factors are added, for example 3 mM tirilazad mesulate (a lipid peroxidase inhibitor), 0.5 µM ciclosporin A (which inhibits the mitochondria transition pore and reduce the Ca^{2+} efflux from ischaemic mitochondria), and 500 µM ac-YVAD-cmk (a caspase inhibitor reducing induced apoptosis). The suspension is injected into the target site for the normal innervation site, the striatum (heterotopic implantation site). Typical graft volumes used in rodents are 2–4 µL, and in humans 20 µL per track. Between 3–9 tracks have been used in clinical settings per side, and in total 120–360 µL have been grafted to patients. The recipients are immunosuppressed using various drug combinations or immunomodulators.

porcine tissue was pretreated with the F(ab)$_2$-antibody fragments against porcine MHC I before implantation to the striatum and this led to enhanced graft survival compared to the untreated group (Pakzaban and Isacson 1994).

Further work is needed, and combination of donor tissue purging, and modification of the tissue either through drug treatment, transgeneic mechanisms, targeted gene deletions are likely to improve on the surival rate, and reduce the risks for rejection. A rational way to assess the efficacy of any intervention is to assess the pattern of cytokine responses in the brain after grafting as summarized in Table 11.2 (Kogure *et al.* 1998; Vine *et al.* 1999; Mirza *et al.* submitted).

11.5 Clinical trials using embryonic porcine tissue

The first clinical trial with pig tissue was conducted in the US as a phase I study, comparing two regiments of immunosuppression, 5 mg/kg ciclosporin A as a monotherapy, versus

Table 11.2 RT-PCR determined cytokine profiles after grafting into the brain

Donor–host combination	IL-1β	IL-2	IL-4	IL-10	TNF-α	γ-IFN
Syngeneic (SD rat → SD rat)	+	+ +	+	+	+	—
Allogeneic • (Lewis rat → SD rat)	+	+ +	+	+	+	+ +
Concordant xenogeneic (mouse → rat)	+	+ +	+ + +	+ +	+	+ +
Discordant xenogeneic (pig → rat)	+ + +	+ +	+ + +	+ + +	+ + +	+ +

From (Mirza *et al.* 2002, submitted).

immunomasking of anti-porcine MHC class I antigens. Six patients each were grafted and followed for 12 months. No PET data have been reported. There was no improvement in the group data, but two patients, were reported to have 15 per cent improvement in clinical rating scales (Schumacher *et al.* 2000). One case came to autopsy at 7 months after grafting and histologically, pig tissue was detected, but only 638 dopaminergic cells, far short of the 80–1 00 000 cells needed for clinical effects (Deacon *et al.* 1997). A second multi-centre phase II study has been performed in the US, with sham-operated control patients. Ten patients were grafted, and eight were randomized as controls and underwent sham-surgery and sham-immunosuppression. PET images may have indicated hot-spots in certain areas, but clinical evaluations have not resulted in any overall clinical improvement, except for a reduction time spent in on with dyskinesias. In addition, 12 patients with Huntington's disease have been grafted with embryonic neural pig tissue (Fink *et al.* 2000). The functional effects have been negative. There have been no complications in terms of host infections nor any demonstrations of anti-PERV antibodies, and negative PCRs for PERV (Dinsmore *et al.* 2000).

11.6 **Stem cells**

Stem cells involve a novel, largely unknown biological principle of controlled, *in vitro* differentiation. There are several types of cells of various origins and developmental phases, as reviewed in Temple (2001). The most immature, and with the largest potential, are embryonic stem cells (ES). There are fears that ES will result in teratomas or other uncontrolled cell growth which are illustrated by animal experiments in which up to 22 per cent of rat recipients developed fatal intracerebral teratomas after grafting of mouse ES. In addition, 24 per cent of the grafts never developed in to any tissue, and the ES cells were probably rejected in spite of immunosuppression (Björklund *et al.* 2002).

The immunlogy of grafted stem cells has not been studied, but is of importance as the cells are either allo- or xenogeneic and secondarily vascularized. It is predicted that rejection is possible, and it is of importance to investigate the fate of the grafted cells in conditions with inflammation and rejections, in which there are multitude of potent cytokine and growth factors around. Even therapeutic cloning, with an enucleated ES cell exchanged with a syngeneic nucleus, will not be exempt from potential immune responses as there is a possibility of minor transplantation antigens being produced and presented in such cells. There cannot be a guarantee that rejection will not occur.

The use of adult progenitors, taken from the patients themselves, may be a future avenue, but requires that the pregenitors are not affected by a disease process as well, or if reimplanted in to a diseased brain after having been differentiated *in vitro* and *ex vivo*, remain stable and differentiated in the implant site and irrespective of a local inflammatory response.

11.7 **Non-neuronal tissue**

Non-neuronal cells cannot be used for the repair strategy, which requires reformation of neuronal circuitries and a controlled synaptic release. Attempts to replace neurotransmittors with transfected cellular 'minipumps' have all resulted only in partial effects. There has not been a complete behaviour recovery with non-neural grafts, as with optimal neural grafts in any model assessed so far (Brown and Dunnett 1989; Dunnett and Björklund 1999).

In neurodegenerative disorders, a lack of adequate growth supporting substances has been suggested to contribute to the degenerative process and therapeutic approaches to supplement these essential growth factors have been suggested in a number of conditions, provided the correct growth/trophic factor has been identified.

The implantation of a genetically modified cell, or direct gene transfer, in order to rescue the remaining neural population at risk for further deterioration, is thus a more appropriate approach. However, there are several examples that such grafts have been rejected in spite of cells that have been transfected have been syngeneic or allogenenic, but after the trasnfection have been rejected promptly, with a need for continous immunosuppression. Even if transcription defective virus vectors have been used, it is clear that intracellular antigens find their way to the surface, or as picked up by host APC and an effective immune response can be mounted. Prior to clinical applications, *in vivo* studies are needed, in pre-immunized animals and the local inflammatory responses assayed. Non-viral vectors are probably to perfer.

Encapsulation of transfected xenogeneic cell lines have been suggested as a way to avoid immune responses, but there are several examples of a non-cellular response against such encapsulated cells resulting in graft destruction (Gray 2001) mediated by toxic factors released by T-cells and activted macrophages/microglia cells. The encapsulation may not protect such cells completely from rejection, but may be of importance to avoid release of tumour cells.

11.8 **Summary**

Immune responses need to be addressed in any protocol for transplantation of tissue and cells into the brain for successful outcome. It is probably possible to circumvent many of the conditions that may result in rejection, without reverting to massive and life long immunosuppression, but in each case this needs to be addressed experimentally prior to implantations are tested in the clinic. The brain is indeed a privileged site for graft purposes, but not except from immune responese.

Acknowledgements

The work was supported by the EU-Biomed II programme BMH4-CT-97-2596 'Development of a xenogeneic donor tissue for neural transplantation in neurodegenerative disorders', the Swedish Medical Research Council grant 12XC-122436, the Medical Faculty at Lund University, the Segerfalk, the Kock, the Wiberg the Bergwall, the Crafoord Foundations, Neurologically Handicapped Organisation (NHR), and the Swedish Society for Medical Research.

References

Aloisi, F., Ria, F., Columba-Cabezas, S., Hess, H., Penna, G., and Adorini, L. (1999). Relative efficiency of microglia, astrocytes, dendritic cells and B cells in naive CD4+ T cell priming and Th1/Th2 cell restimulation. *Eur J Immunol*, 29, 2705–14.

Auchincloss, H. and Sultan, H. (1996). Antigen processing and presentation in transplantation. *Curr Opin Immunol*, 8, 681–7.

Banchereau, J. and Steinman, R. M. (1998). Dendritic cells and the control of immunity. *Nature*, 392, 245–52.

Barker, C. F. and Billingham, R. E. (1977). Immunologically privileged sites. *Adv Immunol*, 25, 1–54.

Barker, R. A., Ratcliffe, E., McLauhlin, M., Richards, A., and Dunnett, S. B. (2000). A role for complement in the rejection of porcine ventral mesencephalic xenografts in a rat model of Parkinson's disease. *J Neurosci*, 20, 3415–24.

Barker-Cairns, B. J., Sloan, D. J., Broadwell, R. D., Puklavec, M., and Charlton, H. M. (1996). Contribution of donor and host blood vessels in CNS allografts. *Exp Neurol*, 142, 36–46.

Bechmann, I., Mor, G., Nilsen, J., Eliza, M., Nitsch, R., and Naftolin, F. (1999). FasL (CD95L, Apo1L) is expressed in the normal rat and human brain: evidence for the existence of an immunological brain barrier. *Glia*, 27, 62–74.

Billingham, R. W. and Boswell, T. (1953). Studies on the problem of corneal honografts. *Proc Roy Soc Ser B*, 141, 392–406.

Björklund, A. and Lindvall, O. (2000). Cell replacement therapies for central nervous system disorders. *Nat Neurosci*, 3, 537–44.

Björklund L., Sanchez-Pernaute, R., Chung, S., Andersson, T., Yin Ching Chen, I., McNaught, K., *et al.* (2002). Embryonic stem cells develop into functional dopaminergic neurons after transplantation in a Parkinson rat model. *Proc Nat Acad Sci USA*, 70, 1–6.

Baron, J. L., Madri, J. A., Ruddle, N. H., Hashim, G., and Janeway, C. A. (1993). Surface expression of a4 intergrin by CD4 T cells is required for their enry into the brain parenchyma. *J Exp Med*, 177, 57–68.

Brabb, T., von Dassow, P., Ordonez, N., Schnabel, B., Duke, B., and Goverman, J. (2000). *In situ* tolerance within the central nervous system as a mechanism for preventing autoimmunity. *J Exp Med*, 192, 871–80.

Brevig, T., Holgersson, J., and Widner, H. (2000). Xenotransplantation for CNS repair: immunological barriers and strategies to overcome them. *Trends Neurosci*, 23, 337–44.

Broadwell, R. D., Baker, B. J., Ebert, P. S., and Hickey, W. F. (1994). Allografts of CNS tissue possess a blood–brain barrier: III. Neuropathological, methodological and, immunological considerations. *Microsc Res Tech*, 27, 471–94.

Brown, V. J. and Dunnett, S. B. (1989). Comparison of adrenal and fetal nigral grafts on drug-induced rotation in rats with 6-OHDA lesions. *Exp Brain Res*, 78, 214–18.

Brundin, P., Widner, H., Nilsson, O. G., Strecker, R. E., and Björklund, A. (1989). Intracerebral xenografts of dopamine neurons: the role of immunosuppression and the blood–brain barrier. *Exp Brain Res*, 75, 195–207.

Cascalho, M. and Platt, J. L. (2001). The immunological barrier to xenotransplantation. *Immunity*, 14, 437–46.

Cumming, P., Danielsen, E. H., Vafaee, M., Falborg, L., Steffensen, E., Sorensen, J. C., *et al.* (2001). Normalization of markers for dopamine innervation in striatum of MPTP-lesioned miniature pigs with intrastriatal grafts. *Acta Neurol Scand*, 103, 309–15.

Czapiga, M. and Colton, C. A. (1999). Function of microglia in organotypic slice cultures. *J Neurosci Res*, **56**, 644–51.

Cserr, H. F. and Knopf, P. (1992). Cervical lymphatics, the blood–brain barrier and the immunoreactivity in the brain – a new view. *Immunol Today*, **13**, 507–12.

Deacon, T., Schumacher, J., Dinsmore, J., Thomas, C., Palmer, P., Kott, S., *et al*. (1997). Histological evidence of fetal pig neural cell survival after transplantation into a patient with Parkinson's disease. *Nat Med*, **3**, 350–3.

Dinsmore, J., Mnahart, C., and Raineri, R. (2000). No evidence for infection of human cells with porcine endogenous retrovirus (PERV) after exposure to porcine fetal neuronal cells. *Transplantation*, **70**, 1382–9.

Duan, W-M., Brundin, P., Björklund, A., and Widner, H. (1994). Sequential intracerebral transplantation of allogeneic and syngeneic fetal dopamine-rich neuronal tissue in adult rats: Will the second graft be rejected? *Neuroscience*, **57**, 261–74.

Duan, W-M., Cameron, R. M., Brundin, P., and Widner, H. (1997). Rat intrastriatal neural allografts challenged with skin allografts at different time-points. *Exp Neurol*, **148**, 334–347.

Duan, W-M., Widner, H., Cameron, R. M., and Brundin, P. (1998). Quinolinic acid-induced inflammation in the striatum does not impair the survival of neural allografts in the rat. *Eur J Neurosci*, **10**, 2595–606.

Dunnett, S. B. and Björklund, A. (1999). Prospects for new restorative and neuroprotective treatments in Parkinson's disease. *Nature*, **399**, A32–9.

Fischer, H. G. and Bielinsky, A. K. (1999). Antigen presentation function of brain-derived dendriform cells depends on astrocyte help. *Int Immunol*, **11**, 1265–74.

Fink, J. S., Schumacher, J. M., Ellias, S. L., Palmer, E. P., and Saint-Hilaire, M. (2000). Porcine xenografts in Parkinson's and Huntington's disease patients: preliminary results. *Cell Transplant*, **9**, 273–8.

Freed, C. R., Greene, P. E., Breeze, R. E., Tsai, W. Y., DuMouchel, W., Kao, R., *et al*. (2001). Transplantation of embryonic dopamine neurons for severe Parkinson's disease. *N Engl J Med*, **344**, 710–19.

Galili, U. (1993). Interaction of the natural anti-Gal antibody with α-galactosyl epitopes: a major obstacle for xenotransplantation in humans. *Immunol Today*, **14**, 480–2.

Galpern, W. R., Burns, L. H., Deacon, T. W., Dinsmore, J., and Isacson, O. (1996). Xenotransplantation of porcine ventral mesencephalon in a rat model of Parkinson's disease: functional recovery and graft morphology. *Exp Neurol*, **140**, 1–13.

Gould, D. S. and Auchincloss, H. Jr. (1999). Direct and indirect recognition: the role of MHC antigens in graft rejection. *Immunol Today*, **20**, 77–82.

Graeber, M. B. and Streit, W. J. (1990). Perivascular microglia defined. *Trends Neurosci*, **13**, 366–70.

Gray, D. W. (2001). An overview of the immune system with specific reference to membrane encapsulation and islet transplantation. *Ann NY Acad Sci*, **944**, 226–39.

Hagell, P. and Brundin, P. (2001). Cell survival and clinical outcome following intrastriatal transplantation in Parkinson disease. *J Neuropathol Exp Neurol*, **60**, 741–52.

Hart, D. N. J. and Fabre, W. J. (1981). Demonstration and characterization of Ia-positive dendritic cells in the interstitial connective tissues of rat heart and other tissue, but not brain. *J Exp Med*, **153**, 347–61.

Hickey, W. H. (2001). Basic principles of immunological surveillance of the normal central nervous system. *Glia*, **36**, 118–124.

Hickey, W. F. and Kimura, H. (1988). Perivascular microglial cells of the CNS are bone-marrow derived and present antigen *in vivo*. *Science*, **239**, 290–2.

Hong, S., Scherer, D. C., Singh, N., Mendiratta, S. K., Serizawa, I., Koezuka, Y., and Van Kaer, L. (1999). Lipid antigen presentation in the immune system: lessons learned from CD1d knockout mice. *Immunol Rev*, **169**, 31–44.

Kogure, K., Tanuma, N., Teramoto, A., and Matsumoto, Y. (1998). Quantitative analysis of pro- and anti-inflammatory cytokine mRNA in neural graft rejection. *J Neuroimmunol*, 87, 114–20.

Kordower, J. H., Freeman, T. B., Snow, B. J., Vingerhoets, F. J. G., Mufson, E. J., Sanberg, P. R., *et al.* (1995). Neuropathological evidence of graft survival and striatal reinnervation after the transplantation of fetal mesencephalic tissue in a patient with Parkinson's disease. *N Engl J Med*, 332, 1118–24.

Kordower, J. H., Styren, S., Clarke, M., DeKosky, S. T., Olanow, C. W., and Freeman, T. B. (1997). Fetal grafting for Parkinson's disease: expression of immune markers in two patients with functional fetal nigral implants. *Cell Transplant*, 6, 213–19.

Larsson, L. C., Czech, K. A., Widner, H., and Korsgren, O. (1999). Discordant neural tissue xenografts survive longer in immunoglobulin deficient mice. *Transplantation*, 68, 1153–60.

Larsson, L. C., Czech, K. A., Brundin, P., and Widner, H. (2000). Intrastriatal ventral mesencephalic xenografts of porcine tissue in rats: immune response and functional effects. *Cell Transplant*, 9, 261–72.

Larsson, L. C., Corbascio, M., Widner, H., Pearson, T. C., Larsen, C. P., and Ekberg, H. (2002*a*). Simultaneous inhibition of B7 and LFA-1 signaling prevents rejection of discordant neural xenografts in mice lacking CD40L. *Xenotransplantation*, 9, 68–76.

Larsson, L. C., Anderson, P., Widner, H., and Korsgren, O. (2001). Enhanced survival of porcine neural xenografts in mice lacking the CD1.1; but no effect of NK1.1 depletion. *Cell Transplant*, 10, 295–304.

Larsson, L. C., Sumitran, S., Holgersson, J., Korsgren, O., and Widner, H. (2002*b*). Complement mediated damage of porcine ventral mesencephalic tissue *in vitro* and *in vivo*. *Exp Neurol*, in press.

Lindvall, O. and Hagell, P. (2000). Clinical observations after neural transplantation in Parkinson's disease. *Prog Brain Res*, 127, 299–320.

Lynch, F., Doherty, P. C., and Ceredig, R. (1989). Phenotypic and functional analysis of the cellular response in regional lymphoid tissue during an acute virus infection. *J Immunol*, 142, 3592–8.

Lövhagen, P., Johansson, B. B., and Nordborg, C. (1994). The nasal route of cerebrospinal fluid drainage in man. A lightmicroscopic study. *Neuropathol Appl Neurobiol*, 20, 543–50.

Maloy, K. J. and Poiwre, F. (2001). Regulatory T cells in the control of immune pathology. *Nat Immunol*, 2, 816–22.

Mason, D. W., Charlton, H. M., Jones, A. J., Lavy, C. B., Puklavec, M., and Simmonds, S. J. (1986). The fate of allogeneic and xenogeneic neuronal tissue transplanted into the third ventricle of the rodents. *Neuroscience*, 19, 685–94.

Merrill, J. E. and Murphy, S. P. (1997). Inflammatory events at the blood brain barrier: regulation of adhesion molecules, cytokines, and chemokines by reactive nitrogen and oxygen species. *Brain Behav Immunity*, 11, 245–63.

Mirza, B., Krook, H., Anderson, P., Cameron, R. C., Korsgren, O., and Widner, H. (2002). Intracerebral expression of cytokines and chemokines after syngeneic, allogeneic, concordant and discordant xenogeneic neural tissue grafting. Submitted to *Exp Neurol*.

Murphy, B., Auchincloss, H. Jr., Carpenter, C. B., and Sayegh, M. H. (1996). T cell recognition of xeno-MHC peptides during concordant xenograft rejection. *Transplantation*, 61, 1133–7.

Pakzaban, P. and Isacson, O. (1994). Neuronal xenotransplantation: Reconstruction of neuronal circuitry across species barriers. *Neuroscience*, 62, 989–1001.

Pedersen, E. B. and Widner, H. (2000). Xenotransplantation. *Prog Brain Res*, 127, 157–88.

Perry, V. H., Hume, D. A., and Gordon, S. (1985). Immunohistochemical localisation of macrophages and microglia in the adult and developing mouse brain. *Neuroscience*, 15, 313–26.

Prineas, J. W. (1979). Multiple sclerosis: presence of lymphatic capillaries and lymphoid tissue in the brain and spinal cord. *Science*, 203, 1123–5.

Poltorak, M. and Freed, W. J. (1991). BN rats do not reject F344 brain allografts even after systemic sensitization. *Ann Neurol*, **29**, 377–88.

Santambrogio, L., Belyanskaya, S. L., Fischer, F. R., Cipriani, B., Brosnan, C. F., Ricciardi-Castagnoli, P., *et al.* (2001). Developmental plasticity of CNS microglia. *Proc Natl Acad Sci USA*, **98**, 6295–300.

Schumacher, J. M., Ellias, S. A., Palmer, E. P., Kott, H. S., Dinsmore, J., Dempsey, P. K., *et al.* (2000). Transplantation of embryonic porcine mesencephalic tissue in patients with PD. *Neurology*, **54**, 1042–50.

Schwarz, S. C., Kupsch, A. R., Banati, R., and Oertel, W. H. (1996). Cellular immune reactions in brain transplantation: effects of graft pooling and immunosuppression in the 6-hydroxydopamine rat model of Parkinson's disease. *Glia*, **17**, 103–20.

Sumitran, S., Anderson, P., Widner, H., and Holgersson, J. (1999). Porcine embryonic brain cell cytotoxicity mediated by human natrual killer cells. *Cell Transplant*, **8**, 601–10.

Stewart, P. A., Clements, C. A., and Wiley, M. J. (1984). Revascularization of skin transplanted into the brain: source of the graft endothelium. *Microvasc Res*, **28**, 113–24.

Streilein, W. J. (1993). Tissue barrier, immunosuppressive microenvironments, and privileged sites: the eye's point of view. *Regulatory Immunol*, **5**, 253–68.

Temple, S. (2001). Stem cell plasticity-building the brain of our dreams. *Nat Rev Neurosci*, **2**, 513–20.

Vine, A. M., Lang, J., Wood, M. J., and Charlton, H. M. (1999). Cytokine gene expression following neural grafts. *Exp Brain Res*, **126**, 281–8.

Wang, T., Donahue, P. K., and Zervos, A. S. (1994). Specific interaction of type I reseptors of the TGF-ß family with the immunophilin FKBR-12. *Science*, **265**, 674–6.

Waldmann, H. and Cobbold, S. (2001). Regulating the immune respose to transplants. A role for CD4 + regulatory cells? *Immunity*, **14**, 399–406.

Wennberg, L., Czech, K. A., Larsson, L., Bennett, W., Song, Z., and Widner, H. (2001). Effects of immunosuppressive treatment on host responses and survival of porcine neural xenografts in rats. *Transplantation*, **71**, 1797–806.

Widner, H., Brundin, P., Björklund, A., and Möller, E. (1989). Survival and immunogenicity of dissociated allogeneic fetal neural dopamine-rich grafts when implanted into the brains of adult mice. *Exp Brain Res*, **76**, 187–97.

Widner, H. and Brundin, P. (1988). Immunological aspects of grafting in the mammalian central nervous system. A speculative synthesis. *Brain Res Rev*, **13**, 287–324.

Widner, H., and Brundin, P. (1993). Sequential intracerebral transplantation of allogeneic and syngeneic fetal dopamine-rich neuronal tissue in adult rats: Will the first graft be rejected? *Cell Transplant*, **2**, 307–17.

Widner, H., Jönsson, B-A., Hallstadius, L., Wingårdh, K., Strand, S-E., and Johansson, B. B. (1987). Scintigraphic method to quantify the passage from brain parenchyma to the deep cervical lymph nodes in rats. *Eur J Nucl Med*, **13**, 456–61.

Widner, H., Möller, G., and Johansson, B. B. (1988). Immune response in deep cervical lymph nodes and spleen in the mouse after antigen deposition in different intracerebral sites. *Scand J Immunol*, **28**, 563–71.

Wood, M. J., Sloan, D. J., Dallman, M. J., and Charlton, H. M. (1993). Specific tolerance to neural allografts induced with an antibody to the interleukin 2 receptor. *J Exp Med*, **177**, 597–603.

Index